INFLUENZA

INFLUENZA

A Century of Science and
Public Health Response

⤳

GEORGE DEHNER

University of Pittsburgh Press

Published by the University of Pittsburgh Press, Pittsburgh, Pa., 15260
Copyright © 2012, University of Pittsburgh Press
All rights reserved
Manufactured in the United States of America
Printed on acid-free paper
10 9 8 7 6 5 4 3 2 1

Library of Congress Cataloging-in-Publication Data

Dehner, George.
    Influenza : a century of science and public health response /
George Dehner.
        p. ;   cm.
    Includes bibliographical references and index.
    ISBN 978-0-8229-6189-5 (pbk. : alk. paper)
    I. Title.
    [DNLM: 1. Influenza, Human—prevention & control.
2. Communicable Disease Control—history. 3. History, 19th Century. 4. History, 20th Century. 5. History, 21st Century
6. Influenza, Human—history. 7. International Cooperation—
history. 8. Pandemics—history. 9. Pandemics—prevention &
control. WC 515]

    616.2'03—dc23   2011048865

CONTENTS

ACKNOWLEDGEMENTS

A project of this duration acquires many debts, and I am pleased to be able to acknowledge the support of the many who aided me. I gratefully acknowledge the professionalism and assistance of the staff at the National Archives and Record Administration, Southeast Region, Tom Love and the Centers for Disease Control, the Food and Drug Administration, the National Institutes of Allergy and Infectious Diseases, Marie Villemin at the World Health Organization (WHO) Archives, Avril Reid at the WHO library (Geneva), and the staff at the Gerald Ford library in Ann Arbor for providing archival material. I also want to thank the efficient staff in Interlibrary Loan at Wichita State University, Nan Myers in Government Documents, Wichita State University for providing funding to travel to the WHO in Geneva, and Northeastern University for financial aid and support. Parts of chapters eight and nine were drawn from "WHO Knows Best?," which appeared in the *Journal of the History of Medicine and Allied Sciences,* and an embryonic form of chapter one appeared in *History Compass* under the title "Flu: Past and Present."

The people I interviewed were uniformly generous with their time and expertise, making the process enjoyable for me and hopefully not too painful for them. My thanks to Walter Dowdle, Ian Furminger, Claude Hannoun, J. Donald Millar, David Sencer, Kennedy Shortridge, and Sir John Skehel. I also want to extend special thanks to D. A. Henderson who both agreed to be interviewed and read and commented on parts of chapter four. In addition, Dr. Henderson was also extraordinarily gracious when I realized, to my horror, that I had neglected to acknowledge his contribution to my "WHO Knows Best?" article in *JHMAS.*

A number of people read various portions of this book, and their critiques helped me shape the final product. My thanks to Edward Dehner, Paul Dehner,

Stephen Dehner, Clay McShane, Day Radebaugh, William Vanderburgh, and Albert Waitt for allowing me to intrude on their time and for their helpful comments. I also want to thank Helen Hundley for translation of some Russian language documents. My editor at University of Pittsburgh Press, Beth Davis, was strongly supportive of the project and willing to move quite fast when my circumstances called for it—for that I am very grateful. Thanks are also due to the editorial team at University of Pittsburgh Press, which saved me from some embarrassing errors. I want to extend my deepest appreciation to Anthony Penna and Patrick Manning for their help and for guiding me along on my career path. No amount of Guinness will settle the debt I owe you both, but I hope that I will able to aid future scholars in similar fashion.

Finally, this book has a twin dedication. First is in the memory of Edwin Kilbourne. I showed up on his doorstep in January 2004 to conduct an interview and he went on to be an advisor and a sounding board for questions I had about influenza thereafter. The more I learned about this tricky virus, the more I came to realize how lucky I was to be able to ask a giant in the field about it. I greatly appreciate his patience and willingness to share some measure of his expertise with a historian. I also want to thank my wife Jodi, without whom I never would have been able to begin this project let alone complete it, and my three boys Brendan, Patrick, and Sean. They might not have liked that daddy had to work, but they are as generally excited as anyone to see the final product.

INFLUENZA

Wagers and Unexpected Outcomes

It all started with a bet.[1]

On 5 January 1976, the U.S. Army base at Fort Dix, in south-central New Jersey, rapidly filled with a mixture of new recruits, advanced recruits, and military and civilian personnel and dependents. The camp barracks and quarters—which had been nearly deserted over the Christmas and New Year's break—quickly crowded with about 19,000 people. Quarters were tight, and none more so than those for the approximately 6,000 basic trainees. These new recruits were grouped into units of fifty and assigned to eight-person rooms. In addition to sharing a common mess hall and repeated training processes, the men were restricted to their barracks for the first two weeks and to the camp for the following two weeks. The combination of close proximity, physical exertion, sleep deprivation, and high stress prompted the rapid circulation of infectious disease, a phenomenon military leaders have long observed.[2] To help forestall such infections, the U.S. military routinely inoculates new recruits against a host of diseases, including influenza, during their initial three-day stay at the reception center. Despite these precautions, the post's medical officer, Colonel Joseph Bartley, anticipated a surge of illness reports, especially of respiratory problems, which readily spread among those housed in close quarters. Col. Bartley was particularly vigilant for adenovirus, which causes mild flulike symptoms. The infection had been reported at a base in Missouri prior to the Christmas break and, more recently, at Fort Meade, just down the highway in Maryland.

In the weeks following the repopulation of the camp, recruits began to complain of fevers and coughs, and a surprising number were put to bed in the camp hospital. In casual conversation with Martin Goldfield, chief epidemiologist for the state of New Jersey, Colonel Bartley reported the suspected outbreak of an adenovirus infection at the camp and warned Dr. Goldfield to watch out for it in the civilian population. Dr. Goldfield listened to the description of the symptoms and suspected that the sudden rise of cases, rapid onset, high fevers, and large number of hospitalized recruits signaled influenza rather than an adenovirus infection. In the course of their friendly banter, Dr. Goldfield wagered Col. Bartley that the illness was influenza. To settle the bet, Col. Bartley sent nineteen samples from sick recruits to the Division of Laboratories and Epidemilogy, New Jersey Department of Health for identification on 29 and 30 January. Eleven samples tested positive for influenza, winning Goldfield the wager. Of these eleven, seven readily reacted to antigens for the prevailing strain of influenza, A/Victoria.[3] The other four positives appeared to be influenza, but of a type that the state laboratory could not identify. Standard procedure called for unidentified viral material to be sent to the Atlanta office of the Centers for Disease Control (CDC) for typing. Goldfield dutifully arranged to have the specimens sent to Atlanta by airplane on 6 February.

Meanwhile, Fort Dix continued to undergo what was now identified as a mini–influenza epidemic. Even so, despite the increased numbers hospitalized on the base, the epidemic had proved to be of minor consequence. All the soldiers had recovered and reported back to duty. However, this status was about to change.

Private David Lewis, a nineteen-year-old recruit from Ashley Falls, Massachusetts, had been fighting what he believed was a bad cold for about a week before he visited the camp dispensary on 3 February. He was given cold medicine and ordered to his bunk for the next forty-eight hours. The next morning—either feeling better or fearful of having to repeat basic training if he missed too much time—Lewis formed up with his unit for a five-mile march to the shooting range. After training all day, the unit reformed for the march back to camp. On the return march Lewis fell farther behind and collapsed, gasping for air. Sergeant Good, who was walking "drag" on the march, came to his aid. Lewis stopped breathing, and Sgt. Good administered mouth-to-mouth resuscitation while the senior drill sergeant rushed Lewis to the base hospital by car. By the time they arrived at the hospital, Lewis was dead. Postmortem testing provided another sample of the unidentified influenza, and this specimen, too, was sped to Atlanta.

The Lewis sample added to the urgency in identifying the unknown influenza strain. Five examples of a new flu strain had been found, one of which killed an apparently healthy nineteen-year-old man. The CDC's testing on 11 February revealed the virus from Fort Dix to be type H1swN1. Retesting confirmed it; the influenza strains were a type of swine flu, the same type believed to be the cause of the infamous Spanish flu, which had killed millions in 1918 and 1919.

The investigation of events at Fort Dix seemed to confirm health officials' worst fears of a pandemic. Goldfield's bet had set in motion what would become a massive immunization program designed to protect every "man, woman, and child in the United States" from a pandemic of swine flu (in 1976 the only protective option against contracting influenza was vaccination).[4] The National Influenza Immunization Program (NIIP)—commonly dubbed the "Swine Flu Program"—sought to produce, purchase, and distribute a protective vaccine for the entire population of the United States (over 200 million doses) before the onset of the next flu season the following September. Despite numerous setbacks, the program successfully injected over 42 million people, more than 31 percent of the population, twice the percentage achieved by any previous influenza program.[5] The program continued until it was stopped in mid-December because of concerns that it might be prompting an obscure neurological disease known as Guillain-Barré syndrome (GBS).

Such an incongruously large response to a comparatively minor influenza epidemic in a military encampment demands explanation. The key to this dramatic response lay not in the events at the camp themselves but in the potential portents of this flurry of infections. The infections at Fort Dix had been seen as a possible opening act to an ensuing influenza pandemic. Public health officials readily acknowledged that the infections might be no more than a curiosity, but the miniepidemic at the camp fit some predictive models indicating a potential for a significantly wider spread. Knowledge of the virus and its transmission pattern suggested that the events at the camp were not likely to remain isolated. Medical researchers were confident in their predictions of a worst-case scenario because of their faith in the science that underlay their assessments. The influenza virus still retained much to confound scientists, but by the early 1970s researchers believed that the tools and techniques of science had cracked the code on the virus and its pandemic spread. And who could doubt their assurance? Influenza researchers in the 1970s were the inheritors of the scientific revolution, and the scientific revolution had provided so many fantastic breakthroughs and solved so many puzzles that no one could suggest their faith was misplaced.

The scientific revolution, as any schoolchild knows, was a dramatic change in understanding how the world works. But this time-worn retelling often overlooks the fact that the revolution, without which our modern technical world simply could not exist, is of surprisingly recent vintage. The value of this new approach was not necessarily self-evident to our ancestors; in fact, it is still not universally accepted today. At the heart of this new science-based model lies the primacy of evidence. In some cases, evidence is produced through carefully controlled experimental manipulations; in others, however, the evidence results from close observations of uncontrolled events to detect changes and determine causal connections. Simply put, many natural phenomena remain too complex to re-create in the laboratory, a problem as true today as it was for our intellectual ancestors. Such systematic observation, whether in poking through cadavers or peering at the heavens at night, has generated data to bolster rational explanations for events. Absent visible data, whether in controlled or uncontrolled settings, it remained difficult to craft a compelling scientific rationale to supplant magical thinking, and competing theories long retained strong acceptance among the learned and unlearned alike.[6] Accepting a rational rather than a mystical explanation for the world required a radical break with the accepted worldview, a true paradigm shift.[7]

Although the term *revolution* generally carries connotations of suddenness, or rapid change, the science-based model for the world developed in fits and starts over centuries. Societies and even individuals held competing interpretations for the world they inhabited.[8] Part of the reason for this comparatively slow transformation from a magical to a science-based orientation (beyond sheer inertia) was the difficulty of uncovering clear evidence to support the new interpretation, and the messy world of biology presented some of the greatest difficulties in demonstrating rational explanations, with scientific accounts of health and illness perhaps being the most difficult to produce.

The question of disease causation was a vexing problem for would-be medical researchers for many years. The failure of observation to explain disease onset—especially rapid and generalized disease onset—hindered the development of effective disease-specific responses until nearly the end of the nineteenth century. Compounding these explanatory difficulties was the fact that a system reliant on the observation of illness—symptomology, in effect—created catch-all categories, such as "fevers" or the "bloody flux," that masked the origin of various sicknesses. Even distinctive diseases such as smallpox were occasionally misdiagnosed as measles or some other dire skin-erupting infection.

This is not to say that close observation did not lend itself to the discovery of some useful strategies for mitigating diseases in the days before the scientific revolution. The feared Black Death prompted quarantine practices whose later use successfully interrupted epidemic spread in some cases. And as was discovered in China (and likely independently in India) as early as the tenth century C.E., variolation offered protection from epidemics of smallpox.[9] But while the proponents of these responses recognized the contagious nature of these infections, they could not fully delineate why their tactics worked in some cases but not in others. Quarantine boosters could not explain why holding suspect ships in the harbor did not prevent cholera from afflicting their cities in the nineteenth century. And if the sanitarians were correct in suggesting that cleaning up the accumulated filth of a town was a healthy idea, it was not because doing so prevented the development of the deadly invisible miasmas for which they were perpetually alert. A truly satisfying determination of disease onset would be able to explain any patterns a disease exhibits and identify its cause.

It is the ability to identify the origins of diseases that made Pasteur and Koch's "germ theory" of disease revolutionary. The germ theory addresses the questions of illness transfer and onset with a testable model that can produce evidence. This radically new concept—namely, that a specific sickness is caused by a discrete microscopic organism and that distinctive illnesses arise only though contamination with particular entities—offered a compelling explanation for observed events. Variolation worked in part because it transferred the smallpox germ from arm to arm. Quarantine worked for the plague but not for cholera because it prevented the transfer of some unknown substance that caused the former but failed to block whatever element was responsible for the latter. The new theory did not immediately supplant the competing narratives for disease outbreaks, but it did provide an empirically verifiable method for describing illnesses. Interested observers were keen to detect evidence to prove or disprove this new theory of disease onset.

In many ways, the story of the promotion and acceptance of a scientific model for disease causation intertwines with the history of influenza pandemics. The first pandemic in the mode of the twentieth century appeared in 1889, when the germ theory of disease was still a matter of fierce scientific debate, generating much study and argument. The identification of Pfeiffer's bacillus as the causative agent behind the flu and the perception of the disease as the mild "old person's angel of mercy" bred complacency over the disease. This complacency was shattered by the catastrophic Spanish flu. Physicians' inability to counteract the disease represented a signal failure in the scientific approach to health. Compounding this failure was the fact that researchers could not even identify the agent causing the pandemic. Strangely, the unmitigated global public health disaster of Spanish flu did not result in the founding of research institutes dedicated to studying the illness. Instead, research on influenza during the interwar years became the province of individual scientists largely working alone. These researchers not only discovered the agent responsible for influenza but also helped propel scientific understanding of the invisible filter-passing elements we now call viruses. Interest in or knowledge about these scientific breakthroughs regarding influenza remained largely confined to a small circle of researchers.

Considering the role influenza research played in the history of science and the drama of global pandemics, it is surprising that, with one notable exception, the topic has drawn little scholarly attention outside the fields of public health and medicine. Some historical geographers focused on the 1889 Russian flu to construct models of disease transmission, and one of these researchers followed the pattern up through the 1957 Asian and 1968 Hong Kong pandemics.[10] But these pandemic years received little examination outside the historical epidemiology focus or medical researchers' studies of the outbreaks.[11] The 1976 Swine Flu Program, however, generated significant interest in understanding how this "fiasco" could have occurred. The incoming secretary of health, education, and welfare ordered a study of the decision-making chain that led to the massive program. The report by the Harvard colleagues Richard Neustadt and Harvey Fineberg was subsequently published as a book, *The Swine Flu Affair,* and it remains a touchstone for any discussion of the program. Its characterization (or mischaracterization) of the decisions and the individuals involved in the ill-fated vaccination program prompted Arthur Silverstein to rebut Neustadt and Fineberg's evaluation in his book *Pure Politics and Impure Science.*[12] Aside from these examples, the story of influenza pandemics and the science surrounding them has been principally the domain of the medical community, with Spanish flu being the sole exception.

In the 1990s and 2000s, Spanish flu became a topic of intense investigation. In fact, if one were to graph the number of books and articles on Spanish flu that appeared in these decades, the result would mirror the steep epidemic rise of the illness they describe. Such a flourishing of interest stands in stark contrast to the relative lack of attention paid to the pandemic in previous decades, at least in published discussions of the event. The 1920s saw a spate of articles and reviews on the disease, including the monumental survey of medical literature undertaken by Edwin Oakes Jordan. In the ensuing decades, however, a curious silence descended on the subject, with little discussion of the event outside the specialist literature, and even there the disaster received scant attention. In 1976 Alfred Crosby's book *Epidemic and Peace, 1918* appeared. To the publisher's good fortune, the book was placed on shelves just as the debates over the Swine Flu Program were dominating the news.[13] Crosby's book retained some interest in the following years and sparked renewed attention when it was purchased and reissued by the Cambridge University Press under the title *America's Forgotten Pandemic* in 1989. However, it was the dramatic recovery of the virus in 1997 and the appearance of bird flu that galvanized interest in Spanish flu. In short order a number of books and articles appeared recounting aspects of the pandemic, including a popular history; a collection of papers from a scholarly conference; a documentation of the U.S. military's encounter with the virus during the war; and even a biographical account of the attempt to recover the virus from frozen, entombed victims of the pandemic.[14] In the present day, any discussion of influenza epidemics is certain to contain some reference to the Spanish flu pandemic.[15]

Reflecting a similar apathy, research foundations, both public and private, seem early on not to have placed a high priority on studying the virus and the pandemics it periodically sparked. Institutional support came comparatively late to the study of the influenza virus. But the model of focused work on the infectious agent was championed by government investment, as has been the case in many other programs of scientific research. It is a matter of no small coincidence that the first well-financed research effort on the diagnosis, treatment, and prevention of the disease came originally as part of the military effort during World War II. Similar to that on other topics of scientific interest, research on the influenza virus was initially part of a government-science partnership that dominated postwar science, especially in the United States. Such focused research efforts produced a number of technologically driven strategies that could be rapidly deployed to safeguard against influenza and a host of other infectious diseases. The state began to shoulder an increasing role in protecting the public's health, and these treatment and prevention programs and practices were at first so successful that they seemed to herald a new age.

As befits federal efforts, the public health plans were national in scope. Protection against infectious diseases, including influenza, was to be obtained by quickly delivering a protective vaccine to those at risk. Emblematic of a heady, optimistic time in public health, massive inoculation campaigns were undertaken to intervene in emerging influenza pandemics in 1957 and 1968. Such large-scale state-directed efforts culminated in the Swine Flu Program of 1976, one of the most dramatic national vaccination campaigns ever undertaken. This universal interventionist approach fell out of favor as the sole option against infectious disease in subsequent years, and attention to influenza infections dissipated as new and newly reemerging afflictions commanded scientific and medical research and dollars. After being crowded out by attention to dramatic new and resurgent afflictions, however, pandemic influenza reappeared as a focus for concern in the twenty-first century, now recast as an emerging disease. Emerging influenza pandemics and research into the virus illustrates the scientific and medical conceptualization of disease that remains the dominant paradigm.

Conceptualizing illnesses as new or reappearing threats that endanger not only individuals but the state itself was an idea that rapidly gained favor in health and policy-making circles. Vigorously promoted by Stephen Morse and Joshua Lederberg at a National Institutes of Health conference in 1989, the model of seeing infectious diseases as both a health and a security problem quickly found traction among a variety of science and policy committees.[16] Studied from this vantage point, the 1976 Swine Flu Program was in fact a preview of this later model.

The 1976 Swine Flu Program can also be read as the climax of a century's worth of investigation into infectious diseases; in addition, the program crystallized a number of public health and scientific issues that had not been contemplated previously. The massive response initiated by the U.S. Public Health Service (USPHS) resulted from a number of trends that came together at this critical moment in history. The first trend was a dramatic series of break-throughs in scientific knowledge about the virus and its behavior. This knowledge, which centered on the intricacies of the virus's genetic code, exemplified the staggering increase in knowledge produced by the scientific revolutions of the twentieth century—revolutions fueled by dramatically expanded government investment in scientific research. Powerful new tools, technologies, and approaches were unlocking a multitude of mysteries across the scientific disciplines. Armed with new information and technical approaches, medical researchers applied their scientific know-how to controlling and eradicating the numberless bacteria, viruses, parasites, and rickettsias that afflict humankind.

In a second trend, a string of successes throughout the twentieth century gave health officials a powerful and abiding faith that science held the key to the imminent extinction of infectious diseases. Many health officials believed that the most important questions surrounding epidemic diseases would be ones of logistics: specifically, how to get the life-saving magic cures into the hands of all. Public health officials sought to create large-scale programs not just to protect against but to permanently eradicate a number of infectious diseases. By 1976 smallpox was well on its way to global elimination, and other massive vaccination programs were under way or on the drawing board.

The events at Fort Dix in 1976 also occurred at a time of long-term change in the field of global public health. As medical science began to demonstrate the extent to which infectious diseases had affected populations in the nineteenth century, nation-states began to recognize the true costs of epidemic disease. National governments realized that the ad-hoc local and regional authorities that sprang up in response to periodic epidemics of yellow fever and other diseases were ineffectual in protecting the public. Governmental officials also disliked quarantine, often suggested as the proper response to pandemics, because it disrupts trade. Accordingly, some state governments began to create more permanent public health organizations, and although not particularly powerful initially, these boards began to strengthen by the end of the nineteenth century.

National governments also began to recognize that threats at home might be better combated by keeping diseases far offshore and that the safety of their populations might be best maintained by cooperating with other states for mutual protection. To some degree this cooperative approach was evident in quarantine responses to plague infections. But such combined approaches were minimal and often evaded by any party that found itself aggrieved in the process. In the nineteenth century, only the arrival of the dreaded cholera truly galvanized interstate coordination. Cooperative action in preventing the interstate spread of the disease was initially hindered by disagreements over the mode of transmission and by stout resistance—especially by the British—to regionwide quarantine efforts in places presumed to be undergoing cholera outbreaks. But the gradual acceptance of the germ theory of disease led to effective international anticholera programs by the century's end. In 1907 a number of powerful (and mainly European) states sponsored an international organization to manage the barricade effort of public health. The Office International d'Hygiène Publique (OIHP) was charged with overseeing quarantine programs designed to keep diseases common to the colonial world—cholera, yellow fever, and plague—from infecting the founders' home states.

Although theoretically an international organization, the OIHP sought resolutely national goals: to keep the sicknesses of "others" away from the home populations. This philosophy also undergirded the creation of a regional organization in the Americas; founded in 1902, the Pan American Sanitary Bureau was implicitly mandated with keeping diseases out of the United States. Such organizations may have been on the pathway to international public health, but they remained staunchly national in focus. This nation-centered emphasis continued up through World War I.

In the wake of the Great War, an internationalist spirit infiltrated the field of global public health. The newly formed League of Nations established its own body, the League of Nations Health Organization (LNHO), whose mandate was to facilitate improved public health for all league members. This internationalist goal contrasted with the nation-centered philosophy of the

OIHP. The powerful European states that benefited from the workings of the OIHP jealously guarded this organization's assets and resisted its incorporation into the LNHO. Starved for resources, the LNHO coexisted uneasily with the OIHP and was forced to rein in its more ambitious global health plans. The LNHO was able to establish a reputation for technical proficiency—especially in the arenas of epidemiology and vaccine standardization—but its fortunes were tied to the League of Nations itself, which succumbed to the bitter nationalist passions that spurred World War II. The dislocations resulting from that war temporarily thwarted the development of a number of international organizations. But, as Akira Iriye points out, not even the caustic nationalist sentiments of the two world wars could reverse the trend toward an increase in the number of intergovernmental and international nongovernmental organizations. An intricate network of state, quasi-state, and private international organizations continued to develop.[17]

As the planet recovered from the trauma of World War II, a reinvigorated spirit of internationalism bloomed anew. Just as the LNHO had been a manifestation of global health concerns for the League of Nations, so too was the World Health Organization (WHO) an outgrowth of the United Nations. Like the LNHO, the WHO was unable to completely separate itself from nation-centered health organizations. But unlike the LNHO, it was able to carve out sufficient revenue streams to pursue broader international health goals and to fold national or regional health systems into a global health system.[18] The method of achieving international health goals by relying on national health resources resulted in some tensions, but generally issues of global health harmonized with those of national health, for, as national public health officials realized, quarantine or barricade efforts were impractical in an era of rapid and widespread global commerce and travel. Also like the LNHO, the WHO adopted technical solutions to health issues, a hallmark of its predecessor's approach. Such technical methods suited the interests of the WHO's primary backer, the United States, which provided the largest share of financing and was also the major source of the organization's leaders and experts via the Centers for Disease Control. In the early decades of its existence, the CDC strongly favored technical approaches to safeguarding health.

The CDC evolved from coordinated programs created during World War II to protect troops against malaria, a deadly and debilitating infection. In the postwar period, the organization continued its mosquito eradication programs around the nation to break the chain of malarial infection. Having stamped out malaria in the continental United States, however, the CDC was left without a clear mandate. Under its two eminent leaders—Joseph Mountin and Alexander Langmuir—the organization reinvented itself as the nation's epidemiology and public health laboratory par excellence. Under the leadership of David Sencer, its director during the 1960s, the CDC had steadily increased its global reach, its staff members working sometimes as experts invited by other states but more often within WHO programs. The CDC provided the leadership and expertise in the smallpox eradication effort; it also reorganized malaria control after the failed global malaria eradication effort of the 1950s and 1960s.[19] The CDC's technical solutions to health objectives meshed well with, and in some respects dominated, many WHO programs.

In the 1970s and continuing through the 1980s, the WHO roiled with debate as more and more member states pushed for broader public health programs rather than technically based, disease-specific approaches. Such debates over the WHO's proper emphasis in improving health led to fractious coalitions and bitter funding clashes. Further complicating matters in the late twentieth and early twenty-first centuries was the appearance of richly funded private organizations, such as the Bill and Melinda Gates Foundation, that sought to craft independent programs of global health. In the present day, responses to infectious diseases still highlight the sometimes contradictory goals of national and international health, a legacy of the comparatively recent change in health protection models.[20]

The convergence of these trends in 1976 helps to explain why the United States responded so quickly to a novel influenza strain at Fort Dix. But that does not explain why it was virtually the *only* government to respond with a massive vaccination program. Like all highly transmissible infectious diseases, influenza does not respect borders or nationalities. Since vaccination was the only protective option against influenza in 1976, it is surprising that no other nation joined the United States in immunizing its citizens against this new flu. Only Canada took steps to create any type of crash immunization program. Experts at the WHO evaluated the same evidence as did those at the USPHS but recommended a policy best described as watchful waiting. The U.S. program was labeled a "fiasco" when no swine flu pandemic occurred, and this assessment remains the popular perception of the effort, while the cautious WHO recommendation has been held up as the wiser course of action.[21]

A close examination of the Swine Flu Program illustrates one of the key themes of public health and this book. Events in 1976 laid bare questions that public health policy makers continue to face in the present day. What should be done? What can be done? What should not be done? In 1976, influenza scientists and USPHS officials weighed the likelihood of a pandemic, the capabilities of the nation's surveillance and vaccine manufacturing capacity, and the cost of a pandemic in human and economic terms and then recommended a massive vaccination campaign to protect the nation's citizens. Officials at the

WHO, drawing on the same evidence, addressed the same issues and recommended a "wait-and-see" policy for their member states. Both groups based their decisions on partial and contradictory evidence, and in both cases, the answers to what *could* be done shaped the assessment of what *should* be done.

The USPHS and WHO officials in 1976 were addressing the problem of risk analysis, a component of every health decision. In the case of influenza, weighing the various options is further complicated by the unpredictable behavior of the virus. Misjudging the pandemic potential of the particular strain had tremendous potential costs to be measured both in the sickness or deaths of millions of people and in billions of dollars in health expenses and lost income. Mounting a large but unnecessary vaccination campaign can waste millions of dollars in itself, but further potential costs lie in adverse reactions to the vaccine and disruptions both to everyday life and to other public health programs. An additional complication in predicting the possible course of any novel influenza strain is the fact that a decision must be made quickly because of the highly transmissible nature of the virus and the laborious vaccine-manufacturing process. Judging the likelihood of adverse reactions to be low, U.S. public health officials in 1976 believed that the worst outcome would be the expenditure of public funds to prevent a pandemic when no such threat ever truly existed. The officials at the USPHS opted to risk the dangers of an unneeded vaccination campaign, which they viewed as gambling with dollars, not lives. Officials at the WHO, however, had wagered that the virus would not develop into a pandemic, at least not in the near future. When the fall came and there was no pandemic, the U.S. program was condemned, and the WHO decision lauded. Nonetheless, such a simple summation of the actions pursued in 1976 fails to acknowledge the complex elements that formed the calculated decisions. The Swine Flu Program was labeled a fiasco not because of mismanagement or a failure to develop the program but simply because the pandemic never developed.

The USPHS's and the WHO's conflicting policies regarding the new influenza strain illustrate the core weaknesses of national health programs that attempt to serve both national and international health goals. Events in 1976 also illustrate the WHO's uneven mixture of international and national capacities. The surveillance program for detecting novel influenza viruses was a truly global entity, with national organizations providing data for an international constituency. Founded in the days after World War II, the system had steadily increased its reach and sophistication as more national programs entered into sentinel roles. The surveillance system was an exemplar of the technical approach to health. National health laboratories around the world collected samples, but the process of typing the strains was done at a small

number of labs (two in 1976, since expanded to four) that possessed the technology to differentiate between the viral types. However international the
surveillance system might have been, though, the response to novel influenza
strains remained a resolutely national program. The WHO had no resources
for producing or distributing vaccine. Any vaccination campaign would be
a purely national affair and thus limited to those states with the resources to
mount crash immunization efforts. Such limited national responses to universal pandemic threats clashed with "health for all" mandates that were attract-
ing the interests and attention of a number of delegations to the WHO. What
good was a global health net if it benefited only a handful of states?

The Swine Flu Program remained a cautionary tale for public health
officials throughout the later twentieth century and dampened the enthusiasm for interventionist pandemic flu response for nearly two decades. That
changed when a series of headline-grabbing events prompted a reassessment of
influenza pandemic preparedness. In the spring of 1997, Jeffrey Taubenberger
announced that his laboratory had successfully recovered and sequenced a
portion of the genetic code of the infamous Spanish flu.[22] Hot on the heels
of Taubenberger's announcement, health officials uncovered cases of human
infection with an avian influenza strain (H5N1). Eighteen people were infected
by contact with live poultry, and six died. In dramatic fashion, local health
officials ordered the slaughter of all poultry in Hong Kong and banned the importation of chickens from surrounding areas. The Hong Kong wet markets
were supplied with live poultry both produced in farms within Hong Kong
territory (subsequently to be termed the Special Administrative Region when
sovereignty was transferred to the Chinese by the British) and imported from
Guangdong and other provinces in the People's Republic of China. In fact,
roughly 80 percent of the birds supplied to the market came from mainland
Chinese farms. After bird importation had been halted, the birds on hand
destroyed, and the markets closed for several weeks for cleaning and disin-
fecting, Hong Kong government officials—working cross-border with PRC
officials—developed an import and farm inspection plan to detect a reoccur-
rence of the deadly virus. The procedure appeared to break the chain of infection from birds to humans.[23]

The combination of these two events—new research into Spanish flu and
the pandemic threat posed by avian flu in 1997—galvanized both national and
international public health officials to reexamine their plans for countering influenza pandemics. Shortcomings in the two major components of pandemic
responsiveness, surveillance and manufacturing, provided additional spurs
to this reexamination early in the twenty-first century. On 11 February 2003
China reported to the WHO that it was experiencing an outbreak of "atypical

pneumonia." This illness, subsequently dubbed severe acute respiratory syndrome (SARS), had been occurring for over two months before the Chinese reported it.[24] The SARS virus spread globally before it was controlled, ultimately infecting over 8,000 people and killing at least 774.[25] The outbreak and reaction cost billions of dollars and illustrated the weakness in global disease surveillance. If a nation could not or, as in the case of China, would not report an epidemic, the infection might spread widely before it could be stopped.

The second major component of pandemic planning is manufacturing protective vaccines. In 2004 the limitations of influenza vaccine production were starkly illustrated. That year vaccine regulators in the United Kingdom condemned the entire production lot of influenza vaccine from Chiron, one of two influenza vaccine producers for the U.S. market. The loss of almost half the vaccine supply for the United States prompted a shortage and desperate attempts to make up the shortfall.[26] Only limited amounts of vaccine were available to the United States, because the remaining global producers of influenza vaccine had already been operating at basically full capacity; they could produce no more.

Also in 2004, Vietnamese officials reported observing an avian influenza similar to the strain that had appeared in Hong Kong in 1997. This highly pathogenic virus circulated through domestic poultry flocks throughout Southeast Asia. Most alarming, the virus had periodically infected humans, with a high percentage of mortality. At last count, 565 people have been positively identified as being infected with avian influenza, and 331 of those infected have died.[27] Adding to the concern about the spread of avian influenza was the fact that the virus had been detected in migratory waterfowl whose migration routes link all the continents to one another. Combined with the international poultry trade, this meant that the avian influenza virus would have ample opportunity to spread globally.[28]

In the light of these events, national and international health organizations quickly moved to assess response plans for an influenza pandemic. The results were not encouraging. Few nations had any concrete plans to respond to an influenza emergency. Recognizing the "general lack of preparedness," the World Health Assembly called on nations to create national response plans, and the WHO pledged to strengthen global surveillance.[29] The WHO realized that reliance on purely national programs had failed in the past and would not be of interest to nations that could not participate in such vaccination efforts. A new approach was needed to complement national vaccination programs. In response to these new demands, the WHO created its "Global Influenza Preparedness Plan" in March 2005 to coordinate national and global response to an emerging influenza pandemic. This vital document provides a blueprint both for responses to influenza pandemics and for the future of global public health.

In 2005 the WHO also issued its revised International Health Regulations (IHR), a plan that radically transformed the reporting duties of states facing epidemic threats. As Lorna Weir and Eric Mykhalovskiy point out in their study *Global Public Health Vigilance,* the new regulations discard the mandatory disease-specific reporting mechanism—limited to cholera, plague, smallpox, and yellow fever in a 1969 revision—for a broader requirement to report "public health events" that could provoke an "international public health emergency." Previous IHR plans going back to the founding of the WHO gave sovereign states the responsibility for reporting their incidences of these "notifiable" diseases. As Weir and Mykhalovskiy demonstrated, the short list of reportable diseases combined with a state's desire to hide these inconvenient outbreaks—cholera being the most common example—meant that the WHO was notified of outbreaks only rarely, and even then, the reports were not filed in a timely fashion. These factors combined to give the WHO only a limited role in epidemic disease prevention. Drawing on the work of the international law expert David Fidler, Weir and Mykhalovskiy argue that the new regulations have broadened the effectiveness of the WHO reporting mechanism and, combined with powerful new surveillance systems (they favor the Internet-based Global Public Health Intelligence Network), have created a "global emergency vigilance system" and a "world on alert." This new reporting system holds out the promise of a more active and effective role for the WHO in epidemic prevention.[30]

While there is much to recommend in Weir and Mykhalovskiy's examination, their focus on a formal top-down approach fails to capture the workings of the WHO below the level of officially reported disease outbreaks. For example, from the organization's founding in 1948 up through the IHR revisions of 2005, influenza was not classified as a reportable disease. Despite this gap in the prevailing IHR guidelines, however, the WHO influenza surveillance system was an active international health organization and, as I will show, much more than just a clearing house for information. Moreover, the officials monitoring influenza constituted just one of a number of expert groups dedicated to crafting WHO policies for threats to global public health that did not fall under the mandated reporting requirements. Under Weir and Mykhalovskiy's approach, even the massive WHO-coordinated malaria eradication program of the 1950s and 1960s would not appear as a WHO-sponsored assault on epidemic outbreaks, for malaria was not a reportable disease. The WHO's international health programs involve more than just the official interstate relations created by its constitution. The WHO operates at a variety of levels in detecting and protecting against epidemic diseases. An examination only of the officially notifiable diseases misses much of the organization's work in communicable disease protection. That said, revamping the IHR to broaden the WHO's role as an epidemiological clearinghouse for global health issues was long overdue.

The reassessment of public health preparations for pandemic influenza and the revision of the IHR immediately proved their value when an emerging pandemic strain of influenza did appear, even though it was not the one to which the global influenza plans had been geared. In the spring of 2009, the WHO's pandemic plan got its first real-world challenge. While participating in a test of enhanced influenza surveillance, USPHS officials in San Diego detected a new influenza strain infecting two children with no apparent connection to each other. On 21 April 2009 the CDC announced that the children were infected with a novel strain of influenza, typed as H1N1 swine flu. By 24 April 2009 the CDC was able to link the novel strain with an influenza-like illness that Mexican health officials had observed in March and early April of that year. Faced with the information that a novel influenza strain was circulating in their country, Mexican health officials quickly installed social distancing measures, closing schools and restaurants and banning public gatherings in the hopes of forestalling a wider spread. It was too late. By 6 May 2009 the swine flu had been identified in twenty-one additional countries aside from the United States and Mexico. The WHO quickly escalated its influenza pandemic alert system to level 6, its highest, which confirmed that the virus was causing "sustained community level outbreaks" in countries in "two or more WHO regions." In short, the virus was a pandemic.[31]

The sudden appearance of H1N1 confounded influenza experts. The virus's surprising genetic makeup, its unusual pattern of summer spread in the Northern Hemisphere, and its explosive infection rate in the Southern Hemisphere prompted a desperate race to produce protective vaccines for the Northern Hemisphere's coming fall flu season. The pandemic turned out to be mild, although at this writing its full impact cannot yet be gauged. In any case, the programmatic responses to this novel epidemic strain taken by national and international health organizations have unquestionably been shaped by responses taken and not taken during more than a century's worth of experience with pandemic influenza, and as it has in the past, the virus behaved in unexpected ways.[32]

Contemporary public health officers and policy makers struggle with the same sets of questions about influenza that have bedeviled their predecessors: Will the new virus prompt a pandemic? How deadly will the pandemic be? How will the pandemic affect things economically? Socially? Politically?

What can be done to mitigate or stop it? The answers to these questions are necessarily tentative, since formulating them requires us to predict an unpredictable virus. In 1918 medical researchers were unable to detect the organism responsible for the pandemic. In 1976 USPHS officials weighed the available evidence, assessed their capabilities, and judged a massive vaccination campaign to be both necessary and possible. In 2011 the public health landscape has again changed. Our ability to detect and describe novel influenza viruses has increased dramatically; conversely, our ability to protect the public through the production of vaccines and antivirals has failed to keep pace with burgeoning populations. Consequently, public health officials have had to develop new strategies to deal with influenza pandemics.

The new approach developed by the WHO builds on successful elements of the organization's influenza surveillance system while recognizing the limits of nation-based vaccination efforts. The key element that thwarted previous vaccination campaigns was the mismatch between a speedily transmissible virus and a laborious and slow manufacturing and distribution process. Simply put, the virus infected populations before a vaccine could be developed, manufactured, and delivered in any quantity. The increasing volume and speed of travel and trade are likely to further widen the gap between pandemic and protection for the foreseeable future. In response, the new approach seeks to reverse the process of surveillance by giving sentinel sites powerful new tools for rapidly identifying new strains. And once a strain is identified, the new plan—enshrined in the WHO's Pandemic Preparedness Plan (the new name for the Global Influenza Preparedness Plan) and facilitated by a new version of the International Health Regulations—calls for the delivery of influenza experts to the site of the new viral strain.

The new WHO influenza pandemic plan represents a reversal in the traditional surveillance structure because instead of waiting for the satellite laboratories to send samples from the outbreak to the experts, the experts are to rush to the site of the outbreak and immediately begin a program of pandemic disruption. The WHO influenza experts would be armed with either "barricade" vaccines—a small stockpile of general, family-wide vaccines that offer at least partial immunity—or rapidly produced doses of experimental vaccines against the specific new virus. These vaccines would be combined with widespread antiviral treatments given with the intent of choking off the new strain before it efficiently adapts to its new human host.[33] Such a program relies on effective surveillance for quick detection of a new virus and international cooperation of influenza experts and resources. The new model creates a hybrid approach to public health that may finally move the WHO closer to its idealistic health mandate. It harnesses technical sophistication to identify a potential pandemic but relies on a combined global approach rather than a nation-centered solution. As the 2009 H1N1 swine flu pandemic demonstrated, this new approach is hardly foolproof, but it offers the current best hope for protecting against an emerging influenza pandemic.

The story of influenza pandemics is ultimately a story about the natural world, too. The preceding decades of study and observation of the virus have revealed many of its secrets. While no scientist could claim mastery over the subject, medical researchers became increasingly confident of their ability to predict the behavior of the virus, and with prediction came the ability to control its impact. Nevertheless, as the virus demonstrated in 1976 and over the ensuing decades, the infection operates in random, unexpected ways. This is hardly unusual, however, for the natural world still offers much to surprise and confound us. The emergence of new diseases, such as AIDS and SARS, and the reemergence of old infections, including tuberculosis, suggest that the long-running war between humans and the infections that plague us has no foreseeable end. The search for deeper understanding of infectious diseases continues, but perhaps with a greater appreciation of the difficulty of the task.

The struggle between science's ability to understand and predict nature and the natural world's stubborn unpredictability played out across the long twentieth century. This back and forth between science and nature forms a second theme of this study. Emerging influenza pandemics and institutional responses to real or perceived pandemics present a unique window on a number of processes evolving over the course of the twentieth century. The 1889 Russian flu appeared during the ascendancy of the germ theory, and the tracking and tracing of the infection bolstered those who asserted this model of pandemic spread, even though researchers had mischaracterized the agent responsible for the illness. The catastrophic Spanish flu shook the complacent confidence of the medical establishment, eventually leading to the proper identification of the virus responsible for the affliction. Sustained, institutionally supported research has unraveled many mysteries of the virus, leading to the point where extinct strains can be resurrected and every letter of a current strain's genetic code can be scrutinized for hints of future behavior. But even our increased knowledge of the influenza virus has proven unequal to the task of protecting the public from influenza pandemics.

In a related fashion, the narrative of influenza outbreaks from the 1870s onward reveals the increasingly interconnected world we inhabit. Russian flu was truly an international affair exploiting transportation networks to infect residents of every region of the world. Spanish flu roared around the planet in four months, its speed of transmission amplifying its devastating impact. In 1957 and 1968 small localized outbreaks of a new influenza strain were uncovered around the world. Scientists call this process of low-level distribution "seeding," and when conditions are right, a seeded virus can burst into epidemic spread around the globe. In recent times the rapid cycling of 2009's H1N1 swine flu into pandemic status underscored the reality that we are all citizens of one global disease environment.

A final theme of this book is that a close study of influenza pandemics casts light on the evolving role of organizations and their responses to health emergencies. Weak public health organizations had little to offer in 1889, and a lack of accurate knowledge and techniques rendered medical responses to Spanish flu useless at best and dangerous at worst. Mirroring a pattern of research support across many fields of science, military investment in influenza prevention generated some important protective breakthroughs. The wedding of governmental support and academic research that evolved from the war effort built on these advances and continued to contribute to increased scientific knowledge of the virus and its properties. A reincarnated global health agency, now known as the World Health Organization, expanded on the approaches first developed by its predecessor, the League of Nations Health Organization. In some arenas the WHO managed to foster the development of truly global approaches that combined national and international goals, the influenza surveillance system being a notable example. But the organization remained fundamentally reliant on national health organizations and the resources they were willing to extend to achieve global health. Such a reliance on national resources carries with it the seeds of conflict, for priorities and capabilities may differ markedly among states. The national vaccination campaigns of the 1957 and 1968 pandemics illustrate the great mix of capabilities and resources found in various health programs. In the fallout from the 1976 Swine Flu Program and (as will be detailed) the accidental and artificially produced epidemic of 1977, interventionist pandemic planning was placed on the shelf, soon to be eclipsed by new global health emergencies. The overall effect of twentieth-century responses to influenza pandemics was to illustrate the limitations of national responses to international health threats. Successful programmatic responses would need to draw on new models.

Any new approach to international public health must recognize the central conundrum at the heart of previous antipandemic programs. Quickly detecting spreading infections demands a global surveillance net, but the technical capability for responding rapidly to detected threats is limited to a mere handful of states. Accordingly, any effective new program would permit a greater variety of nation-states to participate and benefit from the new system. High-tech approaches favored by technologically advanced states remain key, but low-tech systems have their value, too. The surveillance system adopted to track bird flu embodies this hybrid approach: the sudden die-off of domestic chicken flocks serves as an early indicator that bird flu may be circulating and that enhanced strain surveillance is needed. Such a blending of high- and low-tech tools can serve as a template for new international health tactics that offer greater chances for success and the ability to utilize the capabilities of an increased number of states.

This book's central thesis is that the new influenza pandemic response model represents a template for a truly global public health system. This new model, promoted by an assertive WHO, was crafted by drawing on successes and limitations in earlier epidemic years. As increasing scientific knowledge of the mutability of influenza virus suggested, and the failed national interventionist efforts of 1957, 1968, and 1976 demonstrated, nation-centered vaccination efforts cannot protect citizens from influenza pandemics. For the foreseeable future, only the close international cooperation of health experts and organizations manifested in the WHO Global Influenza Preparedness Plan offers the hope of thwarting an emerging pandemic and protecting the public's health. National health programs will continue to play an important role in protecting citizens' health, but protection against epidemic diseases in this interconnected, global world requires greater investment of time, talent, and money in health programs with a global focus. Such a rapid, collaborative approach offers the only opportunity to derail pandemic threats and so provide safety for all.

In a very real and demonstrable sense, any individual's health is intimately tied into the health of all. Influenza pandemics starkly illustrate this reality. Influenza experts can tell us that the virus has periodically mutated into pandemic strains that caused massive illness, suffering, and death. Based on that history, it is highly probable the virus will do so again. But as events in 2009 remind us, they cannot tell us when; that determination is up to the virus. Only by acknowledging the shared nature of the threat and strengthening rapid international responses can we hope to limit the impact of an influenza pandemic.

CHAPTER 1

Influenza:
Virus and History

By any measure, the scientific and medical breakthroughs of the late nineteenth and twentieth centuries are truly astounding. For millennia, human societies attributed their sickness and afflictions to angry gods, misaligned cosmological events, evil witches, or any number of other supernatural causes. It is stunning to consider that the knowledge that most diseases are caused by discrete, invasive microscopic agents (or "germs") is only about 150 years old. Not until the early twentieth century did people finally abandon the idea that diseases can be caused by malodorous vapors, or miasmas. Medical knowledge about illnesses and the organisms that cause them has increased at a dizzying and breathtaking pace.

Scientific research began as an individual pursuit, undertaken largely for its own sake. As such, it was a comparatively slow-paced endeavor, for beyond the few who possessed enough resources and leisure to permit full-time scientific inquiry, the people conducting it had to squeeze it into their spare time. In addition, the exchange of data, information, or ideas—the lifeblood of science—was often blocked and almost always excruciatingly slow. Such limitations make the achievements of individuals such as Harvey or Lavoisier all the more heroic and those places where free scientific inquiry held sway, such as tenth-century Baghdad and sixteenth-century Padua, all the more glittering.

By the nineteenth century, research was still an individual avocation, but the exchange of information was beginning to flow much more freely and rapidly. Advancement in science still relied on heroic soloists such as Louis Pasteur and Robert Koch (though by now such individuals typically worked in academia), but their breakthroughs quickly stimulated debate and inspired others to expand on their discoveries.

By the turn of the twentieth century, financial support and interest in scientific research had begun to draw more attention from powerful states. State-supported research had traditionally focused on useful implements for war—da Vinci had peddled siege engines and defenses against them for Italian city-states, and Archimedes had bent his genius to protecting Syracuse from the besieging Romans—but institutions were now increasingly developing around research areas removed from or at least only tangentially connected to national defense. By the twentieth century, a number of state-supported and independent entities were pursuing a host of research avenues.

At first these state-supported organizations competed with the institutions and researchers of rival nations, each trying to outdo the others in advancing science, but eventually the most technologically advanced states began to coordinate and cooperate on mutually beneficial goals. Transnational and international committees of experts began to form, and once they did, they began to develop their own goals and directions. Even as these international organizations pursued their own, technical agendas, however, their reliance on nation-states for support and financing kept an inherent tension alive. Some powerful independent organizations of the present day, such as the Gates Foundation, command vast resources of their own, yet this tension between international goals and national financing remains an issue.

It would be remiss to suggest that the history of scientific advancement resulted from a logical progression of new information and ideas and that global institutions naturally evolved from national organizations. Instead, science progresses in fits and starts with numerous blind alleys followed and numerous competing hypotheses and theories advanced. Over time compelling information and models win out, but the process is necessarily messy and discordant. The study of the influenza virus and influenza pandemics illustrates this larger pattern of scientific development; in fact, because of the difficulties in studying this virus, scientific research on influenza provides a compact narrative mirroring the larger process of scientific advancement.

In some ways, the study of the influenza virus had a late start. Initially the illness was misattributed to a bacterial infection. As late as the 1930s, the fact that the disease is caused by a virus remained unknown. In the decades after the discovery of the influenza virus, however, increasingly powerful technologies and tools were used to crack its secrets. Today scientists can speak confidently about the behavior of the virus, discuss its interactions with the human immune system during the course of infection, and study the genetic makeup of viral strains to the last base pair. Nonetheless, despite this wealth of information, predicting the distribution pattern of influenza viruses in the human population remains an uncertain proposition.

Before embarking on an examination of the long-twentieth-century history of influenza, a brief summary of the virus and its course of infection is in order. The following few pages provide a quick overview of the current knowledge of the virus, its transmission properties, and the responses of the human immune system. Although brutally truncated, this discussion is an essential prelude to any effort toward tracing pandemic influenza.

Science of the Virus

The influenza virus is a member of the family Myxoviridae.[1] There are three types of influenza—A, B, and C—named in the order of their discovery. Type C rarely causes human infection and is relatively unimportant in the study of human infections. Type B can cause epidemics, but the course of infection is milder, and the spread of the virus is slower, with less impact on human society. Type A, which poses the greatest threat to human health, is the one associated with an explosive spread and high rates of morbidity and mortality. This book focuses on pandemic influenza type A, and any subsequent references to influenza should be understood as designating this type if not otherwise noted.

The influenza virus is a single-stranded, generally spherical RNA virus whose virion comprises eight segmented sections. Like all viruses, those causing influenza must infect a living cell to replicate; the influenza virus generally attacks the epithelial cells that line the respiratory tract from the nose to the lungs in humans. The virus contains six genetic segments that code for specific tasks, such as replication, though the full functions of the virus's various components are not completely understood. Two components of the virus's genetic code make up its outside shell and are believed to be responsible for binding with and entering epithelial cells and with cutting loose the daughter cells that bud out from infected cells. The virus includes proteins known as hemagglutinin (H), which forms spiky extensions and constitutes about 90 percent of the outside shell. These hemagglutinin spikes latch on to a type of receptor on the outside of respiratory cells that binds preferentially with sialic acid. The virus docks on this outside receptor and induces the cell to coat the virus in a membrane and transport it into the cell. Once inside, the virus undergoes a process in which it hijacks the cell and causes it to produce new copies of the virus. These new viruses use the other major component of the viral surface—known as neuraminidase (N)—to shut off the sialic acid receptors. Neuraminidase proteins are mushroom shaped and make up the remaining 10 percent of the virus's outside shell. New viral copies bud out from the infected cell, and the neuraminidase cuts them free so that they can seek out new cells to infect, starting the process all over again. Ultimately the influenza virus destroys any infected cell by destroying the outer layer. The daughter cells that infect adjoining epithelial cells quickly produce many millions of copies of the virus.

The regular pattern of hemagglutinin and neuraminidase on the viral shell provides a signature shape. The pattern and shape of the hemagglutinin and neuraminidase underlie the categorization of subtypes. Sixteen types of hemagglutinin and nine types of neuraminidase have been located in the animal world, but thus far only three types of each have been found to readily infect humans; these are labeled H1, H2, and H3 and N1, N2, and N3, respectively.

The human immune system is not an idle bystander to this process; in fact, it has evolved two types of responses to foreign invaders.[2] The first, or primary, response to foreign substances occurs within the innate, or nonspecific, immune system. White blood cells known as phagocytes continually circulate through the bloodstream. These cells have the simple ability to identify "self" from "nonself." When a phagocyte encounters a nonself entity, it envelops the foreign matter and releases powerful enzymes to digest it. (The failure to distinguish self from nonself gives rise to autoimmune diseases, including multiple sclerosis.) Injuries to the organism, whether from physical trauma or from toxins produced by microbial invaders, result in localized swelling. Fluid is rushed to the site of the injury, bringing with it increasing numbers of phagocytes and natural killer (NK) cells. Natural killer cells identify cells infected by nonself viral invaders and release a toxin destroying the infected cell. The NK cells target infected cells fairly broadly and frequently end up damaging or destroying surrounding cells. As the phagocytes digest this foreign matter, they secrete a chemical known as interleukin-1, which is detected by the hypothalamus. When a threshold concentration of interleukin-1 is reached, the hypothalamus induces a fever, raising the temperature of the body. The immune system works more efficiently at higher temperatures, at which point most viral replication is slowed.

In the case of an influenza infection, this battle between the innate immune system and the viral invader occurs in the epithelial cells that line the respiratory tract. The debris of cell and virus destruction is bound up with mucous, which the cilia that line these cells sweep downward for expulsion by coughing or sneezing. The coughing or sneezing expels mucous, cellular and viral debris, and new copies of the influenza virus, all of which are ejected into the surrounding environment. Both the speed of replication—a cell can be infected and begin producing copies within an hour—and the volume of viruses created quickly outstrip the innate system's ability to control the invader. Fortunately, the human immune system has another line of defense.

The second line of immune response is known as the cognate, or specific, response. The foreign invader's exterior proteins and structures mark the entity as nonself and are called antigens. As the innate immune system response wreaks its carnage, it produces numerous fragments of the destroyed invader. Special cells known as antigen-presenting cells scoop up these segments, stick them onto their exterior surfaces, and transport them to the lymph nodes. The lymph nodes are packed with T and B cells (*T* here stands for immune system cells produced in the thymus; *B,* for those produced in bone marrow). If the antigen (small pieces of the antigen are known as epitopes) comes from an invader the immune system has encountered before, it will be presented to a memory B cell; upon recognition, this cell immediately begins massive production of antibodies to neutralize the invader. These antibodies are specifically designed to latch on to the exterior of the invader, preventing it from binding with cells and slowing it down for capture and destruction by the phagocytes. The speed with which the invader is identified and neutralized explains why the immune system prevents or foreshortens reinfection with the same virus or microbe.

If the invader is a novel one for the human organism, then no memory B cell for it will exist. The lymph nodes, however, are packed with a host of nonspecific B and T cells, and in this case B and T cells matching the antigen or epitope fairly closely are stimulated to produce antibodies. Over time a B cell that fits the invader exactly will be selected and will produce antibodies to neutralize the virus or microbe.[3] Numerous copies of the B cell circulate in the blood immediately following the successful eradication of the invader. But eventually the number dwindles just to a memory B cell that stands ready to crank out antibodies if the same foreign entity returns. Each individual's immune system is therefore unique, carrying a record of the infections successfully eradicated. If influenza were a stable or slowly evolving virus—like smallpox, for example—an individual would undergo a limited number of flu infections in his or her life, and a small number of influenza vaccinations could provide lifetime protection. The yearly recommendation for the flu vaccine and the regular "flu season" suggest that influenza is not a stable virus.

In fact, the influenza virus has developed two tricks to evade the immune system. The first relies on a penchant common to RNA viruses: they introduce replication errors when copying the original code. Because RNA replication lacks the ability to check the newly created code for errors, as DNA replication can, daughter cells formed by RNA replication possess numerous coding errors. Most of these mutations have no effect or are detrimental to the virus itself and are extinguished. Some mutations, however, offer competitive advantages of some sort, and these are passed on to subsequent generations. In other words, RNA viruses have a mutation rate about three orders of magnitude higher than that of organisms that use DNA replication; that is, there are about one thousand RNA mutations for each DNA mutation. In the case of influenza viruses, these copying errors subtly rearrange the pattern of hemagglutinin and neuraminidase jutting out from the exterior. This process of rearranging the surface pattern—known as viral drift—can provide a competitive advantage in the Darwinian world of the human immune system. These drifted viruses escape the antibodies designed to neutralize them and thus are propagated, through coughs or sneezes, into the environment to infect the next person.

The virus's second evasive trick relies on the segmented nature of its genetic code. During replication in an infected cell, a given virus will readily swap a genetic segment (or "packet") with one from another influenza virus. If an individual is infected with two types of influenza, this reshuffling of genetic packages creates a spectrum of new strains with anywhere from one to seven new genetic components being combined. This "swapping process" is known as recombination (though it's more fun to call it viral sex), and the resulting genetic variation is referred to as a viral shift. These combinations create new viruses with which the immune system may have no experience. Recombination is generally considered to be responsible for pandemic strains. In 1957 the prevailing viral strain, typed H1N1, was replaced by a new strain, typed H2N2. This new strain, called "Asian flu," was a shift from the prevailing strain and rapidly spread around the globe. In 1968 another shift occurred with the new "Hong Kong" strain then circulating rapidly; it was typed H3N2. Both 1957 and 1968 were pandemic years, and it was retrospectively determined that these pandemic strains were the result of a reassortment of human and avian strains. In 1957 an avian donor provided new hemagglutinin and neuraminidase genetic segments; in 1968 only a novel hemagglutinin was inserted.[4] An estimated two million people died from the flu in 1957, and one million perished in 1968.[5]

Recent investigation of the virus responsible for the 1918 Spanish flu suggests a third possible route for the pandemic outbreak of influenza. Genetic study of the recovered virus suggests it to be an avian strain that developed a few key mutations that enabled it to infect a human population. The largely avian character of the virus may account for its stunning ferocity and heightened mortality in the human population.[6] This direct transfer from an avian population to a human population is an apparently rare event. Generally the influenza virus moves into the human population only via an intermediate host or hosts.

As the preceding discussion suggests, the influenza virus has an animal reservoir. In fact, many animals may catch or transmit influenza, including pigs, waterfowl, seals, whales, horses, and humans.[7] It appears that the oldest animal reservoir is the aquatic avian population. In fact, all sixteen known hemagglutinin types and nine neuraminidase types can be collected from waterfowl.[8] The influenza virus appears to be ubiquitous in the waterfowl population, with strains having been recovered from all around the globe during all seasons. Wild ducks have been a particular focus of avian influenza virus research; tests reveal that up to 30 percent of the juvenile fledgling population is infected with influenza. Moreover, an influenza infection causes little apparent ill effect on the birds, resulting in only a few days of (literally) ruffled feathers and decreased feeding.

The fact that the influenza virus has such a large, active, and mobile reservoir ensures that the virus cannot be eradicated as a potential threat to the human population. Strategies of containment and eradication are impractical because the virus has unquantifiable opportunities for jumping from its natural hosts to other species, including humans. Instead, solutions to pandemic influenza must lie in other tactics for quickly identifying and managing infections and some commonsense plans for minimizing intermingling of wild bird and domestic animal populations so as to limit the opportunities for species transfer.

Influenza is an alimentary infection in birds. Again, the epithelial cells of the intestinal tract are lined with sialic receptors to which the hemagglutinin binds. The sialic acid receptor site in birds is called alpha 2,3. The virus replicates and is excreted in high concentrations in the birds' feces. Since the birds suffer few ill effects, the virus takes wing along with the birds and thus circulates widely, to be deposited in lakes and ponds the birds visit. In fact, the virus has been recovered from the cold water of sampled lakes several weeks after birds have migrated on, presumably infecting other transients at the site. Because the virus circulates so readily through waterfowl, there are few evolutionary pressures, and the virus is remarkably stable in this population. Though the virus is prone to replication errors, the resulting mutations offer few competitive advantages, so that the code of circulating avian strains changes very slowly.

Fortunately for us, the relative stasis of the influenza virus in the avian population hinders its transfer to the human population. The influenza virus is supremely adapted for transmission in the bird host, attaching readily to the sialic acid receptor in the intestinal lining. Humans, too, have sialic acid receptors that line the epithelial cells of the respiratory tract (in this case, alpha 2,6), but the shape of these receptors, or docking ports, differs from that of avian receptors (alpha 2,3). Humans do have some alpha 2,3 receptors, but they are located deep in the lungs. Avian influenza strains rarely infect humans directly because they cannot effectively latch on to cells to begin replication, but even if they do, the cells are located so deep in the lungs that the infected person cannot readily cough out the infection and thus does not transmit the disease to a new host.[9]

Since influenza is a human disease with many millions of cases per year, and has been so for hundreds (and maybe thousands) of years, the virus did find a way to infect humans. Although we will never know definitively, it is highly probable that an intermediary host facilitated the virus's passage from an avian to humans, with pigs being a likely candidate for that intermediary role. In addition to being longtime companions of humans (they were domesticated around ten thousand years ago), pigs have epithelial cells with sialic acid receptors. These epithelial cells line the respiratory tract just as they do in humans, but these cells contain receptor structures for both alpha 2,3 and alpha 2,6. Thus pigs can readily catch and transmit both bird and human flu strains; to put it another way, the pig provides an environment that offers a competitive advantage for a mutation that allows the influenza virus to bind to an alpha 2,6 site. Whether pigs played a role in originally transferring influenza viruses into the human population is unknown and unknowable, but they clearly serve as a stepping stone for avian influenza viruses today. Because this animal, and even its individual epithelial cells, can be infected with strains of both avian and human flu, the individual segments of the viral code can be jumbled together when the infected cell is co-opted into producing copies of the virus. The result is an array of new viruses combining up to seven components of the other virus. Those new, shuffled viruses combine the ability to replicate in a human host with a novel appearance that evades immune system response, giving them a competitive advantage. The new virus constitutes a viral shift from the prevailing strain. In 1957 five human gene-coding segments were combined with three avian segments; in 1968, seven human virus gene segments were combined with one avian segment. Both strains sparked pandemics.[10]

The scientific knowledge of the influenza virus just presented was hard earned, and most of it resulted from fairly recent research. Before they reached this point, however, researchers followed a number of false steps that marred scientific investigations of infectious diseases in general and influenza in particular. To fully appreciate how far medical knowledge has come, it is useful to examine the scale and scope of research on disease causation prior to the late nineteenth century. The transition from magic to science required some difficult conceptual breakthroughs and often bitter debate. The history of human interaction with and research on influenza pandemics highlights the turmoil involved in conducting science.

The Virus and Human Populations

The length of time the influenza virus has been circulating in the human population is unclear, but the epidemiological symptomology and rapid spread of this highly infectious and transmissible disease permit some educated guesses.[11] For one thing, this rapid diffusion and course of infection means that the virus needs a large population to sustain its chain of infection. Since it is primarily transmitted through respiratory droplets, it needs a relatively densely distributed population. Therefore, influenza—like many other diseases—is a disease of dense, large populations. When influenza infects a nomadic band or even a small city, it quickly runs through the hosts, and the chain of infection is broken. But as the human population began to grow and urbanize, and those urban areas began to have contact with other urban areas, the population of hosts for influenza expanded. William McNeill calls this growth and interconnection in the ancient world the confluence of disease pools, which he dates as beginning around 500 B.C.E.[12] Consequently, it comes as no surprise that some medical historians see a depiction of an influenza outbreak in descriptions from Hippocrates in 412 B.C.E. and an account from Livy detailing an infection among Roman soldiers. The telltale epidemiological pattern of an influenza outbreak—rapid, widespread onset of a disorder marked by fevers, body aches, respiratory distress, and prostration, coupled with a low mortality rate, primarily among the very old and very young—is suggested by several accounts throughout the Middle Ages in Europe. Several scholars follow the lead of the nineteenth-century historian August Hirsch in pointing to an epidemic in 1173–1174 C.E. as the first clearly identified influenza epidemic. Ancient chronicles, however, are notoriously imprecise in their depiction of symptoms and diseases, rendering many of these retrospective diagnoses open to debate. Nonetheless, given that even ancient times had large interconnected Eurasian and African populations living closely with their domestic animals, including waterfowl and pigs, and that people writing then offer descriptions of infectious respiratory diseases, influenza has no doubt been circulating periodically through the human population for some time. We cannot determine how widely or rapidly those epidemics spread, however, or, of course, what type of influenza strain caused them.

By the Renaissance observers had begun providing descriptions of the symptoms and courses of diseases that allow for more confident identifications of influenza outbreaks. In fact, an outbreak in Italy provides us with the name *influenza*. The sudden, community-wide infection prompted observers to search for a cosmic source of the disease; as was done for many of the diseases at the time, they chalked it up to the baleful *influenza* (influence) of the stars.[13] Beveridge quotes a classic account from a 1562 letter from Lord Randolph to Lord Cecil describing how the disease "Called the newe acquaintance" had run through Queen Mary's court with a "plague in their heads . . . soreness in their stomaches, with a great coughe. . . . The queen kept her bed six days. There was not appearance of danger, nor manie that die of the disease, except some olde folks."[14]

Still, most medical historians feel confident in positively identifying as influenza only outbreaks that occurred during the Enlightenment or later. The richness of the accounts, the clinical accuracy of symptom descriptions, and the geographic reach of Enlightenment sources has led medical historians to identify and sketch a number of pandemic outbreaks.[15] Pandemics are marked by a sudden, community-wide outbreak in which all or almost all the people in a population are susceptible to infection. The number of infections multiplies rapidly, quickly reaching an epidemic peak, and then almost as rapidly drops off. Graphing the sharp increase in cases produces a distinctive wave pattern in which the time from initial cases to decline can be as short as six weeks. Subsequent waves of the pandemic reappear at later times and are generally (but as we shall see for 1918, not always) milder. The medical historian is able to chart the pandemic's movement and tentatively identify its origin by comparing accounts of the infection's first appearance in each locality. From 1700 to 1900 pandemics were generally traced back to Russia or China.[16] In the 1700s there were true pandemics (from the Greek *pan*, meaning "all," and *demos*, meaning "people") circulating to virtually all continents on the globe. Beginning with the European explorers in the late fifteenth century, people across the globe were brought into increasingly closer contact. "The Columbian exchange," as Alfred Crosby terms it, knitted together the world's people, although this knitting was often a violent and deadly affair. As the Europeans tightened their colonial reach and transportation sped up and expanded, pandemic influenza became a regular visitor to all populations.[17]

Physicians or researchers interested in disease causation faced a number of conceptual and technological barriers that prevented them from escaping the mystical or humoral imbalance paradigms that passed for medicine. Part of the difficulties lay in the fact that much of the evidence on which physicians relied was anecdotal, making it difficult to get an idea of the scale and scope of infectious diseases. The new scientific approach to inquiry differed from other explanations, then, in its reliance on objective, quantifiable, and replicable methods of data collection. Above all, statistics helped scientific investigators focus on the general rather than the particular, and statistical measures would prove to be central for understanding the effects of an influenza pandemic.

The impact of these influenza pandemics has traditionally been difficult to determine. The overwhelming majority of those afflicted recover with apparently few ill effects. In the 1840s, the English health statistician William Farr developed a key concept in appreciating influenza's impact. Having examined mortality records, Farr determined a seasonal pattern to the deaths in a given year. Because the total number of deaths was regular across years, within certain parameters the statistician was able to craft a model of expected deaths for any particular time period. Any sudden surge in the number of burials would point to some new force causing the deaths, generally some epidemic outbreak of a disease. The number of "excess deaths" illustrated the impact of the disease. This statistical measure turned out to be important in assessing influenza epidemics because it was (and is) difficult to definitively state that influenza kills someone. In some cases it is clear: the person catches influenza, develops pneumonia, and dies. In other cases, however, another cause, such as heart attack or stroke, is directly responsible for killing the patient. Few death certificates have identified influenza as the cause of death. For example, people died all the time from pneumonia in the nineteenth century; who could definitively identify the triggering cause as an influenza infection? In fact, until Spanish flu brutally disabused people of this notion, influenza was considered the merciful agent that gently escorted the elderly from life. Even now, some dismiss the potential threat of influenza pandemic because, being young and healthy, they feel they have nothing to fear.

Farr's graphs of actual burials against expected burials mirrored the steep curve of a pandemic peak. Taken in conjunction with contemporary descriptive accounts, such charts allow present-day medical historians to retrospectively identify pandemic years with a great deal of confidence. Although virulence does vary, in general the number of dead suggests the number of people infected. Indeed, counting up the number of extra dead is still the measure used to identify a pandemic today.[18]

William Farr was honing his statistical tables—indeed, he was laying the groundwork for the field of epidemiology—during a tumultuous time in medical research.[19] Enlightenment-era scientific observation had increasingly undercut supernatural explanations for epidemic disease, but no clear substitute definition had emerged to account for the multitude of early deaths that plagued the nineteenth-century world. Some learned people were "contagionists," who asserted that epidemic diseases were spread to a population

by some infected individual. These contagionists could point to the examples
of smallpox and bubonic plague as clearly demonstrating a disease's commu-
nicability through infected people. The mechanism for transfer from the sick
to the well remained a mystery, however, despite the tantalizing observation
of "wee beasties" seen through the primitive microscope of Anton van Leeuwenhoek in the 1670s.[20]

A counterexplanation of disease causation asserted some sort of environmental source of affliction. The classic example used for this type of explanation was malaria, which (as its name reveals) was ascribed to the "bad air" of
swampy or wet regions, where the disease was prevalent. This environmen-
tally mediated appearance of a disease seemed to satisfy the vexing problem
of the sudden widespread eruptions of diseases such as yellow fever. The 1793
yellow fever outbreak in Philadelphia served as a prime example. This abrupt
and panic-inducing outbreak drew the attention of scientists influenced by
Enlightenment values. Contagionist physicians including William Currie observed that the outbreak began shortly after the arrival of ships from the Ca-
ribbean, where the illness was an acknowledged scourge. But this contagion
explanation was undermined by the fact that the epidemic had not followed
the 20,000 or so citizens who fled the city (including the fledgling federal government under the new U.S. constitution). An alternative interpretation of
events was promoted by the renowned physician Benjamin Rush. Rush postulated that the generalized filth of eighteenth-century Philadelphia produced
a dangerous disease-causing miasma. In his investigation of events possibly
precipitating the yellow fever outbreak, Rush determined that a large load of
spoiled coffee beans had been dumped on the docks and left to rot. The combination of general insanitary conditions and the rotting coffee sparked the
deadly outbreak of yellow jack, he argued, which spread via an invisible noxious cloud all throughout the city. By the later nineteenth century, miasmists
conceded that yellow fever was transportable but insisted that the true cause of
the disease was a combination of heat, filth, and moisture.[21]

Support for an environmental role in disease eruption came from the mid-
nineteenth-century statisticians Louis-René Villermé, Lemuel Shattuck, and
most important, Edwin Chadwick. These public health pioneers gathered a
host of statistics, including measures of mortality and morbidity, from Paris,
Massachusetts, and England, respectively.[22] The statistics detailed shocking
disparities in sickness and death among various regions, with the highest rates
of death and disease centered in the poorest, most squalid sections of industri-
alized cities. These men thus argued that the way to ameliorate the effects of
disease was to clean up the accumulated filth and drain the noxious pools and
ponds of effluent that marred urban areas.[23] The views of these "sanitarians"

gained support from local and then-expanding national governments, which saw the value in promoting a healthier and more productive workforce and in limiting the economic dislocation that invariably followed disease outbreaks.

In addition to harboring concerns about keeping a healthy laboring population at work in the expanding industrial factories and workhouses of mid-nineteenth-century European and American cities, the wealthy and powerful were all too aware that diseases in the poorer areas of town threatened them, too. Not even the aristocracy was safe, as the death of Queen Victoria's husband, Prince Albert, demonstrated in 1861 (he purportedly died of typhoid fever).[24] These fears of diseases spreading from poorer areas to threaten the "better sorts" crystallized in the global spread of a scourge from the exotic East: cholera. In the mid-nineteenth century, the dramatic pandemic waves of cholera laid bare the issues of contagion and sanitation, the inequalities in living conditions for the wealthy and the poor, and the unexpected implications of imperial and economic connections. In the late nineteenth and early twentieth centuries, the concept that poorer regions constitute the seedbeds of dangerous infections was expanded to include entire geographic areas. Part of the underpinning of tropical health was to prevent the deadly diseases of the imperial periphery from contaminating the metropole.

Cholera, as we now know, is an enteric disease caused by a bacterium of the genus *Vibrio* that is spread via fecal contamination of water and food sources.[25] The apparently ancient affliction is generally considered to have its origins in the Ganges River watershed, where it remained confined aside from sporadic transfer to China. The debilitating nature of the illness limited its easy exchange. In the nineteenth century, technological advances in the speed and volume of transportation from India combined with the colonial concerns of imperial Britain to facilitate cholera's emergence from its traditional limits. The year 1817 was marked by an eruption of cholera infection that traveled east into Southeast Asia and China and as far north as the Russian steppe. In 1820 British troops from India were rushed to Oman to help quell a disturbance in the kingdom and inadvertently brought along cholera, which infected the local population and, more dangerously, pilgrims traveling to complete their hajj.[26] This first transfer of cholera eventually smoldered out and spread no farther globally, but in retrospect, we can see this episode to have been a precursor to the dramatic cholera pandemics that swept the nineteenth-century world. Transportation, trade, and colonial concerns facilitated the disease's spread. In addition, European authorities linked the spread with religious pilgrims (especially Muslims), whose purported insanitary and backward ways made them a threat of contagion to "more civilized" states.

The cholera pandemic years of 1832, 1848, and 1866 generated strong public fears and responses and galvanized governments to begin considering international cooperation to protect against global health threats. Cholera was a particularly confounding disease for nineteenth-century scientific experts. It clearly was a contagious disease, for its progress could be traced from region to region as it radiated out from infected areas to new regions connected by water or rail. Indeed, this steady march of infection was what sparked the dread and panic that were fanned by the newspapers of the day.[27] The fear of a deadly disease transferred from an Other (the xenophobia was revealed by the fact that cholera was often referred to as "Asiatic cholera") prompted dramatic responses ranging from strongly empowered local health boards to calls for national days of prayer and repentance.[28] Most perplexing for the contagionists was that quarantine, the traditional method of preventing the transmission of illness, was completely ineffectual. Neither holding ships in the harbor if they came from suspect ports nor isolating infected patients seemed to have any impact on the disease's implacable progress.

Cholera served to bolster the budding sanitary movement, which asserted some sort of environmental component of the illness. The disease often appeared first and most frequently in the squalid sections of a community. In the rapidly industrializing cities of Europe and North America, the cramped and densely populated sectors of the lower classes provided ample opportunity for the affliction to establish itself in a region. Sanitary reformers called for a cleanup of the fetid pools of waste, refuse, and animal carcasses that fouled the city streets. Sanitationists also urged the emptying of privy vaults and the draining of stagnant ponds and cesspools as immediate measures and the construction and maintenance of a comprehensive sewage system as a more long-term step, all with a view toward removing the pollution responsible for Asiatic cholera. Each report of a new cholera outbreak hitting a city prompted its town fathers to engage in an orgy of cleaning the filth accumulated since the last cholera outbreak, flushing city streets with disinfectants to clear the muck and dispel the potentially dangerous vapors.

Some other reformers saw a connection between the disease and what they considered dissolute living in the poorer districts. These reformers charged that the poor led irreligious and immoral lives, which made them susceptible to cholera infections, while sober, moral, and upstanding members of a community faced no danger. If these poorer folks cleaned up their neighborhoods and abandoned their decadent ways, they too could avoid infection. But the unpredictable nature of cholera infection undermined such retributive explanations. While it was true that the blow of cholera fell most heavily on the impoverished and insanitary sections of town, anybody, no matter how apparently upright, might suddenly be stricken.

The first glimmerings of a way out of this morass began to appear around the middle of the century. In a classic epidemiological investigation undertaken in 1848, John Snow demonstrated the relationship between a single water pump (the famed Broad Street pump) and the pattern of cholera cases in a London neighborhood. Snow later followed this report with a study demonstrating a correlation between rates of cholera infection and competing London water companies. One firm (Lambeth), whose customers had a lower infection rate, drew its water from upstream of London. The other (Southwark and Vauxhall), whose clients had a significantly higher disease rate, drew its water from below London. Clearly cholera infection was related to water.[29] Snow's observations were initially not widely reported or accepted, but they steadily acquired support and eventually were validated by the work of Koch and Pasteur.

The global waves of cholera infection also sparked another innovation: international cooperation on disease outbreaks. The clear progression of cholera outbreaks from one region to another and the dismal failure of quarantine efforts convinced governing authorities that interstate efforts might be useful in mitigating or protecting against select deadly diseases. Spurred by the preceding cholera epidemics, representatives from eleven European states and the Ottoman Empire gathered in Paris in 1851 in what was billed as the first international sanitary conference.[30] Although meeting for a remarkable six months, the delegates were unable to agree on a set of recommendations and regulations to govern shared responses on the three obviously transportable diseases of cholera, plague, and yellow fever. Their inability to reach an agreement resulted in part from the confused nature of disease causation. Was disease outbreak a result of contagion, insanitary conditions, or some combination of the two? Another sticking point in the negotiations lay in the fact that some states—Britain in particular—strongly resisted the traditional response of quarantine. Quarantine significantly disrupts international trade, and trade among states and between states and their overseas colonies was escalating at this time.[31] The British also resented the fact that several states blamed their colony of India as the source for many of these scourges and advocated strict limits on travel from this region during disease outbreaks.

This international sanitary conference set a pattern for subsequent sanitary conferences that had both positive and negative implications. On the positive side, to participate in such a conference is to recognize that protecting the public's health at home does not stop at one's border, to acknowledge that your own health and that of your fellow citizens are connected to the health of citizens from other states, wherever they may be. Therefore, it is in your interest to help keep other peoples healthy. Although this idea was not fully developed until later in the twentieth century, its embryonic form is visible in the logic of the conference. On the flip side, however, the meetings can be seen as twelve powerful states meeting to devise effective methods for protecting themselves from the diseases of Others. In this sense, the diseases under discussion (cholera, plague, and yellow fever) became a concern only when they threatened the interests and peoples of the home nation. The notion that people at home needed special protection against exotic diseases drew heavily from the racial perception of disease susceptibility. It was generally believed that white Europeans were not constitutionally suited for novel climates—tropical ones in particular.[32] In the view of nineteenth-century Europeans, unlike the "natives," who were bred to shrug off the heat and illness, whites were simply not racially suited to survive the harsh climates of these regions or to survive the onslaught of these exotic infections.

From the 1870s onward, this tension between inclusion and exclusion remained at the heart of much debate over public health authorities' roles and responsibilities in addressing pandemics. As I will show, selfish national interest held sway in the early the twentieth century, with enlightened self-interest subsequently rising to the fore. Strands of both models, however, continue to vie for support even in the present day.

Five more conferences were held over the ensuing three decades, and all foundered on the contradictory explanations for disease causality. By the 1885 conference in Rome, however, a new radical explanation for disease origin was beginning to dominate scientific discussions on the topic. This conceptual breakthrough resulted from the work of two pioneering scientific giants: Louis Pasteur and Robert Koch. Their discovery, that microbes play a major role in causing illnesses, is known as the germ theory of disease.

The well-known monumental work of Louis Pasteur and Robert Koch in the 1860s and 1870s needs no retelling here, but it will be worthwhile to underscore a couple of salient points for retracing scientific and medical developments in disease incidence. First, Pasteur's and Koch's assertion that ubiquitous microscopic agents, or "germs," cause specific diseases in organisms was only one explanation of sickness among many. The germ theory was slow to gain widespread acceptance, partly because it was a truly new paradigm in the Kuhnian sense, so that adopting it required abandoning tenaciously held interpretations. In addition, the evidence supporting the new theory initially encompassed only a handful of afflictions.[33] Indeed, even as late as 1892, prominent sanitarians such as Max von Pettenkofer asserted that germs were insufficient to cause disease and needed to undergo environmental interaction to do so. In a marvelous bit of nineteenth-century scientific bravado, von Pettenkofer drank a beaker of cholera *Vibrio* bacteria provided by Robert Koch to demonstrate that the bacillus was insufficient to bring about the disease. He suffered only mild intestinal discomfort.[34]

Pasteur's and Koch's work created the field of bacteriology, and researchers (often young and new to science) scrambled to identify the bacilli responsible for many of the deadliest killers of the nineteenth century. In a remarkable flurry of activity, researchers identified the organisms responsible for twenty diseases between 1880 and 1898, including cholera, plague, and tuberculosis.[35] Attempting to be the first to identify the causative agent of a disease became a highly competitive scientific endeavor, with researchers avidly tracking and gathering data on the progress of disease outbreaks, as occurred with the 1889 Russian flu pandemic.

Nonetheless, the race to uncover new disease-initiating microbes was not just an individual competition; it became a proxy for national rivalries, too. The Franco-Prussian War of 1870–1871 had heightened preexisting tensions between French and German scientists, but researchers from many other nations, too, competed to plant the metaphorical flag of empire on every new microbe discovered. Naturally, the most interesting targets for discovery were those exotic diseases of faraway lands whose existence threatened a home nation's population. In the colonial powers of England, France, Germany, and Japan, the new bacteriology and germ theory became bound up with the creation of tropical medicine.

Tropical medicine gave colonial powers a newfound confidence in their abilities to protect against and control the effects of dreaded tropical diseases.[36] During the early twentieth century, medical personnel not only made scientific breakthroughs on the importance of vectors in so-called tropical diseases such as malaria, yellow fever, and the plague but also began to develop an effective arsenal of curative and preventative treatments for these health threats. Bacteria and vectors were things that could be detected, calculated, prevented, and eradicated. In the words of Daniel Headrick, medicine was becoming a "tool of empire."[37]

This new knowledge, however, did not offer benefits for all. The thrust of tropical medicine was to protect "Westerners" when they traveled in the service of empire and to prevent the introduction of these tropical afflictions back to the seat of that empire itself. At the turn of the twentieth century, many still believed that the diseases of the tropics affected local populations less dramatically than they did "white" populations. Girded with the protective armor of the new public health measures, colonial officials could subdue and civilize the colonial hinterland for the benefit of the metropole. Few benefits of the bacterial revolution extended beyond the Western enclaves of colonial administration.

The extent to which medical knowledge has been driven by self-interest was further manifested in agreements and mutual regulations enacted between powerful states.[38] By the early twentieth century, the generalized acceptance of the germ theory of disease allowed such nations to harmonize their efforts in disrupting the transfer of certain epidemic diseases. At international sanitary meetings held in the 1890s at Venice, Dresden, Paris, and Venice again, delegates found congruence on a number of protective regulations. These meetings culminated in a conference held in 1903 at Paris; delegates to this conference established international regulations that ended up governing quarantine until World War II and recommended establishing an international office of public health. Twenty nations signed the agreement, including all the major European colonial powers plus the United States, Egypt, Persia, and Brazil. The Office International d'Hygiène Publique, or the "Paris Office," as it was designated in English-speaking circles, was established in 1907 and survived the two world wars, disappearing only when it was folded into the World Health Organization in 1948.

The overwhelming imperial character of the OIHP reflects its purpose, which was to prevent the introduction of dangerous diseases into the populace of the powerful signatories. Implicit in this mandate was the notion that deadly diseases posed problems only when they traveled. The self-interest of individual nation-states thus drove international public health policy.

During this period of tumultuous scientific debate over the source and nature of disease, influenza had remained relatively quiet. A series of widespread epidemics and pandemics had raged throughout the eighteenth and early nineteenth centuries, but following the 1847–1848 outbreak, the one that had drawn William Farr's attention, influenza subsided into the background. The disease did not disappear—far from it. It continued to circulate each year, causing sickness and death, but no pandemic strains emerged with the characteristic curve of steep epidemic increase and a corresponding subsequent wave of burials. In the years following 1848, connections among the world's regions became tighter and firmer. Industrialization continued and broadened its reach. Transportation quickened and increased in volume. Rail lines connected cities; steamships plied the oceans, outstripping the fastest clippers. Whether they were adherents of the germ theory or not, physicians were little concerned with influenza. It was merely a minor seasonal annoyance. At any rate, there was little a physician could do. The patients usually healed on their own, and those who succumbed generally had already been near death in one fashion or another. The pandemic of 1889, however, demonstrated influenza's power and danger and galvanized researchers in efforts to uncover its causative agent. As they were with regard to other epidemic diseases, medical researchers were confident they could uncover the agent responsible for the infection and provide effective treatment and prevention. But the 1889 pandemic differed from previous epidemics in both the speed and the scope of its spread. Although this pandemic occurred in the nineteenth century, the 1889 Russian flu already illustrated the pattern influenza pandemics would take in the twentieth century.

Russian Flu

In a real sense, the world was smaller in 1889 than it had been in 1848 (the most recent pandemic year). By 1889 most of the blank spaces in the Europeans' maps had been filled in with mines, plantations, markets, or colonies. The imperial reach of colonial powers moved peoples and goods from one end of far-flung empires to another. This was also a year of voluntary mass movement, with hundreds of thousands streaming from Europe for destinations in the Americas or Australia and massive migrations of people throughout Asia. As was already noted, the waves of cholera in the nineteenth century alerted officials and citizens to the border-defying nature of pandemic disease, and statistics revealed the movement of contagions through afflicted populations. The germ theory derived from Koch's and Pasteur's work emboldened those who collected health statistics to gather them as effectively as they could in order to verify or falsify this novel explanation of diseases.

As a result of this activity, medical historians have rich records for the 1889 pandemic. The major European powers kept careful records of vital statistics for both their own nations and their overseas possessions. Several other nations also kept detailed records. In addition, during and after the pandemic, several published compilations of these records traced the pandemic's spread and its likely origin. Finally, many medical researchers of the day sought to uncover the causative agent of the infection in the fashion of Pasteur and Koch.

This unprecedented collection of international data revealed some significant statistical patterns. One concerned the relationship between transportation and pandemic spread. Researchers at the time concluded (and researchers today agree) that the 1889 pandemic can be traced back to Russia.[38] Retrospective analysis suggests an uptick of influenza cases in central Russia during the spring, near the end of flu season that had begun the previous autumn.[40] Flu researchers now call this upsurge of cases a "herald wave"; in it, the new flu circulates through a population and seeds itself. With the onset of the subsequent flu season, the new strain bursts into epidemic and pandemic proportions. In October 1889 the pandemic spread rapidly out of Russia heading west, east, and south. Mapping the movement of the pandemic (according to Patterson, this was the first such mapping)[41] revealed the railroad's role in rapidly spreading the disease. Influenza traveled with infected passengers, and the stops on the rail line served as the epicenters of spread into different regions. The second pattern to emerge from the data tracking the pandemic concerned population distributions.[42] Larger cities served as nodes of spread, with the infection then moving to smaller cities and towns and then into the rural communities. Eventually all regions would be visited by the pandemic, but at different times.

The data showed that steamships, too, played a role in transmitting the disease. The steamships were larger than their sail-powered predecessors, giving them larger populations for sustaining chains of infection; they were also faster, allowing them to deliver people still actively contagious. As a result, they brought the pandemic to every port. These port cities continued their time-honored role of disease introducers, and from them the infection rapidly penetrated the interior via rail and river lines.[43]

The medical and public health establishment was completely unprepared for pandemic influenza. Few physicians then in practice had been around for the 1847–1848 pandemic, and even if they had been, they could have offered little medical advice of any value. And again, the medical establishment considered influenza to be a trivial concern, certainly nothing alarming.[44] As community-wide outbreaks developed, hospitals and physicians were swamped with hundreds of cases of people suffering high fevers, respiratory distress, and a host of other symptoms. Morbidity in some regions approached 50 percent at peak infection. Effective treatment consisted of little beyond palliative nursing care, and in this transitional time in the medical sciences, patients were fortunate if they managed to *avoid* seeing a physician, some of whom prescribed heroic measures such as bleeding or purging. The lack of effective medical care and prevention emboldened a host of quack therapists who suggested a range of remedies "guaranteed" to protect an individual from flu. These nostrums came in the form of liniments, sarsaparillas, extracts, powders, and something known as "electricity in the bottle," to name a few.[45]

The surprising pandemic set medical researchers on a frantic search to discover the element responsible for the affliction. "Pfeiffer's bacillus," a bacterium found in the lungs of several individuals prostrate with pneumonia, was identified as the contagion, and researchers peered through their microscopes hoping to uncover its secrets.[46] Bacteriologists congratulated themselves. They may have been unable to cure or prevent the infection, but at least now they knew the cause. Medical researchers would keep a sharp eye out for the telltale Pfeiffer's bacillus, which they knew would signal a patient was stricken with influenza.

The global mortality of this 1889 pandemic is unknown because record keeping in many areas was incomplete or nonexistent, but some measure of the deaths can be obtained by examining places that did have complete records. A conservative estimate for Europe (defined as land west of the Urals up to the Atlantic, including Britain) sets the deaths at no fewer than 250,000, far higher than the number of those who died in previous nineteenth-century pandemics, including cholera outbreaks.[47] The first pandemic wave in the fall of 1889 was followed by two more waves lasting into 1892. In some localities these subsequent waves engendered even higher mortality than the initial wave had. This high mortality resulted not from any special lethality of this strain of flu (estimates of its mortality rate range from 0.17 to 1.0 per 1,000) but from its high morbidity. There were so many cases of this extremely infectious disease that even its low mortality rate of less than 1/1,000 quickly produced a significant number of deaths.

By 1889, the application of new scientific approaches to medicine and the gradual acceptance of the germ theory of disease causation had led to tremendous strides in understanding infectious outbreaks, and through the use of statistics scientists were beginning to quantify the terrific burden of infectious diseases. Although identifying the toll of an influenza pandemic and (mistakenly) identifying its cause had at this time not yet led to effective treatments, scientists were certain that this information would serve as the basis for producing a cure for the flu.

At any rate, although this influenza pandemic was the first to be recognized as particularly massive and disruptive, it was still a comparatively minor event when measured against the host of epidemic disease threats that had troubled populations. Statistics proved that the typical victims of the 1889 pandemic fell into two categories: the very young and the very old.[48] Graphing mortality against age creates a U shape, with mortality clustering at the low and high ends of the age scale. This graphic representation of influenza mortality accords with anecdotal historical accounts of flu. Many are infected, but only the weak—young and old—are taken. This pattern of mortality was true for the twentieth century and has remained so into the twenty-first. As a rule, influenza is deadly only for the very young and the very old or for those who suffer from a pre-existing malady. But for every rule there is an exception; in influenza studies that exception is known as Spanish flu.

CHAPTER 2

The Forgotten Pandemic
Remembered

One of the small bright spots amid the horrors of warfare is its propensity to stimulate rapid medical advances. Commanders of the imperial armies locked in the ferocious combat of World War I sought to keep their soldiers fit to fight, taking steps that included inducting vast numbers of physicians, nurses, and volunteers to provide medical support for the troops. Of course, the related medical research and experts involved focused primarily on the horrific injuries soldiers sustained in battle or on the fields where the next crop of casualties were being trained. This focus on protecting a nation's armed forces meant that little attention was paid to minor disease threats or to the afflictions of civilian populations. In the case of influenza, it is not clear that earlier detection would have served much good at this time. But influenza would soon demonstrate that it was no minor annoyance. The terrible Spanish flu pandemic killed more people in a shorter amount of time than had any other disease in history.

Spanish flu is not Spanish at all.[1] The combatant governments of World War I censored news about the spreading flu pandemic so as not to demoralize their citizens, but Spain remained neutral in the war and so had no reason to follow suit. Spanish newspapers remarked on the early summer influenza cases infecting many citizens—even the king—and so Spain was tagged as the origin of the pandemic.[2] The true point of origin cannot be conclusively proven, but a compelling argument identifies the United States as the seedbed of the virus.[3]

When the United States entered World War I, it initiated a massive call-up. The nation's military infrastructure was woefully unprepared for this surge of personnel, and the new draftees were crowded into hastily constructed barracks that dotted the countryside. Camp Funston (now part of Fort Riley) in Kansas was one such camp.[4] Fifty-six thousand men assembled there for basic training, primarily drawn from the Midwest. The barracks were drafty, and the quartermaster section had been unable to keep up with the demand for winter clothing. When not drilling or training, the men huddled around the camp stoves for warmth. In addition, for reasons clear only to higher command, soldiers were periodically shuttled from camp to camp around the nation. The situation—young men from diverse areas (countryside, town, and city) crowded together, under the stress of training, and connected to various regions through a steady stream of transfers—was perfect for incubating and spreading a new infection, especially a respiratory infection.

On 4 March 1918 a cook reported to the Camp Funston infirmary complaining of symptoms typical of influenza. Over the next three weeks he was joined by eleven hundred of his fellow soldiers who were sick enough to require a stay in the infirmary. Many thousands of others received treatment or medicine on an outpatient basis and recuperated in their barracks. Soon other camps began to report outbreaks of influenza-like illnesses, and in short order the infection traveled with the recruits who were being shipped to France to join their compatriots in the American Expeditionary Forces (AEF). The illness quickly radiated out from the American base and circulated through soldiers and civilians alike on both sides of the trenches.[5] The "three-day fever" circulated throughout Europe in the late spring and early summer but attracted little attention. Great things were afoot as the German army spilled over the Allied trenches and drove toward Paris. The Allies tried desperately to slow the Germans as the AEF rushed to halt the German advance. Influenza was only a minor annoyance in this grand drama.[6]

Only retrospectively were there signs that this three-day fever was caused by no usual influenza strain. The virus was at times extremely infectious, especially in enclosed places such as ships and hospitals. And although the mortality rate was not high, some of those who succumbed to the infection died quite rapidly with unusual pneumonia features. The war's insatiable demand for men and matériel ensured that the infection traveled back from the western front to the homelands and colonial possessions that fed the engines of destruction. Throughout the mid- to late summer of 1918 (June–August), the number of diagnosed cases of influenza declined in Europe and North America even as they continued to climb in Asia. It appeared that Spanish flu was ending, a presumption that subsequently proved to be tragically premature.

In late August, influenza erupted epidemically in three locations at almost the same time: Boston, in the United States; Brest, in France; and Freetown, in Sierra Leone.[7] The second wave had begun. This was the killer wave of Spanish flu, and the pandemic's unprecedented scale and scope, as well as some of its unusual features, have fascinated researchers in recent years. The second wave was marked both by typical and atypical patterns in elements of influenza infection and by typical elements whose speed and volume made them atypical. For example, Boston, Brest, and Freetown are all port cities: Boston was an important hub for men and matériel shuttling to the western front; Brest was the major landing site for the AEF (almost 800,000 of the 2 million U.S. soldiers eventually deployed disembarked there); and Freetown was a major coaling station serving Europe, Africa, and Asia. And port cities have traditionally been entry areas for spreading infections. But the simultaneous emergence of the second wave in separate locations is unusual. It is possible that the influenza virus underwent three separate and identical mutations at the same time, but highly unlikely.

In addition to the unusual triple outbreak, another unusual feature consisted in the unprecedented speed with which the virus moved through populations. Rapid epidemic increase of infection had always been a hallmark of the virus, but Spanish flu's second wave moved faster and infected more people than had been seen in any previous influenza pandemic. The virus encircled the globe in four months, infecting 30 percent of the human population, approximately 500 million people.[8] The virus spread via every available means of transportation, whether steamer, railcar, horseback, or foot . . . or even dogsled. By the end of September the virus was raging in the forest headwaters of the Gambia River; by October, in the frozen arctic of the Yukon.[9] Soldier or civilian, rich or poor, black or white, no one was immune. Only those who had suffered flu in the spring showed any resistance to the disease.

In a pattern similar to that for other global infections, such as cholera, only operating at warp speed, the virus exploited chains of infection to quickly expose virtually the entire planet's population. The titanic war did not cause globalization, but the demands of the war accelerated the rate and volume of global connections. Spanish flu brought these interactions into high relief, demonstrating the extent to which the world populations had become closely interwoven. These connections are even firmer and tighter today.

Like the pandemic's speed of movement, the course of infection and mortality pattern indicated a different kind of influenza infection, one never before (or since) observed in an influenza outbreak. Simply put, this strain not only infected more people than previous strains had, but it made them sicker and killed them more frequently. The mortality rate was roughly twenty-five times higher than that of a normal influenza outbreak.[10] Some examples will help illustrate this aspect of Spanish flu. Camp Devens was a military post about thirty miles west of Boston. Like all military encampments during World War I, it was swollen with recruits training to fight in Europe. In September 1918 it housed about forty-five thousand individuals. The first cases of Spanish flu appeared among sailors working the Commonwealth pier in Boston on 27 August 1918, but it would soon be transferred to troops at Devens.

As in any large grouping of people, the population at Camp Devens produced a steady trickle of people reporting illness or injury. Military encampments in particular have traditionally served as places where diseases are readily exchanged because they bring people from various regions into close contact with one another. During the first week of September, hospital admissions at Camp Devens had ranged from 31 on 2 September to 95 five days later, when the first soldier stricken with the second wave of Spanish flu reported for sick call. Initially the soldier's high fever, lethargy, and intense body aches and pains were chalked up to cerebrospinal meningitis, but this first patient was soon joined by dozens and then thousands of recruits with identical or even worse symptoms. On 10 September, 142 soldiers were admitted to the hospital. On 13 September, 350 new patients were taken in. Two days later, 705 new patients were admitted. The admissions reached a peak of 1,189 on 16 September, followed in short order by 1,056 and 1,176 on the following two days. These are not cumulative totals but new admissions for each day.[11] The hospital was overwhelmed, and the chaos was compounded because many of the hospital staff came down with the infection as well. These influenza patients were deathly ill, sicker than anyone had ever before seen in influenza victims. In a letter to a friend, Roy Grist, a physician at the hospital at Devens, wrote, "These men start with what appears to be an ordinary attack of La Grippe or Influenza, and when brought to the Hosp. they very rapidly develop the most vicious type of Pneumonia that has ever been seen. . . . One could stand it to see one, two or twenty men die, but to see these poor devils dropping like flies. . . . We have been averaging about 100 deaths per day. . . . Pneumonia means in about all cases death."[12]

The military immediately recognized the danger of this new infection and dispatched their finest and most prestigious medical team to Camp Devens to assess this outbreak. The team included Simeon Walbach, of Harvard Medical School; Rufus Cole, of the Rockefeller Institute; Victor Vaughn, a former president of the American Medical Association; and William Welch, also a former president of the American Medical Association and a prominent member (perhaps the most prominent member) of the Johns Hopkins Medical School, the country's preeminent medical training facility. These men were the cream of the crop espousing the new scientific approach to medicine, and their positions and prestige indicated the dominance of the germ theory of disease. They both resulted from and had helped create the wedding of science and medical research in medical education.[13]

Like their counterparts in certain other fields, physicians were swept up in the late-nineteenth-century trend for creating professional organizations (the American Historical Association, for example, was founded in 1884). This self-selected movement of practitioners sought to craft an assortment of core competencies and standards whose mastery was required for membership in the professional organization. In the case of physicians, the profession and its organization, the American Medical Association (AMA), pressured state licensing boards to stiffen the standards for the legal practice of medicine. These new standards placed greater pressure on medical schools to make training more rigorous. Following the lead of the best medical schools, such as those at Harvard and Johns Hopkins, medical training programs began incorporating more hands-on research in fully equipped anatomy and chemistry labs, as well as instruction in the latest aspects of microbiology. Following a ruthless evaluation of all medical schools that Abraham Flexner undertook in 1910 at the behest of the AMA, a number of medical schools were forced to combine with other schools or close their doors.[14] This restructuring left only those schools that were strongly supported and steeped in research and practice based on the germ theory of disease. In this development, then, lie the roots of the scientific research paradigm that dominates medicine today.

When they arrived, the men on the team were confident that their knowledge and training could adequately address any health task they might encounter. They entered the camp on 23 September and found the hospital to be an anarchic scene, with thousands of soldiers and hospital staff suffering searing fevers, intense body pain, delirium, and for ominously many, signs of pneumonia. Welch himself led the group in autopsy, working in a morgue where the bodies were heaped about him. Welch sliced open the chest of a cadaver and saw the likely cause of death: the lungs were swollen and filled with bloody fluid. The same situation was found in other cases; the victims' lungs were so filled with fluid that the men had literally drowned. This discovery explained a phenomenon many had noted in those who were stricken. The cheeks and even entire faces of those who were at death's door would turn blue or even black. Their bodies had been unable to oxygenate their blood, leading to the discoloration. The tour left Welch shaken, and he groped for an explanation. The disease must be some "new infection," he said, or perhaps "plague." Ultimately, one-third at the Devens post contracted influenza by the end of October, and 787 died.[15] And Camp Devens was a harbinger of things to come.

The explosive rise of infections was not limited to military camps in the United States but quickly spread along the eastern seaboard, and then, as happened in 1889, the virus began to hopscotch along the nation's transportation routes. Hospitals were quickly overwhelmed, and many were forced to limit or halt admissions.[16] Temporary hospitals were formed out of schools, dormitories, and even in tents pitched in public parks. The difficulties in caring for this crushing amount of influenza victims was further compounded by the fact that many doctors and nurses were serving in the war effort and were thus far from their communities. But the sick were not alone in overwhelming the system; the dead, arriving in vast numbers, swamped coroners and undertakers alike. The city of Philadelphia was particularly hard hit. In the third week of the autumn epidemic, 4,597 people died there. The bodies were stacked on the loading dock of the city morgue, and purportedly, in a scene reminiscent of the Middle Ages, a cart trolled the streets collecting the dead.[17]

The havoc resulting from Spanish flu was not at all limited to the eastern seaboard of the United States. Virtually the entire globe suffered the pandemic at the same time. Both Boston and Bombay recorded their peak mortality on 5 October 1918; Philadelphia, Liverpool, Prague, and Madras, on 19 October; and San Francisco, Dublin, Amsterdam, and Rangoon, on 2 November. Australia's stringent quarantine kept the infection at bay until the winter of 1919, but only American Samoa escaped unscathed.[18] Spanish flu was a global disease, and even if the overriding crush of the pandemic's local impact initially narrowed medical researchers' horizons, the universality of the statistics and anecdotes demonstrated the disease's broad reach.

The rapid spread and community-wide involvement with the infection matched the diagnosis of influenza, but the esteemed Dr. Welch was not alone in seeking an alternative explanation for the pandemic. The people flooding into hospitals and doctor's offices were sicker than was normal for influenza cases, and many of those most afflicted had hitherto been in the prime of health. For the most part, however, these facets of the infection remained the objects of impressionistic observation during the pandemic, because anyone with any medical training was put to work treating the stricken. Still, medical researchers not directly involved in frontline care, and those physicians who could spare the time, sought to identify the agent responsible for the new plague. It clearly could not be influenza. Medical science had discovered the cause of influenza in 1889, and its name was *Bacillus influenzae,* commonly called Pfeiffer's bacillus. Researchers around the globe reported their inability to recover Pfeiffer's bacillus from the afflicted. "Therefore," one European scientist concluded, "the disease was 'not influenza.'"[19] The researchers peered through their microscopes, collected numerous bacteria samples in a multitude of cultures, and tried a host of antiserums, vaccines, and almost every known medical compound to cure or prevent the disease, all to no avail.[20]

Facing these failures, medical researchers reluctantly concluded that the illness sweeping the globe *was* influenza, albeit of a power never seen before, and that physicians could offer little in terms of treatment beyond palliative nursing care. The failure of medical research to cure or even identify the agent responsible must have come as a shock to the researchers whose professional career spanned the introduction and successful application of the germ theory of disease. These scientists had witnessed and participated in research that had brought many dreaded killers to heel. The organisms responsible for plague, tuberculosis, cholera, and typhoid, and other terrible illnesses had been identified, and though cures were not always forthcoming, outbreaks of them could be controlled. Even diseases that could not be identified through the microscope, as was the case with yellow fever, were beaten back and in some places even eradicated through close study of the afflictions and their transmission patterns. Nowhere was this confidence of control more prevalent than in the medical leadership in the U.S. Armed Forces.[21] Called to service to protect the troops from the traditional scourge of militaries in history, these prominent physicians were coolly confident that they could protect the soldiers from epidemic diseases. Their stunning failure in the face of Spanish flu haunted these researchers, who either declined to discuss Spanish flu's onslaught or took great pains to emphasize how successful they were in preventing the outbreaks of other diseases. Influenza was a disease these physicians would like to forget. Still, some scientists expressed their despair openly: "Although influenza is one of the oldest known of the epidemic diseases[,] it is the least understood. Science, which by patient and painstaking labor has done so much to drive other plagues to the point of extinction[,] has thus far stood powerless before it."[22]

The pandemic swept the globe throughout the fall and early winter of 1918. In region after region, cases quickly soared to an epidemic peak and just as suddenly dropped off. Many regions were revisited by the flu in the winter and spring of 1919 in a third wave of the pandemic. This third wave of Spanish flu seemed milder only in comparison to the previous catastrophe. As the Massachusetts Commission of Public Health stated: "If the terrific influenza fatality had never occurred this epidemic would have been considered by health officers and the general public alike as an almost unprecedented disaster. In all, 1,660 deaths and about 35,000 cases were reported."[23] Soon after this third wave began to recede, public health officials went about calculating the pandemic's impact as they always did: by counting up the number of extra dead.

The statistics provided breathtaking data to bolster the initial impressions of physicians. First, Spanish flu was far deadlier than any previous recorded flu epidemic had been. Edwin Oakes Jordan, who collected as many state and city mortality statistics as he could, estimated that 548,542 U.S. citizens had died from the disease during the ten months from October 1918 through July 1919.[24] Spanish flu dropped the life expectancy in the United States ten years and probably killed as many men in the military as died in battle during World War I.

Perhaps the most unusual aspect of the mortality was the age group that suffered the worst. Traditionally, influenza—in epidemic and nonepidemic years alike—has had its greatest impact on the very young and the very old. Those most at risk of succumbing from a case of influenza are those with the weakest immune systems, who are unable to fend off the viral invader and its opportunistic cohort. Graphing this typical mortality distribution provides a crude U shape, with mortality dropping steeply beyond the initial few years of age and slowly rising in the older portion of the population. The data on Spanish flu mortality, however, confirmed physicians' impressions: the burden of mortality fell heaviest on young adults, the most immunologically fit people of a community. Graphing Spanish flu mortality against age creates a crude W shape, with the greatest number of the dead clustering between twenty-one and twenty-nine years of age. Mortality was elevated in all age brackets (although apparently less so in those over the age of sixty) but the lion's share occurred in individuals from twenty to forty years old. In South African cities, 60 percent of the deaths fell in this age bracket; in Chicago, the number of deaths in that bracket was almost five times higher than the number for people age forty to sixty. This abnormal mortality pattern appeared to be a global phenomenon.[25]

Because of this heightened mortality in this twenty-to-forty age group, Spanish flu wrought greater social damage than is typical for influenza. First, it robbed society of its most productive and strongest members. In crude economic terms, societies lost their returns on the costs of raising children to adulthood. Second, context could increase the importance of mortality in this age cohort, for if the society was particularly reliant on this group for survival, its loss could lead to especially desperate straits. For example, the pandemic struck Tanzania at the start of planting season. The combined impact of many stricken with influenza across all ages and the loss of the society's strongest members—perhaps as high as 10 percent of Tanzania's inhabitants—resulted in a failure to plant or tend crops. The epidemic was thus followed by a famine that extended into the following two years.[26] The unusual mortality pattern could also have a demographic echo effect, the loss of a society's most fertile members reducing the number of children born later.[27]

The sobering collection of statistics and medical science's failure to mitigate the pandemic chastened the public health community.[28] Edwin Oakes Jordan's encyclopedic examination of the medical literature for Spanish flu led him to conclude, "In the face of the almost certain recurrence some day of another world-wide pandemic, we remain nearly as helpless to institute effective measures of control as we were before 1918."[29]

Jordan's book, published in 1927, was written before it was clear that influenza was caused by a virus. We in the twenty-first century now know more about the Spanish flu virus than Jordan and his contemporaries could have ever dreamed of knowing, and we gained this knowledge through a combination of technological advancement, foresight, and a little luck.[30]

The Recovery of Spanish Flu

Jeffrey Taubenberger led the Division of Molecular Pathology at the U.S. Armed Forces Institute of Pathology, in Washington, D.C. The institute houses the National Tissue Repository, which collects and stores tissue samples collected by military physicians dating back to the American Civil War. The specimens mostly consist of tissue bearing unusual or unknown afflictions that interested or puzzled medical personnel. Many of the samples, taken from various sections of the human anatomy, were treated with formaldehyde and sealed in wax. In 1995 Taubenberger and his assistant, Ann Reid, were concerned about potential budget cuts and so cast about for a way to highlight the laboratory's worth. Taubenberger and Reid decided to search the institute's collection of Spanish flu victims to see whether they could use powerful new gene-amplification technologies to recover the killer virus's genetic code. Taubenberger and Reid were able to extract fragments of the influenza's genetic code from lung tissue stored from a fatal case in 1918 and, using the new technology of reverse transcription–polymerase chain reaction, managed to amplify and sequence the virus's RNA fragments. Taubenberger immediately recognized the importance of this recovery and rushed the initial results to the journal *Science*.[31]

Taubenberger's group was subsequently able to use the collection to recover genetic information from a second source, but despite their tremendous usefulness, these samples had a few drawbacks. First, both had been treated with formaldehyde, which might have altered the specimens. Second, the two samples came from a limited source: two members of the military located on the eastern coast of the United States (coincidentally, both had died on the same day, 26 September 1918). Third, the pathology segments yielded only a fragmentary amount of the RNA's genetic code. Much to Taubenberger's surprise, the solution to all these problems would arrive in the mail.

Shortly after his article was published in *Science,* Taubenberger received a cordial letter from a retired pathologist named Johan Hultin, who asked whether Taubenberger would be interested in additional examples of the Spanish flu virus.[32] Taubenberger of course said yes. Hultin outlined his plan to retrieve tissue from Spanish flu victims buried in permafrost. The idea itself was not far-fetched; indeed, an expansive, and expensive, mission was being prepared to do just that in a cemetery in Spitsbergen, Norway.[33] At first glance, the seventy-two-year-old retired pathologist seemed an unlikely candidate for such an operation, but Hultin had something none of the virologists, geographers, civil engineers, and modern technicians involved in the Spitsbergen expedition could boast: experience. Hultin had done it before.

In 1949 the Swedish-born Hultin was studying virology at the University of Iowa when he went to lunch with the well-known virologist William Hale. Hale mentioned in passing that the key to understanding Spanish flu might reside in the corpses of victims buried in the permafrost. The task would require the identification of Spanish flu victims' burial sites and a familiarity with excavating in permafrost. Hultin, an avid outdoorsman, had recently returned from a summer recreational trip up the Alaska Highway, where he had met and befriended Otto Geist, a paleontologist at the University of Alaska. Geist had established friendly relations with many residents of isolated villages in his frequent forays for artifacts. Hultin had spent several weeks that summer traveling with Geist and aiding him on his digs. Hultin realized that his experience studying influenza (he was working under Albert McKee at Iowa) and his knowledge of remote Alaskan terrain combined with his connections with Geist made him a perfect candidate for just such a project. Hultin approached McKee, who suggested he explore the feasibility of the project, and Hultin contacted Geist, who was immediately enthusiastic. Geist provided an introduction to Lutheran missionaries who gave Hultin access to church records of outposts that had suffered Spanish flu outbreaks. Hultin narrowed the list to a few likely places where accurate records of victims had been kept and where burial sites lay north of the permafrost line. Hultin sought funding from the National Institutes of Health, which denied his request. Not discouraged, Hultin, McKee, and the University of Iowa pathologist Jack Layton arranged university funding and traveled north, where they were joined by Geist.

The NIH's denial of Hultin's funding request provides an interesting view into the changing world of medical research after the war. Through his department chair's congressional connections, Hultin found out that his grant had been denied because the U.S. Army thought it was a great idea and wanted to recover the virus for its own uses. The chair, Roger Porter, acquired the funds for the expedition from the university, and the trio of Iowa researchers beat the military to the site. Although the military was, and remains, a major source of funds for scientific research, the availability of other funds suggests that the military dominance of scientific and medical research was ending. At any rate, however, Hultin and his mentors determined that the permafrost from the location listed in their application was unsuitable for their project and that they needed to find another burial ground.[34]

A location called Brevig Mission did meet all the criteria: bodies there had been rapidly interred following the Spanish flu pandemic (seventy-two of eighty villagers succumbed that awful winter, and their bodies had been buried at least six feet deep by hired gold miners), and the permafrost remained intact. After receiving permission from the town council, the four men began digging. Wearing gauze masks and limiting the number of people in the excavating trench, the team disinterred several of the bodies and retrieved slices of lungs, kidneys, spleen, and brain from the frozen corpses. After packing the samples, the team returned to the University of Iowa laboratories, where Hultin tried, without success, to grow live virus. Apparently the cold had destroyed the fragile virus. Interestingly, the team was able to grow both Pfeiffer's bacilli and pneumococci.[35]

Hultin never forgot this unusual expedition, and when he read Taubenberger's *Science* article, it fired up his desire to try again. Two weeks after sending the letter to Taubenberger, Hultin was on his way to Alaska, intending to revisit Brevig Mission. In contrast to members of the lavishly funded, media-spectacular assault on the graves of Spitsbergen, Hultin traveled by himself, on his own dime, carrying a pair of garden shears purloined from his wife. Hultin reasoned that since he had been unable to retrieve live virus in 1951, the possibility that cadavers still contained viable virus in 1997 was extraordinarily remote, but he realized that genetic fragments of the virus might still reside entombed in the tissues of the frozen dead.

Upon arrival in Brevig Mission, Hultin asked the mayor for permission to exhume the bodies. His appeal was greatly aided by the fact that several village members recalled the story of the previous expedition. The village elders again granted him permission, and Hultin, with four local youths hired for the task, set about digging up the mass grave. The initial discoveries were not favorable; most of the bodies were skeletonized. Then Hultin uncovered a body he dubbed "Lucy." Lucy was a large woman, and so her corpse had retained most of her body mass. When he snipped open her chest with the garden shears, he saw two swollen and intact lung sacs. Hultin cut a few sections from the lungs and retrieved samples from several other organs. He then packed the lot into insulated flasks and reburied the bodies—even reconsecrating the gravesite with two wooden crosses he constructed to mimic two crosses he recalled from forty-six years earlier that had subsequently disappeared.

Returning to San Francisco, Hultin divided the tissue samples into four separate packages, which he then addressed and mailed to Jeffrey Taubenberger—two by one private shipping company, another by a second private shipping firm, and one by the U.S. Postal Service. In a testament to the efficiency of all three delivery services, the four samples arrived at Jeffrey Taubenberger's lab. As expected, none of the samples contained viable virus; a significant amount of genetic material was included, however, and the Brevig Mission sample was almost an exact copy of the South Carolina and New York samples. The same virus had killed the soldiers on the East Coast and the unfortunate Lucy in Alaska. A similar paraffin-stored sample was later retrieved from British sources, and even some fragmentary material from the Spitsbergen expedition was recovered. From this mixture of genetic material, the laboratory was able to re-create the entire genetic code.

The cracking of Spanish flu's genetic code has led to research experiments designed to unlock the mysteries of the virus's unusual killing pattern. Using this genetic code and the technology of reverse genetics, the various segments of the virus have been reconstituted and examined for their relationships to other influenza virus segments. These experiments culminated in the fall of 2005 when the Spanish flu virus was reconstituted in its entirety, perhaps the first time it existed in complete form since 1920. Under strict biosafety precautions, the Spanish flu virus was experimentally introduced into mice. Various combinations incorporating segments of the Spanish flu virus were found to heighten effects on the animals—for example, combining the hemagglutinin gene from Spanish flu with seven genetic segments of a laboratory strain of influenza produced measurably higher courses of infection. But by far, the most devastating course of infection occurred when the Spanish flu virus was introduced intact. That is, the constellation of all eight Spanish flu genes was the most deadly infection; indeed, all the infected mice died within a few days of exposure to it. The report of this experiment stated: "In fact, no other human viruses that have been tested show a similar pathogenicity for mice 3 to 4 days after infection."[36] Exactly why Spanish flu is so deadly remains unclear.

Nonetheless, a second set of experiments utilizing the re-created Spanish flu virus does offer some suggestions as to the virus's enhanced lethality. A report in the journal Nature described the experimental introduction of Spanish flu into a number of cynomolgus macaques. The monkeys infected with the

1918 strain of influenza suffered a significantly more violent course of infection than did the control monkeys infected with a recent laboratory strain of influenza. The animals infected with the re-created 1918 flu strain were extremely sick, some so ill that they had to be euthanized several days ahead of schedule. The animals had high viral loads, meaning that they shed a lot of virus, making the virus more transmissible. In addition, the infection spread rapidly through the individual, infecting other organs beyond the respiratory system, including the heart and spleen. It was the lungs, however, that showed the greatest impact of the viral invader, and the course of infection in the macaques mirrored that found in historical descriptions of Spanish flu victims. The monkey's lungs were severely damaged, swollen and filled with bloody discharge that hampered the vital gas exchange in oxygenating the blood. Just as was described in 1918, the monkeys were drowning in their own fluids.[37]

Examining the monkey's lungs on autopsy provided an answer for the death of the animals and a possible hypothesis for Spanish flu's unusual mortality pattern in humans. The damage to the lungs did not directly result from the influenza infection; that is, the replication of the virus itself did not cause the widespread damage to the lung cells. Rather, the innate immune system was what destroyed the lung cells. The infection prompted an overreaction, dubbed a "cytokine storm," where the immune system rushed an excessive amount of fluid and first-line immune-system defenders into the infected lungs, damaging not only virus-infected cells but also many cells surrounding the infected ones. This violent response may occur in part because Spanish flu inhibits the body's ability to shut off this first-line innate defense. The second reason for the widespread damage to the lungs lay in the strain's ability to replicate. In the macaques the Spanish flu virus replicated very rapidly, and the increasing numbers of infected cells thus prompted greater damage by the innate immune system as it sought to repel the infection.

A second feature of the Spanish flu virus's duplication capabilities further increased the proportion of lung cells liable to infection. Macaque lungs are similar to human lungs in that the epithelial cells that line the upper tract of the lung have both alpha 2,6 sialic acid receptors and, deep in their lungs, alpha 2,3 sialic acid receptors. As I noted previously, avian-type influenza virus binds preferentially with alpha 2,3 sialic acid receptors, and human influenza virus strains bind with alpha 2,6 receptor. In the macaques, the virus replicated in both the upper and lower portions of the lung, making the infection in the lungs much more widespread. The result of this widespread destruction of the lung surface is known as Acute Respiratory Distress Syndrome (ARDS).[38] Physicians at the western front during World War I were familiar with this particular lung distress; it was an effect of blistering agents, such as mustard gas.

The experimental infection of mice and macaques provides the basis for a retrospective hypothesis about mortality patterns and a potential warning for future influenza pandemics. The ill effects of an overactive innate immune response suggest that, perversely, those with the strongest immune systems will suffer the worst effects of a Spanish influenza infection. The innate immune system's rapid and massive response to the widespread and escalating virus results in greater damage to the lungs, so that victims will drown in the resulting cellular and fluid debris. In the human population, young adults have the fittest immune systems. This influenza hypothesis also fits anecdotal accounts that this segment suffered the direst Spanish flu infections.

Examining the recovered Spanish flu virus also offers an ominous portent to strains circulating in the present. Spanish flu is almost entirely avian in character, and it likely had a limited circulation in the human population before erupting into a pandemic. Indeed, a small number of mutations—perhaps as few as two—were needed to change this virus from a poorly transmitted human infection into the pandemic known as Spanish flu.[39] In 2009 the avian influenza H5N1, dubbed "bird flu," circulated predominately throughout Southeast Asia, but it has been found in an increasing number of cases in Europe and Africa. The virus has thus far proven to be poorly transmitted from human to human. The vast majority of cases have been contracted directly from poultry or waterfowl.[40] There is presently no way to determine the number of subclinical or mild infections of bird flu, data that, if added, would surely lower the mortality percentage; as it stands, however, the mortality rate of those infected approaches an alarming 60 percent. Victims infected with bird flu have had violent responses, with great damage to the lungs. The virus has not mutated into one readily transmitted to humans, and odds are that it will not, but the situation requires close monitoring.

Despite the unprecedented insight into the way Spanish flu kills, we will never be able to specify how many it killed. Part of the difficulty lies in assigning death to an influenza infection. Recall that since William Farr, the method of calculating the human impact of an influenza epidemic (or any disease outbreak) is to count the number of dead above a predicted threshold. The easiest place to identify the mortality impact of an influenza impact is in the "Pneumonia and Influenza" records, the so-called P and I figures. These numbers soar in lockstep with the number of cases of influenza diagnosed. But as Farr discovered, and other researchers have verified, mortality rises in other causes too, such as heart attacks, strokes, or that catchall phrase old age. As a statistical trend, the rise of mortality is easy to graph; on the case-by-case level, the cause of death may not be so clear. In the Spanish flu pandemic, the chaotic deluge of cases swamped bureaucracies in many areas, with record keeping suspended and many hospitals forced to limit their admissions, leaving the rest to recover—or not—at home. Estimating mortality in places where records are kept poorly or intermittently is difficult; doing so where they are not kept at all is highly speculative.

Therefore, a completely accurate account of Spanish flu's impact is impossible, but several intrepid researchers have fearlessly set sail into a sea of statistics. The first attempt, as previously stated, was by Edwin Oakes Jordan. Relying on city and state health reports and statistical estimates from government reports, as well as extrapolating known rates to regions with no data, Jordan estimated that 21.6 million died from the three waves of Spanish flu.[41] Jordan's 1927 estimate was widely cited in the subsequent decades, even though local and regional demographic studies based on records and information unavailable to Jordan began to uncover figures much larger than the ones used to calculate his global total. In 1991 K. David Patterson and Gerald Pyle crafted a global synthesis drawing on local estimates accrued in the preceding decades.[42] Using the most conservative estimates, Patterson and Pyle estimated mortality to have been between 24.7 and 39.3 million people globally, with 30 million being their best guess. Finally, in 2002 Niall P. A. S. Johnson and Juergen Mueller tapped an even greater set of local and regional studies and utilized new models to calculate deaths associated with influenza, generating an estimate of 50 million dead globally. But as the authors admit, even this large figure may be an underestimation, perhaps by as much as 100 percent. This means that the global total could range as high as 100 million dead.[43]

Whatever the death toll, 21.6 million or 100 million, the 1918 pandemic seems destined to have become a memorable event. The sudden appearance, the millions killed, the many more millions sickened, the overwhelmed hospitals and public health personnel, the temporary tent cities, the commandeered public buildings, all happening in the span of a few months—such chaos is hardly the sort of thing to easily fade from memory. Yet the most notable historical aspect of Spanish flu is how little it was discussed, at least until the last few decades.[44] The tragedy did not make it into history textbooks, and autobiographies and biographies of leading figures of the age scarcely mention it; it rarely appears in the literature or songs of the day. Public health and political figures were briefly roused to appropriate funds to study influenza, but this interest soon waned, and there were no great institutes established to uncover the mysteries of the illness, no crusades to stamp out flu. A lingering concern with influenza played some role in the creation of the National Institutes of

Health in 1928, and the World Health Organization organized its influenza surveillance network in 1947 to identify an emerging pandemic in its earliest stages, but Surgeon General Rupert Blue's hope for creating a permanent organization in the USPHS to respond to health emergencies such as pandemic flu was quietly ignored in the years following Spanish flu.[45] A curious, public silence grew up around the pandemic.

No generalized statement is completely accurate, however, including this one. If the collective memory had forgotten Spanish flu, the same could not be said about the memories of individuals. These memories of friends, families, and strangers with blue-black faces struggling for breath were stored and handed down to descendants and had a power to evoke strong responses when triggered, as occurred in 1976. And though no scientific institutions or funding streams were dedicated to the study of influenza, that did not preclude the efforts of individual scientists. In the ensuing decades monumental strides were made in understanding the virus and its actions. Finally, there was one institute that held vivid memories of Spanish flu's impact. When the clouds of global war gathered again, the U.S. military invested heavily in studying and preventing influenza infections. The disparate strands of these research approaches began to come together, and talented scientists began to focus on cracking the mystery of influenza pandemics. In the ensuing decades, researchers would unlock many of the influenza virus's secrets.

Nature had humbled scientists again. Influenza was not a bacterial disease but something else, and an influenza pandemic had the ability to kill a staggeringly large number of people, especially young adults. The experts' ostensible knowledge about the illness was called into question, and researchers would have to go back to their laboratory benches to uncover the disease's cause.

CHAPTER 3

Breakthroughs

Spanish flu was arguably the worst pandemic in human history, but as the catastrophe receded from memory, few medical researchers worked on the agent responsible for the disaster. In the interwar years, the study of influenza was largely an individual pursuit rather than an organized research field. During World War II, however, and in the years following it, organizations for systematically tracking and studying the influenza virus began to emerge. One such organization, the World Health Organization, developed a surveillance system that both drew on previous health systems, such as the League of Nations Health Organization, and maintained a narrow focus on technical issues. Sustained, well-funded research on the influenza virus began to yield important breakthroughs. But the methods of studying and responding to it became increasingly technical. In some ways this technical focus helped break down the intense national interests in pursuit of science, but in other ways it created a sharp dichotomy between those who could engage in science and those who could not. Technical programs began to dominate public health efforts. Global public health began to develop in new ways.

Exactly why the medical establishment and historians largely turned their back on unraveling influenza's secrets in the years following the Spanish flu epidemic is a bit of a mystery. Perhaps it was, as Howard Phillips and David

Killingray suggest, a matter of wounded pride: "As the Spanish flu amounted to an enormous rout in the war against disease for the medical profession, it was not a subject to hold much appeal for the triumphalist brand of medical history then in vogue, thanks to medicine's stream of successes since Pasteur."[1] And perhaps the rout occurred because it is difficult to identify what you cannot see. By the end of the Spanish flu pandemic, the medical community had concluded that Pfeiffer's bacillus was not the cause of influenza. As early as 1918, some researchers had begun claiming that influenza was caused by a filter-passing element called a virus (the Latin word *virus* means "poison"), but there was no consensus on the causative organism.[2]

Viruses had been a perplexing riddle for medical researchers. In the frenzied search for the germs that caused diseases, budding bacteriologists identified a host of organisms responsible for various afflictions, but they soon realized that some disease-causing entities resisted identification. Complicating matters, a set of experiments (the first run in 1876 on the tobacco mosaic disease) demonstrated that infectious matter of certain sorts can be passed through even the finest bacterial filters and still cause infection. By 1903 Pierre Roux, successor to Louis Pasteur as the director of the Pasteur Institute, codified this mysterious subgroup of disease-causing material. Roux proposed three characteristics common to the causative entities: they were filterable, invisible via light microscopy, and nonculturable (on known bacterial growth mediums). The nature of these "filterable viruses" would remain a mystery until the invention of the electron microscope in 1938 and the discovery of the double helix structure of DNA by James Watson and Francis Crick in 1953.[3]

To test the viral theory of influenza infection, scientists attempted to use very fine porcelain filters to screen out bacteria but still induce the infection in experimental animals and human volunteers. Probably because of sloppy techniques, none of the experiments were conclusive, and researchers wrongly concluded that the illness was not caused by a virus. Without a method to positively identify the causative agent, medical researchers were forced to rely on identifications based on symptoms. Unfortunately, influenza's symptoms—fevers, cough, body aches, and exhaustion—are common, in various degrees, to numerous respiratory infections. Influenza was easy to see on the community level but difficult to identify in the individual.

Compounding the difficulties of accurate diagnosis was the issue of immunity or resistance to influenza infection. A bout of influenza offered little or even no resistance to the disease in succeeding years. Researchers recognized that this phenomenon sometimes reflected merely an earlier misdiagnosis of influenza infection, but they suspected that something else was going on as well.[4] Some scientists posited remarkably prescient hypotheses about influenza despite their limited knowledge of the virus and its behavior. Edwin Oakes Jordan concluded: "It seems to me at least a plausible hypothesis that the coming into existence of a peculiar strain of influenza virus different from the strain or strains of endemic influenza is the cause of the pandemic mani-festations."[5] But most researchers agreed with the gloomy assessment of two leading medical textbooks of the age: one of them asserted, "There is not the slightest shred of evidence that the disease is due to a so-called filter passing virus"; the other concluded, "There is little hope that they [the difficulties of identification] will ever be overcome in the case of influenza."[6]

Influenza defied identification at least in part because there was almost no institutional support to research the disease. Several factors account for this lack of research focus. Until the nineteenth century, scientific research was conducted individually, generally by knowledgeable members of the wealthy class. Governments and other institutions provided little support for it. Task- and business-oriented research support began to become more prevalent toward the later nineteenth century, but little of this funding ex-tended to medical or health issues. Into this void stepped newly created private philanthropic entities such as the Rockefeller Institute for Medical Research (founded in 1901) and the later Rockefeller Foundation (in 1909).[7] These lav-ishly endowed private organizations were a tremendous boon to medical re-search, funding laboratories, international studies, and eradication campaigns. But even Rockefeller's and Carnegie's deep pockets needed careful husband-ing, and the philanthropic trusts were selective in choosing where to place their money. The Rockefeller Institute invested heavily in yellow fever and polio research, and the International Health Division of the Rockefeller Foun-dation supported research and mitigation efforts concerning hookworm and malaria. In many ways such research efforts into selected diseases mirrored the tropical disease research supported by European colonial governments. Programs to eliminate or modify hookworm and malaria infestations were designed to make local populations healthier and more productive, hence in-creasing the profitability of factories and plantations located regionally (in the American South) and globally (e.g., in South America or the Philippines).

Private funding remained an important component even for educational programs in medicine. Medical schools organized around microbiology and laboratory work required expensive equipment and supplies and generally depended on the generosity of individual benefactors and philanthropic or-ganizations. Public health programs, too, required private funding. The first public health school opened in Baltimore on 1 October 1918 with input and critical funding from the Rockefeller Foundation. The Johns Hopkins School

of Medicine immediately became (and remains) one of the preeminent institutions for public health scholarship and research.[8]

Governments generally eschewed funding research outside a few narrow
areas. As was previously discussed, colonial governments funded tropical medicine to support their colonial ventures, much as the U.S. military supported
research on yellow fever during the imperialist Spanish-American War. The
German government supported chemical and manufacturing research to facilitate industrialization, and German and French institutes in medicine attracted
the best and the brightest medical students imbibing the latest bacteriological
techniques.

The laissez-faire business attitude that held sway in late-nineteenth-
century U.S. government circles was a strong tonic against investment in
medical research or facilities. The scarce exceptions of the time—the Hygiene
Laboratory, established under the Marine Hospital Service in 1887, and the
Massachusetts-funded Lawrence Experiment Station, created in 1886—hardly
undermine the rule.[9] Progressive-era reforms, however, did give the federal
government modest roles in supporting research concerning matters related
to public health. For example, the Biologics Control Act of 1902 and the Pure
Food and Drug Act of 1906 elevated the U.S. Department of Agriculture's Bureau of Chemistry, putting it in charge of testing and overseeing the nation's
food and drug sources. But this predecessor of the Food and Drug Administration (FDA) was poorly funded by Congress.[10]

The relationship between government funding and research changed dramatically as a result of World War I, in which science and warfare interacted
to an unprecedented extent on the deadly fronts of Europe. World War I has
been called a "chemist's war," for chemicals were widely used both as weapons themselves and in the industrial production of war matériel. Prior to this
conflict, many of the chemicals and dyes used in various industrial processes
came from Germany. With the outbreak of hostilities, several nations had to
scramble to replace their usual suppliers. Coming out of the war, many governments recognized the vital role that chemistry, and the sciences in general,
had played on the battlefield. Accordingly, greater state investment in scientific
research was now seen as not only desirable but necessary. Although it would
be dwarfed by the government support for research that followed World War
II, the connection between state money and scientific and medical research
was forged in the cauldron of the Great War.[11]

Surprisingly, considering the impact of Spanish flu, influenza research attracted little government funding, at least in the 1920s and 1930s, and little
attention within state-run entities. Instead, such investigations were left to in-

dividual scientists. One of these scientists, Richard Shope, became interested in the phenomenon of influenza transfer in pigs.[12] Shope was aware of a recent series of experiments that had transmitted infections by intranasal delivery of mucus from pig to pig, though the experimenters had been unable to transmit the illness after filtration (again likely because of the crudity of the filters). Moreover, Shope was aware of an obscure footnote to the Spanish flu tragedy. An Iowa veterinarian named J. S. Koen (who worked for the Federal Bureau of Animal Industry) had observed an outbreak of sickness in the pig popula-tion that he believed was the same influenza pandemic then occurring in the human population. The pigs showed signs of fever, respiratory distress, nasal discharge, and exhaustion. Koen claimed the pigs were suffering from Span-ish flu and that they likely received it from humans, because the outbreak in the swine herd trailed the outbreak in the human population.[13] Since 1919 this seasonal affliction had circulated continuously through the pig population of the Midwest. Shope hypothesized that this disease was influenza and that if he could identify the agent that was infecting pigs, he would be able to identify the causative element of influenza. Shope traveled to the Midwest, where he gathered mucous samples from sick pigs. He then returned to his laboratory at Princeton, where, using state-of-the-art bacterial filters, he was able to infect pig after pig with this filtered fluid, thus proving that the pig infection was caused by a filter-passing agent—namely, a virus.

But Shope's experiments had merely demonstrated the existence of a virus causing an influenza-like illness in pigs. Determining that a virus caused influ-enza in humans would require further proof. Shope's work was published in 1931, and two British researchers working at the National Institute for Medical Research in London happened to read it.[14] The two researchers, Christopher Andrewes and Wilson Smith, were studying all types of viruses with an eye to protecting animals from infections. The British researchers had managed to acquire money for research on viral infections of animals but not of humans, so that their investigations into human influenza technically lay outside their funding mandate.[15] In January 1933, however, an epidemic of influenza struck England. Andrewes and Smith were aware of Shope's hypothesis that influ-enza was caused by a virus, and they hoped to identify a virus as the cause of human influenza. The medical researchers tried inoculating a broad assort-ment of experimental animals with fluids from influenza sufferers in the hopes of inducing the disease in an animal to study, but without success.

During the course of those unsuccessful experiments, Andrewes and Smith received word that researchers involved in canine distemper research at the Wellcome Institute in London had observed that their ferrets had de-veloped something that looked like an influenza infection, exhibiting fevers, coughs, and nasal discharge.[16] Smith decided to attempt to induce influenza in ferrets. Recalling Shope's method of transmitting infection, Smith took throat washings (rinsing the throat with saline solution) from Andrewes, who coincidentally had caught a case of influenza, and dripped the virus-laden solution into the noses of their ferrets. Within a few days the infected animals came down with the flu. Andrewes and Smith then passed the discharge of those sick ferrets through a filter and were able to infect healthy ferrets. Then, in a fortuitous accident, a sick ferret sneezed into the face of a new research assistant (Charles Stuart-Harris, who later went on to a prominent career in medical research). The assistant subsequently developed influenza.

Ferrets, as it turns out, have a respiratory system similar to the human system, and their epithelial cells contain alpha 2,6 sialic acid receptors. The transfer of the infection from human to ferret and back to human again demonstrated that the illness was the same in both species (accidentally fulfilling Koch's postulates) and provided an experimental animal model for further research. Subsequent work transmitted influenza to mice, making research both cheaper and easier than working with ferrets, which are notoriously ill tempered.

The same laboratories at the National Institute for Medical Research produced another important breakthrough in studying influenza. Wilson Smith discovered that he could grow large quantities of the influenza virus by injecting it into fertilized chicken eggs and storing them in an incubator. Within two days a sizable amount of the virus could be retrieved from the allantoic fluid. Here, then, was a way to grow sizable quantities of virus cheaply. This development was a boon for those seeking to study the virus and for those seeking to create a vaccine. In fact, current methods of manufacturing vaccine strains of influenza continue to grow the virus in eggs.[17]

It is easy to overlook the importance of such minor events as developing a method to infect cheaper laboratory animals, but these developments yielded important consequences. Because both eggs and mice are relatively inexpensive, more researchers could work on the influenza viruses, and this expanded circle of investigators produced the research that rapidly expanded knowledge of the influenza virus over the next few decades. In contrast, consider the case of the polio virus, which attracted far more sustained financial support prior to World War II than influenza did. In 1909 the medical researcher Simon Flexner (brother of Abraham, who wrote the scathing report on medical schools for the AMA) successfully infected rhesus monkeys with the filterable virus causing polio. Flexner determined that polio was transmitted through the nasal passages, since this was the only method by which he managed to infect the animals. Flexner was wrong. Polio in humans is an enteric disease spread by fecal contamination of food and water that an individual ingests. Flexner inadvertently compounded this error by repeatedly passing the viral strain through the nasal route in the monkeys, in the process accidently creating a strain that could *only* be spread via this method. Flexner's MV strain became an often-used source of polio experiments. Partly because of his status as the director of the Rockefeller Institute and partly because of the exorbitant cost of using monkeys in research, no scientists conducted experiments to challenge this basic mistaken assumption about polio transfer. Only in 1948, when John Enders grew polio on tissue cultures, were experiments challenging Flexner's assertions undertaken and Flexner's error uncovered. Nearly forty years of research had been stymied by this one mistake.[18]

Researchers around the world picked up on the importance of this ability to grow endless supplies of influenza virus cheaply and began working to further understand the virus. In the late 1930s, Tommy Francis, at the Rockefeller Institute in New York, produced another breakthrough. Francis discovered that influenza exists in multiple types. The first type of influenza virus was dubbed influenza A; the second, influenza B. A decade afterward, in the late 1940s, a much rarer third type—influenza C—was independently discovered by two groups of researchers.[19] The ability to distinguish these two different types of influenza allowed researchers to identify an influenza strain with a test that could be fine-tuned to react to a specific strain.

By the eve of World War II, medical researchers had made tremendous strides in studying influenza outbreaks. They had concluded that the infection is caused by a virus that attacks people through respiration and that it spreads by oral and nasal discharge from infected individuals. Also, numerous experiments could be conducted simultaneously on animals. Viral types A and B could be identified using a fairly simple test. All these developments, largely uncovered by individual scientists working independently, set the stage for the next step in studying influenza: learning how to prevent it.

Although generally forgotten by research institutions after World War I, influenza remained on the minds of many in the U.S. military who vividly recalled how Spanish flu had affected their operations, especially the virus's affinity for killing young adults. Officials in the armed forces recognized that their organizations' special circumstances—troops crowded together in camps, aboard ships, or along various fronts—left the military population vulnerable to respiratory infections. More to the point, the military high command recalled how influenza had interfered with the "business" of war. At the height of the Spanish flu pandemic in October 1918, troop transports to France were cut 10 percent, and even the draft was temporarily suspended in a futile attempt to slow the spread of the infection.[20] The outbreak of war in Europe in

September 1939 spurred the United States to prepare for possible involvement. These preparations included expanding the medical corps, for disease was an age-old companion of soldiers.

The gathering of men under arms has always provided a fertile environment for infectious organisms, and much to the chagrin of battlefield commanders and strategists, these organisms have often been more influential than the leaders in deciding the outcomes of battles.[21] The desire to limit the impact of infectious diseases on strategic forces spurred the development of tropical medicine for European powers and the eradication of mosquitoes both in the occupation of Cuba and during the construction of the Panama Canal. During World War I, the new science of microbiology provided medical officers with powerful new tools to protect health in the armed forces, and these officers were given the authority to intervene widely in the lives of military personnel, controlling everything from living arrangements to sexual relations.[22] Medical corps on all sides of the trenches achieved notable successes against many of the scourges of armies from the past, but as has been discussed, these medical men and women were spectacularly ineffective against Spanish flu.[23]

In addition to fostering the disaster of Spanish flu, the chaos and dislocation of the war created the environment for another epidemic disease to flower. The disintegration of the Russian and Austro-Hungarian empires, coupled with the vicious violence of the civil war between red and white Russians and the widespread movement of desperate refugees and demobilized soldiers, created a perfect environment for a typhus outbreak. Typhus, apparently ensconced in eastern Europe, is a louse-borne disease that flares up in times of distress or insanitary conditions. It had devastated Napoleon's armies on their march into and desperate retreat from Russia in their disastrous winter of 1812; it erupted again in the disorder following the titanic conflict of World War I. Just as typhus trailed behind Napoleon's army during its campaign in France, the soaring number of cases in 1920 threatened the victorious Allies along with their defeated foes.[24]

The exhausting end of World War I brought with it an intoxicating spirit of internationalism. Many pinned their hopes on the proposed League of Nations as the entity that would solve the vicious nationalist problems the war had laid bare. This new organization would offer collective solutions to age-old vexing interstate issues. One of the most natural outlets for this international approach was the field of public health. Proponents of public health saw the opportunity to create an international organization to safeguard the health of populations and to combine the resources of many states in attacking the health problems of its membership. Although this new arrangement—the League of Nations Health Organization—failed to live up to the optimistic dreams of its creators, in many ways it set the foundation on which the World Health Organization would build when that new health edifice was constructed after World War II.[25]

The proponents of the LNHO envisioned the organization as an international public health service, with already existing health organizations, such as the OIHP, being folded into it. The executive board of the OIHP had other ideas and resisted folding their organization into the LNHO. They received surprising support in this rebuff from the United States. The permanent committee of the OIHP was dominated by a cadre of senior and mostly European national public health officials who had long served in the organization; some had even participated in founding it in 1907. These men still considered the primary business of public health to be keeping dangerous epidemic diseases at bay while mitigating any impact on international trade and commerce, an insular view at odds with the more ambitious schemes of the LNHO's supporters.

Two sources gave rise to the U.S. representatives' unexpected support in the move to maintain the OIHP's independence. First, the United States wanted to maintain the independence of the regional health organization it dominated, the International Sanitary Bureau, founded in 1902 (later named the Pan American Sanitary Bureau and then the Pan American Health Organization when it was incorporated as a regional office of the WHO). Health officials in the United States feared that a strong LNHO would supplant regional organizations. Second, and more important, the United States was already a member of the OIHP, but the Senate had declined to authorize participation in the League of Nations. If the OIHP was incorporated into the LNHO, the United States would be forced to resign from the organization, leaving it no role in international health. This contingency was considered to be intolerable.

The parochial nature of independent health organizations undercut the grander dreams of a true international health service. Their multiplicity gave rise to duplicated efforts through overlapping programs and services; in addition, the LNHO competed for resources with the older, more established health organizations, which jealously guarded their revenue streams. The scarcity of funds prompted LNHO planners to scale back their grandiose plans for a multinational public health program, and financial constraints continued to limit the organization throughout its entire existence. The League of Nations' inability to assert dominance in the field of international public health meant that global or transnational efforts would be fragmented or underfunded and often held captive to nationalist priorities.

Nonetheless, the LNHO did meet notable success in the field of epidemiology and epidemic response, which grew out of the first health crisis the organization faced in the wake of World War I. As was mentioned earlier, epidemic

typhus erupted in the disordered regions of Eastern Europe and Russia following the suspension of hostilities.[26] People and governments of other European
states rightly feared that the disease would spread to their own. The nascent
League of Nations quickly formed a typhus commission—later named the Epidemics Commission—and sent the members to Poland to assess the epidemic.
The commission's reports of a mushrooming typhus epidemic combined with
scattered cases of cholera and relapsing fever and an incipient famine alarmed
European health officials.

The scale of the calamity overwhelmed the Polish government and the
independent relief operations undertaken by the United States, Britain, and
the International Red Cross. It was suggested that an international effort to
coordinate health programs was required and that the League of Nations was
the mechanism to effect this coordination. Accordingly, representatives to the
League of Nations voted the chair of the Epidemics Commission as the person
to oversee league efforts to corral and mitigate the typhus outbreak.

The Epidemics Commission adopted a two-pronged strategy. First, it
would work with local government officials to establish a *cordon sanitaire,* halting any further transmission of the disease to noninfected regions by delous-
ing travelers and baggage. Such quarantine efforts fit traditional antiepidemic
practices and addressed the primary concerns of European states. Second, the
commission would work with local officials in setting up emergency hospitals
and clinics to aid the afflicted and provide expertise and supplies in Poland
and any other states that requested assistance, including the new Soviet Union.
The Bolshevik state suffered the greatest impact of the epidemic, with an estimated 25 to 30 million cases in 1922, prompting Vladimir Lenin to state, "Either socialism will defeat the louse or the louse will defeat socialism."[27]

In sum, the Epidemics Commission sought to assist states by providing
technical and logistical support and supplies, working with state governments
(and not with volunteer organizations) in delivering this aid and administering
the programs. Ludwik Rajchman, a member of the commission who helped
organize the relief effort in Poland, strongly recommended that the program
be administered through the local states, arguing that it was "the duty of the
government to bring assistance and not mere relief."[28] This role of technical
support for state public health programs provided the pattern for subsequent
LNHO activities in the following years; the WHO, too, adopted it when that
organization was formed following World War II.

The LNHO would be hampered by financial pressures and participants'
reluctance to surrender their national goals for inclusive international societies. These problems were not limited to matters of health and eventually undermined the idealistic dreams of the League of Nations.[29] The LNHO did

carve out some modest successes, especially in technical matters. The organization standardized the collection of statistics and reporting, which is vital to epidemiology, and attracted a cadre of dedicated scientific and medical experts who served in various functions on commissions and committees. Although league efforts outside Europe were limited, the organization achieved a reputation for technical proficiency and high scientific standards, creating a model of partnership and support that sought to broaden LNHO programs to other states. The organization generated a way for people to identify themselves as experts working in a shared field, not officials of this or that state, and while this new model did not replace that of national identity, it offered the potential for true international health.

By the onset of World War II, however, the international League of Nations had disintegrated under national stresses. In the coming conflagration medicine would again become part of the war effort. Troops could be felled by diseases as well as by bullets, and during World War I the biggest killer had been influenza. In the United States, the military took steps to prevent this from happening again.

In January 1941 the Preventive Medical Division of the office of the Surgeon General of the U.S. Army created the Board for the Investigation and Control of Influenza and other Epidemic Diseases in the Army. As the name suggests, the board was charged with studying infectious diseases—chiefly influenza—in order to protect the troops from epidemics.[30] The army appointed Tommy Francis, the American researcher who had discovered influenza type B and then among the world's most prominent influenza researchers, to a position on the board.[31] During the war years the Army epidemiological board skimmed the cream from the current generation of medical researchers, with Jonas Salk, Albert Sabin, and John Paul all serving under its auspices. Salk worked directly with Tommy Francis. The military was concerned that influenza might incapacitate the troops at a crucial moment in the war and thus wanted a protective vaccine. This vaccine would have to be safe, effective, and amenable to large-scale production. Tommy Francis and his group took the lead in developing an inoculation program.

Francis continued a series of techniques on which both he and British researchers had been working prior to the war. The process involved growing the virus in fertilized chicken eggs, killing the virus with a chemical (formalin or formaldehyde), concentrating the material, and injecting it into the arms of soldiers. In 1943 Francis mounted a large-scale test of the procedure, injecting one group of soldiers and leaving a second group uninoculated as a control. A widespread and relatively severe influenza season developed in 1943. Vaccinated soldiers suffered significantly lower rates of infection, later equated to a 70 percent protection rate (i.e., 70 percent of those vaccinated were protected from infection). The experiment was judged a success, and by 1945 virtually all military personnel were being vaccinated. Shortly thereafter, influenza vaccines were licensed for use in the United States.

Although effective, these new influenza vaccines were rather crude. First, the vaccines tended to include various components—mostly proteins from the egg—that resulted in strong systemic reactions to the foreign material. Second, the vaccine concentrations tended to vary, with some preparations having high levels of the targeted virus and others having low levels that offered little protection. The introduction of high-speed centrifuge machines (initially the Sharples and later the zonal centrifuge) allowed the production of highly concentrated and very pure vaccines, resulting in much lower numbers of adverse reactions to the injections.[32]

Throughout the war years and in 1946, the concentrated vaccine proved effective in protecting recipients from influenza infection. In 1947 the vaccine failed, and that failure provided important information about the influenza virus. But that year also saw the promulgation of a carefully considered but mistaken theory about pandemic influenza. Unfortunately, this mistaken theory became an important element in the 1976 Swine flu decision.

Vaccine Failure, 1947

In the early months of 1947, a sharp epidemic of influenza appeared, striking equally among the vaccinated and unvaccinated.[33] In some locations (e.g., the eastern coast of the United States), the epidemic was intense—especially in military encampments. A young assistant chief of medicine at Fort Monmouth (in New Jersey), Lieutenant Edwin Kilbourne, vividly recalls the impact of that influenza outbreak: "I took care of people with high fever who were laying on gurneys in the halls[;] . . . it made an impression on me as a severe epidemic."[34] Influenza researchers decided that the vaccine had failed because the virus had changed. The scientists dubbed this new strain of influenza "A Prime." In reexamining epidemiological data from 1946 and 1947, medical researchers determined that the new subtype had appeared in Australia toward the end of 1946. In March 1947 this influenza strain spread widely in the United States. The failure of the 1947 vaccine provided two valuable lessons: (1) influenza strains change, and (2) the new type arises in one geographic locality and proceeds to spread. As A. M.-M. Payne noted in a 1953 article: "In retrospect that was a most important observation because if we had known then what we know now, there would have been time to prepare a vaccine before the 1947 outbreak."[35] Initially believed to be an example of genetic shift, it was later determined that the 1946 and the 1947 viruses both belonged to the

H1N1 family of viruses.[36] The vaccine failure of 1947 thus taught influenza researchers a valuable lesson about the behavior of the virus. But unlike the situation during the 1920s and 1930s, this time there would be significant institutional support for investigating it.

As it did for many other medical and scientific topics, the extremity of war spurred rapid development of new technologies and research regarding influenza. And though the war's end prompted a rapid demobilization that affected common soldiers and scientists alike, the partnership between government and researchers continued, far more so than it had following World War I, and nowhere with greater importance than in the United States. Vannevar Bush, who had served as director of the Office of Scientific Research and Development during the war, drafted a report titled *Science—the Endless Frontier,* which called for extended government support for scientific research. The National Institutes of Health snapped up unfinished contracts for medical research commissioned by the military, helping to cement the connection between the federal government and university research centers; ultimately, the National Science Foundation was created. The United States had the means and the will to continue federal support for scientific and medical research in the postwar period. In addition, the experience of the global war had broadened the horizons of researchers who had been charged with solving problems on very large scales and with understanding connections across great geographical distances. Flush with the successful conclusion to the war and possessing the ability and desire to use its position in the global arena, the United States entered a period some historians label a time of "grand expectations."[37]

These demobilized researchers did not all come from the United States. The British influenza researcher C. H. Andrewes had been released from his wartime service and continued to pursue his studies. The events of 1947 cemented his belief in the need for a surveillance system,[38] and Andrewes now realized two things. First, any viable surveillance system would have to be global. New influenza strains could pop up anywhere, and because the infection is so transmissible, local outbreaks can quickly spread around the world. Second, only a relative handful of laboratories had the requisite expertise to definitively compare strains of influenza. Andrewes concluded that the health branch of the newly chartered United Nations was perfectly suited to perform this global surveillance. On 3 April 1947, a Dutch representative at the third session of the Interim Commission of the World Health Organization suggested that the problem of pandemic influenza should fall within the WHO's bailiwick. The idea of a WHO role in tracking influenza was viewed favorably, and the executive secretary sent a representative to the Fourth International Congress on Microbiology, in Copenhagen, to sound out the assembled experts' views on the proposal. Forty-five people attending the microbiology congress met on 25 July to draft a plan for creating a surveillance system. Andrewes prepared a memorandum on the structure of the organization and placed it before the WHO interim commission in September 1947. Thus, before the WHO was even officially chartered (the WHO constitution was ratified on 7 April 1948), the World Influenza Centre (WIC) had begun work.

Borrowing laboratory space at the National Institute for Medical Research in London (coincidentally a wartime surplus hospital donated by the United States), Andrewes began tracking and identifying influenza strains. Eventually the influenza research centers of the United States were given the responsibility for typing samples from the Americas. The National Institutes of Health managed the program in the United States and served as a liaison with military influenza researchers (who maintained a sizable surveillance system relying on overseas military bases) and the WIC in London. The surveillance system was rapidly expanded; by 1953 there were two influenza reference laboratories (London and Bethesda, Maryland) and fifty-four designated influenza centers in forty-two nations.

As with the scramble to identify new microbes at the turn of the twentieth century and the tensions that limited the effectiveness of the LNHO, national and personal jealousies marked the formation of this international system of influenza surveillance. Andrewes had been part of a British team that had made important breakthroughs in studying influenza in the middle to late 1930s. But British attempts to create an influenza vaccine had failed. Successful vaccines were instead created by the American military under Tommy Francis. Furthermore, the U.S. researchers had created a sophisticated surveillance network in the Americas and on military bases around the globe. In addition, both Andrewes and Francis were reported to be headstrong men, and it appears that the competition between their laboratory groups went beyond the "friendly" variety. Andrewes's initial formulation of tasks in the WHO influenza program did not include a substantive role for U.S. researchers, an oversight that was remedied in December 1947 when the U.S. surveillance network was invited to contribute to the laboratory work of identifying influenza samples. Researchers in the United States, however, complained that official WHO reports underplayed U.S. contributions both to the program and to the study of influenza in general. There was a strong suspicion on the other side of the Atlantic that scientists at the laboratories run by Francis and Salk were not inclined to speed samples to their partners in London. In 1952, concerned by this friction, the newly appointed coordinator of the "Research Section" of the WHO's Division of Epidemiological Services, A. M.-M. Payne, sought to smooth over the ruffled feathers so as to facilitate the workings of the surveillance system.[39]

The WHO surveillance system was not just a tracking system; it was a system with a purpose. Surveillance was designed to catch a novel or growing epidemic strain of influenza early so that protective vaccines could be manufactured. This goal of protective vaccination was included in the original call for a WHO surveillance system:

> WHEREAS the outbreak of an influenza pandemic in the recent future should on no account be considered an imaginary danger;
>
> WHEREAS it might perhaps be possible to prevent a world-wide spread of the disease by means of prophylactic immunization;
>
> WHEREAS there might also be a possibility of preventing complications and diminishing the number of deaths in applying modern therapeutics;
>
> WHEREAS measures pertaining to influenza will only have the desired effect if they are taken as soon as possible after the identification of the initial cases;
>
> The Representative of the Netherlands considers it urgent for the Interim Commission of the World Health Organization to appoint a small committee to carry out the required preparatory work.[40]

By 1954 not only was the WHO tracking novel influenza strains, but its expert committees were issuing a list of "strains recommended for current production" to be distributed to vaccine manufacturers.[41] The WHO was now an integral part of vaccine manufacturing.

The reincarnation of the League of Nations dream in the form of the United Nations was a conscious attempt to both learn from the league's failures and retain the elements that had been successful. The biggest failure, of course, had been the league's inability to restrain the pursuit of national interests instead of the common good. One avenue where the League of Nations had achieved some measure of success consisted in fostering international efforts in matters of technical and scientific expertise. Nowhere was this success more evident than in the LNHO.

The belief that membership in a technical and scientific elite transcended national boundaries and served as a model for emerging international formation was known as "functionalism," and prominent functionalist thinkers were involved in drafting the constitution of the United Nations.[42] The relatively successful technical operations undertaken by the LNHO served as a pillar for the WHO and suited the interests of the WHO's biggest benefactor, the United States. The U.S. government and academic hierarchy favored technical solutions to complex problems, and the ideas of Walt Rostow's "modernization theory" held pride of place in U.S. governmental policy making.

In some ways, the surveillance system for influenza that Andrewes proposed harked back to the national self-interest model instrumental in OIHP thinking. The sentinel sites around the globe were designed to funnel timely information to the laboratory in London, which would then issue an alert to initiate protective vaccine production in Europe.[43] But the colonial structure that governed tropical medicine sanitary regulations was fast collapsing, and formerly dependent colonial possessions were rapidly—and sometimes violently—becoming new nation-states. The ship of global public health would soon be pulled by new currents and conflicts as the competition that marked the cold war intruded into science and medical research and policies, but these conflicts lay in the future.[44] In the first decade of the WHO, U.S. interests, U.S. expertise, and most of all, U.S. money dominated the WHO agenda. Andrewes's effort to marginalize U.S. participation in the influenza surveillance system was quickly shunted aside, and influenza research funded by the U.S. government began to shape the WHO and its surveillance system.

The influenza surveillance net expanded its reach throughout the 1950s, with more laboratories in more nations joining the system and a steady increase in the number of samples shipped for identification to the United Kingdom and the United States. Yet the system had yet to receive its first real-world test of a pandemic; it faced no new strains that threatened a global epidemic. But that day was coming. In 1957 a new strain appeared and rapidly circled the globe in pandemic spread. In this first exercise of pandemic preparedness, both international and national health systems failed to mitigate the pandemic and protect their charges. In the aftermath of the 1957 outbreak, public health researchers and administrators learned vital new information about pandemic influenza; international surveillance; and vaccine production, distribution, and inoculation. To their surprise, the experts involved in the WHO system discovered that the technical approach to protecting against influenza was widespread but that very few nations had the production infrastructure necessary for rapidly administering vaccinations. Influenza researchers recognized the global nature of influenza pandemics, but they failed to appreciate the speed of the virus. Successful efforts to protect against the next pandemic would have to be faster.

CHAPTER 4

Setbacks

Based on Christopher Andrewes's observations of influenza B in 1946 and the vaccine failure in 1947, influenza researchers had determined that a new influenza virus arises in one location and then rapidly circulates into the wider world. The scientists did not yet understand the mechanisms of new strain formation—what we now call antigenic drift and antigenic shift—but they recognized that new strains had a competitive advantage in serial human transfer over older strains. This observation about the behavior of the influenza virus provided the logical underpinning for the World Influenza Centre and its role in surveillance. But the surveillance system was not just about observation; instead, the point was to identify a novel strain as it began to be transmitted and thus allow the development of a protective vaccine. The quicker a new circulating strain was identified, the quicker vaccines could be produced and the greater the number of people who would be protected from unnecessary sickness and death—exactly what public health programs are charged with doing, or so goes the theory. But since its founding by delegates of the soon-to-be-incorporated World Health Organization, this proposed procedure had not been put to the test. There had been no great pandemic, like Spanish flu, or even elevated infection rates, as occurred in 1947 (the A Prime, or FM 1, strain, as virologists called it). Instead, the influenza identification centers in the

United Kingdom and the United States marked only the incremental changes now known as viral drift. As the King James Bible says, however, judgment comes as "a thief in the night," and so it was with the sudden appearance of a new pandemic strain in the spring of 1957. The 1957 Asian flu pandemic presented the surveillance system its first trial, and in this test the WHO's early detection plan failed.

Asian Flu, 1957

On 17 April 1957 Maurice Hilleman sat in his office at the Walter Reed Army Institute reading the *New York Times*.[1] Hilleman was no ordinary reader of the paper. He was not only an expert on influenza but also the director of the institute's Central Laboratory of Viral Surveillance. He sat at the center of the vast global surveillance web operated by the U.S. military. Coincidentally, Hilleman had been part of the military's effort to recover Spanish flu virus from the Alaskan permafrost. While reading the newspaper that April morning, Hilleman spotted a "filler," a four-paragraph article that barely made it as "news fit to print." The article was datelined Hong Kong, 16 April 1957, with a headline reading, "Hong Kong Battling Influenza Epidemic." Quoting an unnamed health official, the article stated that thousands of cases of influenza had appeared in the previous few days and called it "the worst epidemic outbreak in years." The article estimated that 250,000 of the colony's 2.5 million citizens were receiving treatment. Hilleman, half a world away outside Washington, D.C., put down his paper and said, "My God . . . this is the pandemic. It's here!"[2] Hilleman recognized that such a large number of patients falling ill in such a short time meant that a new strain of influenza was spreading epidemically, and neither the WHO nor the American military's surveillance system had detected it. Hilleman cabled military bases in Asia, telling staff there to collect samples immediately and send them to Walter Reed. The virus had gotten the jump on the researchers.

As Hilleman had presumed, the WHO surveillance system, too, had failed to detect the rapidly spreading virus. On 5 May 1957 a member of the WHO surveillance system in Singapore, Dr. Hale, sent a telegram to the head of epidemiology for the WHO (Dr. Payne) that read, "Extensive outbreak influenza Singapore. Stop. Not notifiable, definite statistics unknown. Stop. Strains isolated will forward World Centre."[3] Andrewes forwarded the cable to WHO headquarters in Geneva with an extract of a letter from a colleague in Kuala Lumpur. In the letter, dated 30 April 1957, the colleague wrote: "[At least] one ship has passed here enroute for Britain from Hong Kong with the supposed 'influenza' on board. My information about Hong Kong is entirely from the press which state there has been a large epidemic of 'influenza.'"[4] No samples had arrived in London as of that date, and so far the WHO had taken no action. Apparently the "heads-up" telegrams had not aroused much alarm. Indeed, as the novel influenza strain emerged into a pandemic, some member states expressed their anger at the influenza system's slow response. Writing to WHO headquarters on 21 May 1957, the regional director for Southeast Asia, Dr. C. Mani, reported that the government of India "expressed its concern that WHO had not informed it concerning the extent of the influenza epidemic in Singapore et al." and that it had expected the organization "to be more active and alive with regard to their intelligence system."[5]

Meanwhile, Hilleman waited impatiently for the samples from the Pacific to arrive at Walter Reed.[6] A doctor at the 406th Medical General Laboratory in Japan had gathered samples from Hong Kong and Singapore and forwarded them to the United States. The samples reached Hilleman on 17 May 1957, and he worked the next five days and nights typing them. He tested the influenza strain against sera from hundreds of military personnel to see whether any produced antibodies to the new strain. None did. Next he tested the sera from hundreds of civilians. None of those samples produced antibodies. Hilleman now knew that he had a novel strain of influenza in his hands, that this strain was spreading widely in Asia, and that none of the hundreds of people whose blood he tested produced protective antibodies. In short, he knew a pandemic of influenza was looming.

In 1957 the only protective procedure against influenza was vaccination. Once he was certain of the danger of this new influenza virus, Hilleman took several immediate steps. First, he sent samples of the virus to the WHO, the United States Public Health Service, and laboratories at the army's epidemiological board to confirm his results. Second, he issued a press release predicting that the United States would suffer a flu pandemic in the fall of 1957, going so far as to state that the epidemic would arrive in the first week of September "on the second or third day of the opening of school." Finally, Hilleman took a step that seems unbelievable in the bureaucratically hardened, litigious society of today. He bypassed the Department of Health, Education, and Welfare's (HEW) Division of Biologic Standards and contacted the heads of the six U.S. vaccine manufacturers directly. His message was simple. "Don't kill your roosters." As a farm boy growing up in Montana, Hilleman had learned that farmers sell their roosters for stewing pots at the end of the spring hatching season. Because of his years working with the influenza virus, he knew that vaccine manufacturers produce their vaccine in fertilized chicken eggs. To produce vaccine on the scale Hilleman was envisioning would require a massive amount of fertilized chicken eggs. Manufacturers would need every rooster they could get. Recognizing that time was of the essence, Hilleman followed up his phone calls by shipping samples of this new strain to each of these six manufacturers for vaccine production on 22 May 1957. Initially dubbed "Far East influenza," the virus was later named Asian flu.[7]

The heads of the other research laboratories to which Hilleman had sent the influenza specimens were initially skeptical of his prediction for a fall pandemic in the United States. But their own testing data, combined with the continued steep epidemic rise of cases in Asia, soon convinced them of the imminent threat. Health officials were relieved to see that Asian flu was thus far not mimicking Spanish flu's mortality pattern, but they recognized that influenza in general could be costly and deadly. On 28 May 1957 the U.S. Department of Defense's chiefs of preventative medicine attended a hastily called meeting to discuss the military's plans to deal with Asian flu.[8] A delegation of USPHS officials attended as observers. The military officials quickly agreed that the troops would immediately need a protective vaccine and authorized the procurement of a monovalent vaccine against Asian flu, leaving open the possibility of later combining this vaccine with other strains to create a polyvalent vaccine. The military eventually settled on an order of 2.65 million doses of monovalent Asian flu vaccine, with full delivery to be made by 1 September 1957. Manufacturers had their first orders.

Public health officials faced a different set of problems. They recognized that Asian flu presented a pandemic threat, but unlike the military, they were unsure whether they could or should compel civilians to get protective vaccines. The military had a captive audience, as it were. Military personnel were routinely ordered to submit to a host of injections, including influenza vaccines, which they had been receiving since Francis's experiments in 1943. In addition, these people tended to be younger and healthier than those in the general population. For its part, the public health services had to determine whether the same vaccine could be given to an eighty-year-old grandmother and her four-year-old grandson. In addition, the Department of Health, Education, and Welfare under the Eisenhower administration was not an activist organization.[9]

In the days following the military's decision to vaccinate the troops, the USPHS debated what, if anything, it would recommend for the general public.[10] On 31 May General W. Palmer Dearing, the current acting surgeon general (Leroy E. Burney was traveling outside the country), sent a memorandum to a select group of influenza experts debating the USPHS's recommendation suggesting quick action:

> [If] there [is] even a possibility of a widespread epidemic next fall, the investment of the few million dollars necessary to develop and dissemi-

nate vaccine as widely as possible would be the logical step to recommend. Certainly, if the outbreak should occur, and the Public Health Service had simply counseled "wait and see" without having proposed utilization of the technical tools available, our position would be hard to defend. . . . If [the current influenza situation] is unusual, or almost unique, the burden of proof would seem to be on those who oppose the recommendation to press for a mass immunization against the new strain with all possible vigor.[11]

Clearly the USPHS agreed that the evidence for a fall pandemic was strong and the potential for an epidemic required some public health response. In fact, its officials correctly feared what could happen if they just decided to "wait and see." Deputy Surgeon General Dearing felt so confident of the likelihood of a fall influenza epidemic that he considered the burden of proof to lie with those opposed to some public health action. But what that response should be was far from clear. Should the government initiate a federal effort to inoculate citizens? If so, who should receive the shots? Should the government subsidize private medical involvement, by either purchasing or coordinating vaccines? Should the government adopt a hands-off policy and let the market procure and distribute the vaccine? These same questions continue to face public health officials today, for they lie at the heart of the issues that the field must address. In 1957, Surgeon General Burney sought to address them by calling for a meeting of public health experts to craft recommendations for the USPHS.

The meeting was held on 10 June 1957 and was chaired by Surgeon General Burney. The experts included representatives of state health departments, the American Medical Association, the armed forces, and public health services. The meeting began with a summary of the armed forces decision, including the level of potency recommended (200 cca), which Dr. Frederick Davenport admitted was no more than an educated guess. Next the USPHS detailed its actions to date and outlined its future plans for screening travelers coming into the country. Alex Langmuir of the CDC reported that all members of the newly created Epidemic Intelligence Service had been instructed to immediately report any small localized outbreaks of influenza. Finally, Dr. Roderick Murray of the HEW Division of Biologic Standards reported on the current status of vaccine production, including production rates, availability, and time schedules.

With these reports in hand, the influenza experts met to agree on the recommended response for the USPHS. The experts faced many complex questions, which they had to answer using highly uncertain evidence. It seemed likely that the United States would experience an epidemic of influenza, but it was by no means certain. The likely mortality rate was similarly unknown (Spanish flu loomed as a worst-case scenario). Initial reports from Asia suggested those who contracted Asian flu suffered relatively mild symptoms, although all the health officials knew that no complete accounting of the epidemic could be made until the number of extra dead in the populace was calculated. At any rate, Asian flu was certainly no second wave of Spanish flu . . . thus far. In the end, the reluctance to challenge the prevailing system of profit-driven manufacturers and private practitioners combined with evidence of the strain's mildness proved decisive. The committee issued a seven-point recommendation that called for the creation of a new monovalent vaccine, requested that private physicians report influenza cases, and promised that the USPHS would study and track the new virus. The seventh point summarized the key to the recommendation: "At present, the situation does not justify (a) establishment of civilian priorities, or (b) consideration of governmental subsidy in production of vaccine."[12] In private consultation with manufacturers, the Public Health Service promised to publicize the need for a protective vaccine; the USPHS would provide the demand if the manufacturers would provide the supply. Beyond that, the service eschewed a leading role. Officials there felt that private industry and the medical practice were best equipped to handle this outbreak.

The limited activities of the USPHS reflected the Eisenhower administration's conservatism and, more broadly, the government's reluctance to impose itself in the pharmaceutical marketplace. Government regulators generally declined to intervene in medical sales unless some tragedy—such as the patent medicine scandals of the early twentieth century and the "Elixir Sulfanilamide" tragedy of 1937—compelled their intervention. Even when administrators favored greater regulatory practices, their paltry budgets and small staffing levels hindered effective action. The Cutter disaster of 1955 was a signal event in the realization that pharmaceuticals needed careful policing to protect the public.[13]

Like the United States, the WHO hurriedly tried to play "catch-up" with the now spreading epidemic. On 24 May 1957 the WHO sent a memorandum to all influenza centers: "The virus isolated in Malaysia is evidently a new variant of type A differing in several respects from recently isolated strains. . . . Although this is not certain it appears to be so different from previous strains that existing vaccines would probably not give protection. It is therefore being distributed to vaccine manufacturing firms as well as to Influenza Centres."[14] Hilleman had teamed with Harry M. Meyer (who worked in the Department of Virus Diseases at Walter Reed) to pen a 28 May 1957 letter and report that bolstered this characterization of the virus as a new variant, stating that the new virus was going to be a "health problem in the U.S. A. and probably much of the world."[15] The evidence for a pandemic was mounting.

Despite its apparently sluggish start, the WHO had actually been making preparations for the emergence of a new pandemic strain of influenza for several years. After all, its World Influenza Centre had been created precisely to detect newly emerging strains of the virus, but in addition, the WHO had conducted a large exercise to test the feasibility of creating protective vaccines on a crash basis.[16] In 1951 the WHO had conducted a "dry run" exercise to test vaccine production methods and to gauge the quantity of injectables that would be produced. The WHO Influenza Study Program distributed seed virus of the "London" strain, a newly emerged drifted variant of the prevailing A prime group. The organization tapped the National Institutes of Health in the United States to oversee this exercise and sent seed stocks to the NIH on 19 January 1951. The NIH distributed the seed stock to six manufacturers who agreed to prepare 1,000 cc (at potency levels of 200 cca per dose) of a protective vaccine.[17] These vaccines would have to pass tests of sterility, inactivation of the virus, and safety. The first lot of vaccine was delivered to the NIH on the twenty-second day, and all but one of the vaccine lots had been received by the thirty-seventh day. Further, the exercise asked the companies to estimate how long it would take to produce a million doses. The estimates ranged from five to fifty weeks.

This dry run of vaccine production nicely illustrates how U.S. interests dominated the WHO. During a time when the Soviet Union and many eastern bloc nations were boycotting involvement with the WHO, the technical solution that the United States favored was the policy of the WHO.[18] The simulated program was aimed at establishing technical benchmarks: How long would it take to produce vaccine production strains? How long to deliver them for certification? How long to produce a million doses? In addition, the session was administered through the NIH and involved six U.S.-based manufacturing companies.

The practice vaccine production exercise helped establish protocols and channels of interagency cooperation for a real emergence of a novel influenza strain. The USPHS considered the report—especially the production figures—of this vaccination exercise helpful in early discussions regarding the proper response to Asian flu. Speed was of the essence if vaccine was going to protect people from the emerging pandemic.

The WHO recommended that all its member states begin preparations for a protective vaccine as soon as possible, and the organization distributed seed stock of the virus. Many nations responded to this recommendation by creating protective vaccines. Not only large nations with highly developed vaccine-producing firms, such as the United States, Great Britain, and Australia, but also smaller nations, such as Iceland, Egypt, and Israel, created and distributed inoculations in 1957. The amount of protective material produced globally is unclear. It appears that the WHO was not even sure who could make vaccine, never mind the quantity, but aside from a few large producers in the United States and a few other nations (e.g., the Netherlands and West Germany), manufacturers appear to have managed only low production levels.[19] In such small-scale manufacturing, vaccine is produced "at the bench," largely by scientists at research labs.[20] In the first example of one major problem confronting health officials whenever an influenza pandemic looms, the WHO recognized that vaccine would be available to only a small percentage of the world's population.

The limitations on vaccine production were of two sorts. First, the technique itself comprises several steps that require a sophisticated level of precision. The virus is injected into fertilized chicken eggs, harvested, inactivated (or "killed") through the use of a chemical additive, purified to remove extraneous material, diluted to dose strength, shipped, and delivered for injection, all the while maintaining sterility. Second, few facilities could produce the material on the large scale. Many nations had the requisite technical capacity—which is why research laboratories could make the vaccine "at the bench"—but lacked the infrastructure for mass production. In addition, the initial Asian flu strains proved to be difficult to grow in the eggs, so that only a limited amount of vaccine could be harvested from each individual egg.[21]

Solutions to several problems of production and delivery lay in the use of vaccines based on live rather than inactivated virus, and in 1957 several eastern bloc nations—especially the Soviet Union—claimed to have solved the problems of live-virus vaccines and to have used them safely on a large scale. Live-virus vaccines work on the principle of selectively weakening (attenuating) the virus to the point where it prompts the creation of protective antibodies without causing illness. The attenuated virus needs to be stable so that it neither passes on through a population nor reverts to virulence. One technique for limiting person-to-person transmission of live-virus vaccine strains was to select only viruses that replicate at lower temperatures. These "cold-adapted" seed viruses do not propagate well at the warmer temperatures of the human body; in consequence, there should be little or no transmission from those inoculated to other contacts. The major difficulty in creating such strains lies in the influenza virus's high mutation rate, which undermines these engineered replication features.

Influenza researchers continued to pursue the creation of live-virus vac-

cines because they offered potential for higher levels of production in the case
of a pandemic. Live-virus vaccines can be produced in greater quantities (because the inactivation stages are skipped), utilize a smaller dose to induce immunity, and are more easily delivered (because the vaccines are inhaled rather
than injected). The Soviet Union claimed to have safely inoculated millions
of its citizens with live-virus vaccines, which its leaders proclaimed were "the
best flu prophylactic."[22] In 1957 it was difficult to obtain independent verifica-
tion of Soviet claims, and the Soviets released neither detailed data nor samples
of the attenuated flu strains. Researchers in the United States would have a
difficult time in creating stable attenuated viruses for the next thirty years, and
as I will discuss, the WHO had reason to seriously doubt the claimed stability
of the eastern bloc live-virus vaccines in the ensuing years.

The vaccination efforts of the many nations that sought to protect their
citizens largely ended in failure, with benefits accruing only to a comparatively small handful of people who received timely injections. The United
States had by far the largest vaccination effort, and while that nation had some
peculiar features to its campaign (e.g., its reliance on a voluntary distribution
system), the reasons behind the vaccination effort's failure there are instructive for understanding the general failure of vaccination efforts in the past and
challenges that face pandemic response in the present.

The Vaccination Campaign of 1957 in the United States

The overwhelming challenge that confronted organizations that attempted to
protect citizens from the pandemic lay with the virus itself. The highly transmissible infection spread rapidly, thereby making it difficult to get ahead of the
virus. As manufacturers geared up to produce the new protective vaccine, the
Public Health Service began to track the spreading pandemic. This surveillance task fell to the CDC (then known as the Communicable Disease Center).
The CDC in the 1950s was not the preeminent global health organization that
it is today. The organization was created to spearhead malaria eradication during World War II, but as was mentioned previously, its success in eradicating
the disease in the United States left it without a clear mandate. Under first
Joseph Mountin and then Alexander Langmuir, the organization had steadily
expanded its role in tracking and studying infectious diseases. Capitalizing
on cold war fears of biological warfare, Langmuir had created the Epidemic
Intelligence Service (EIS), which he staffed with medical students serving a
two-year hitch in lieu of the requisite two-years' service in the military during
the peacetime draft. Langmuir shrewdly recognized that although expanding
public health training might not readily attract funding, military needs always
would. He pitched the idea that a trained cadre of epidemiologists in state pub-

lic health departments, working with a centralized laboratory, would be an excellent sentinel system if the United States was attacked with biological and chemical weapons. Langmuir knew, of course, that trained epidemiologists would be useful in investigating and tracking disease and sickness not related to biological and chemical warfare, too. Between 1949 and 1970, 672 people completed the EIS training course.[23] In 1955 the CDC had garnered acclaim in the public health community by using EIS personnel to quickly track and trace dangerous polio vaccines produced by Cutter Laboratories in 1955. The investigation had demonstrated the CDC's epidemiological expertise.[24]

Langmuir had promised Surgeon General Burney that EIS investigators would make tracking influenza their number-one priority. Organizing responsibilities for the surveillance system fell to D. A. Henderson.[25] The key to tracking the spread of influenza was obtaining timely information, and so Henderson set up a reporting mechanism modeled on the mimeographed bulletins the CDC had been distributing on hepatitis and diphtheria.[26] The reports were brief summaries of the suspect influenza cases around the nation, sometimes issued as frequently as every three days. The goal was to get information into the hands of public health professionals, so the reports included cases that were untyped or in the process of being typed. The reports reveal both the rapid spread of the new virus and its capriciousness.

Almost as soon as Hilleman had definitively typed the new strain of influenza, cases appeared in the United States. On 2 June 1957 five cooks aboard the USS *Barry* (a destroyer docked at the naval shipyard in Newport, Rhode Island) reported to the dispensary with influenza-like complaints. They were subsequently joined by twenty-five of their shipmates on 3 June and twenty more the following day. By 11 June ninety-nine sailors had reported to sick bay. The likely source of the *Barry*'s outbreak was the Pakistani ship *Mahmood,* which had left Karachi on 14 April for a goodwill tour of Boston, Newport, and Norfolk. An estimated 35 percent of the *Barry*'s crew reported symptoms, and within a few weeks 112 ships docked at the naval base had reported at least one illness among their crews. By 30 June the six other destroyers in the *Barry*'s group were reporting various stages of the outbreak (increasing, decreasing, or subsiding), with the USS *Greenwood* estimating 45 percent of its crew having been infected with the virus. Although there were some reports among workers at the base's infirmary, no widespread epidemic was detected among Newport's civilian population at this time.

A similar sudden outbreak appeared on a military base on the other side of the continent about the same time. A steep epidemic outbreak was identified at the naval base in San Diego, where an astounding 70 percent of naval recruits reported symptoms (the recruits were housed in tight quarters during training). The rest of the base's personnel suffered a 7 percent attack rate. The outbreak appeared to have been triggered by the USS *Washburn's* return from a ten-day training voyage on 11 June 1957. "Far East" (as the USPHS referred to the virus at that time) influenza was subsequently recovered from crew members on this vessel, although it is not clear how they encountered the new strain. Once again the infection seemed to be restricted to the base, for the surrounding city did not experience a similar epidemic.

The first cases of Asian flu to be documented in the United States occurred on military bases, though it remains unclear whether that reflects something about the prevalence of the disease in military living conditions or was just an artifact of superior surveillance and reporting there. Nevertheless, it was inevitable that civilian epidemics would appear. The following three cases in the general public illustrate both the explosiveness of an influenza outbreak and the perplexing nature of the virus.

On 21 June 1957, 391 high-school girls descended on the campus of the University of California, Davis, for a ten-day conference. The girls were housed dormitory style, two to a room, and collected into twelve groups for their conference activities, with all the girls sharing a common dining area. Over the course of the conference 225 of the girls developed symptoms of respiratory illness, including the abrupt onset of head and body aches, sore throats, and fevers, some reaching as high as 104 degrees. Several blood samples were later typed as containing Asian flu, though at the time it was impossible to distinguish which girls had contracted the new flu strain and which, if any, were suffering some other respiratory illness. Compounding the difficulty of diagnosis, on 25 June conference officials announced that anyone who was ill would not be allowed to go home until the person had recovered. Whereas 113 cases had been reported the previous day, the number complaining of symptoms dropped to 9 on this day. As the conference ended, the girls were allowed to leave the campus. All the stricken high-school girls recovered, but a fifty-seven-year-old adviser died on 4 July.

One apparently healthy attendee of the U.C.-Davis conference left the conference to travel to Grinnell College, in Ames, Iowa, for an international church conference. The conference, slated to begin on 26 June 1957, brought together 1,688 participants from forty-three states and ten nations. While en route to the conference in a special chartered rail car, the U.C.-Davis attendee began to complain of influenza-like symptoms. Subsequently other members of the hundred-member California delegation began to complain of similar symptoms. The church conference was crowded, and the California delegation was split up and dispersed among several dormitories. Within a few days a respiratory disease similar to that at the University of California conference had broken out across the Ames conference. The Grinnell organizers initially dedicated a single dormitory as an infirmary to house the stricken, but as the cases continued to mount, they opted to disband the conference and send the participants home on 1 July. While en route or shortly after arriving at home, several participants at the church conference were hospitalized with influenza-like complaints. Over the following few weeks several clusters of Asian flu cases could be traced to participants returning from Grinnell.

The U.C.-Davis and Grinnell college examples illustrate how common and ordinary events can serve to amplify a novel infection. In both cases, the public health community could do nothing except reconstruct events, because they were not alerted until the outbreaks were already in full swing. But the public health community did have a slight lead time prior to another large-scale grouping of people. An international Boy Scout jamboree was scheduled to begin 12 July 1957 at Valley Forge, Pennsylvania. An estimated 53,000 scouts from around the world were anticipated at the weeklong festival of camping and activities. Henderson was alerted to this event just a few days prior to its kickoff, and he and other health officials fretted over what to do. Thousands of people were on their way or already there, and health officials were getting reports that the California delegation—halfway into a seven-day cross-country train ride—had dozens of scouts complaining of fevers, body aches, and fatigue. Eventually, 200 of the 950-member California delegation would be recorded as having reported symptoms. After much discussion and debate, the officials decided to allow the jamboree to be held as scheduled, reasoning that because the majority of activities would occur outside and the scouts were housed in two-person pup tents rather than dormitories, the crowded conditions present at Davis and Ames would not exist. The CDC and the Pennsylvania health departments jointly set up a special infirmary tent for suspected influenza cases, segregated the California delegates (and those who shared a train with them) in a remote region of the park, and crossed their fingers. Although several hundred scouts eventually visited the special infirmary, nothing like the two previous epidemics occurred. On 18 July 1957 the jamboree began to disperse, and the park was emptied of scouts by the twenty-first. For a while, it appeared that the USPHS had dodged a bullet, but it was later determined that several scouts had served as carriers, inadvertently delivering the infection to their home communities.

Although the Davis, Ames, and Valley Forge gatherings sparked some secondary cases of influenza, the total was surprisingly small, and this fact puzzled health officials. The virus could spread explosively; once postconference victims were tabulated, the group at U.C.-Davis was retrospectively determined to have suffered an 89 percent attack rate. Yet despite intense follow-up by

EIS officials, no large outbreaks in the communities to which the infected had returned were detected. This lack of secondary spread was true for even most close household contacts. This new influenza virus was dramatically transmissible in enclosed communities, such as military barracks or dormitories, but thus far seemed unable to transfer in more dispersed populations. Either the virus was not well-adapted for human transmission, or the summer weather did not favor chains of infection. The evidence for epidemic spread in Asia, however, suggested this lull was only temporary. Although there had not been any sustained community-wide outbreaks in the United States, the recorded and unrecorded cases around the nation suggested that the United States was well-seeded with the virus. Some change in transmission or circumstances was likely to spark an epidemic there.

When Maurice Hilleman had issued his 22 May 1957 press release warning of an impending influenza pandemic, he boldly predicted its onset in the first week of September, two or three days after the schools open. In schools, numerous students from dispersed locations crowd together, returning home to their extended families at the end of the day. This pattern, combined with the relatively unhygienic practices of children, make schools ideal locations for the circulation of infectious diseases, especially respiratory ones. Hilleman's logic was correct, but his timing was slightly off. The first community-wide sustained outbreak began not in September but early August in Tangipahoa Parish, Louisiana.

Tangipahoa Parish is an agricultural area stretching from the northern end of Lake Pontchartrain to the border with Mississippi. In 1957 this region grew strawberries, which are harvested there in the late winter and early spring. Accordingly, the schools were closed at that time to allow students to help in the harvest. To make up for that lost school time, the schools opened in early July. In mid-July 1957 a smattering of influenza-like cases began to appear in the student population.[27] Suddenly, in the last of week of July, the epidemic exploded, reaching a peak on 5 August. The rapidly escalating number of cases and the large number of absentees prompted officials to close the schools, but it was too late. Even though ten of the parish's twelve schools were closed, the epidemic continued to spread. Soon neighboring regions, including Baton Rouge and the border regions of Mississippi, were experiencing epidemic growth of influenza.

By late August it was clear that the Louisiana outbreak was a signal to what would most likely occur nationally when the rest of the nation's schools opened in September. Were the public health organizations prepared for the pandemic? At a special meeting with health officials from all the states and territories of the United States, Surgeon General Burney explained the circumstances of Asian flu and the decisions that the USPHS had made.[28] Burney discussed how the disease had appeared unexpectedly in the Far East during the spring of 1957. He detailed how the Walter Reed Army Medical Center had quickly typed the virus as new. Burney discussed how the virus had continued to spread rapidly out of Asia and observed that, although it caused a "mild" course of infection, the simultaneous infection of 10–20 percent of the population would be disruptive. Accordingly, the Public Health Service had crafted a response with five major components. Government officials had approached influenza vaccine manufacturers, who had agreed to produce 60 million doses of vaccine by 1 February 1958.[29] The USPHS promised to mount a publicity campaign to encourage citizens to purchase the injections and had ramped up its epidemiological and influenza study programs. The surgeon general proposed that the manufacturers create a "voluntary allocation system" to equitably distribute vaccine so that each state would get a fair share according to its population. Finally, the Public Health Service was working with medical and hospital authorities to prepare contingency plans to handle potential cases if a large-scale or more deadly epidemic became a reality. Health officials recognized that these plans were likely to be inadequate if the pandemic took off in early September because of vaccine supply limitations. They also realized that the decentralized nature of the distribution system could be problematic, but in the Eisenhower era, there was little government appetite for federal program management.

By early September vaccine production was in high gear. The manufacturers had managed to increase their yield per egg but were still projecting 1 February 1958 as the target for delivery of the 60 million doses they had promised. Events in Tangipahoa Parish suggested that this would likely to be far too late. Manufacturers would not store their vaccine until that date, of course, but rather release production lots as soon as they were certified by the government. However, these earliest stocks were already claimed. The defense department had contracted for 2.65 million doses for its personnel. This request would come right off the top of the vaccines produced by the six manufacturers (Lederle; Lilly; Pitman Moore; National Drug; Parke, Davis; and Merck, Sharpe and Dohme). In addition, as an unnamed pharmaceutical executive had suggested to the USPHS in response to the voluntary allocation plan, many manufacturers had "already accepted a number of orders in good faith from [their] regular customers all over the country, and these [would] have to be given some consideration in any allocation system set up."[30] Many of those "regular customers" were large industrial concerns (Ford and AT&T were specifically mentioned). The Common Cold Foundation, a voluntary health organization, consulted with industry, and its representative Nadine

Miller met with the USPHS on 2 July 1957. Miller was sufficiently impressed by the potential for an influenza pandemic that she recommended to participating industry groups that they preorder vaccine as soon as possible. Most corporations took her advice.

The USPHS had declined to assert a federal role in distributing vaccine because it believed that the free market was the best means for distributing the vaccine as quickly and efficiently as possible. The USPHS wanted to ensure that it was distributed equitably, too—and also that certain select groups received priority vaccinations. The surgeon general had worked with manufacturers to agree to a voluntary allocation plan. One aspect of the plan was an allocation of the vaccine to those providing services "'imperative for the care of the sick' and to essential workers in the communication, transportation, and utility industries."[31] Although the terms *imperative* and *essential* were left undefined, the USPHS estimated the total to meet this need at about 12 million doses. Clearly this was a large demand front-loaded toward industrial manufacturing.

In addition to cobbling together a voluntary allocation plan and to tracking and studying the new virus, the USPHS had promised to publicize the need for the public to get a protective vaccine, an effort at which it succeeded. A 23 September 1957 Gallup poll revealed that 92 percent of the adults polled had heard of Asian influenza, 76 percent knew there was a protective vaccine, and 65 percent planned to get that vaccine.[32] If the pandemic held off until late winter, then a fair number of people would be vaccinated and hence protected from the virus. But if the pandemic arrived early . . . The first test would come when the schools reopened after summer break.

Hilleman, of course, was right. When the schools reopened, the number of influenza cases exploded. It was Tangipahoa Parish writ large. First, the number of cases with "flulike" symptoms soared among student populations, followed by similar complaints among family contacts and finally community-wide spreads. The pattern was duplicated all around the nation. The vaccines were not ready. On 4 September 1957, the day most schools reopened, only 3.7 million doses had been released. Of that total, 1.4 million were earmarked for the Department of Defense. By 24 September it was clear that the pandemic had arrived, and the public clamored for vaccine, but there was none to be had. Only about 7 million doses had been released for use. By the 19 October epidemic peak in the United States (as measured by new cases), fewer than half of 60 million projected doses required had been released. But even this number is deceptive, for after the government released it—meaning the lots had passed tests of sterility and purity—the vaccine still had to be distributed through various layers of wholesalers and distributors until finally reaching the offices of private physicians, who then injected the vaccine into patients. Those inoculated do not achieve full protection until almost two weeks after receiving the shot, which means that even among the people who received the shots, only a few million obtained any protective benefit from them.

As was predictable, the voluntary allocation system was a disaster. The sudden surge of demand for the vaccine combined with the lack of any centralized plan for distribution rapidly overwhelmed the priority system. As the sales manager at Merck, Sharpe and Dohme put it, "You got twenty-five people wanting apples and you got only one apple. So who gets the apple? The guy who's got his hand out first."[33] In many cases these were the large industrial firms that had preordered. By 26 September 1957 the American Medical Association was complaining that the bulk of the vaccine seemed to be going to industrial concerns, and private physicians were obtaining only small quantities, if they obtained any at all. Under the USPHS plan, distributing the vaccine to the general public fell to private physicians. There were widespread reports that people such as the clerks at Dun and Bradstreet and even the football players for the San Francisco 49ers and at Stanford University and the University of California had received shots, but not the municipal police and firefighters.[34]

The federal government's promotion of a vaccine that was not available prompted frustration and even fear among the public. Stories circulated of a thriving black market for the vaccine. Others hinted darkly that the government was conspiring to make obscene profits for pharmaceutical companies. Sadly, even some members of the health profession espoused such theories. At a widely reported meeting in San Francisco, some leading California medical experts suggested that there was public "hysteria" on getting the flu vaccine and that the demand was driven by a deliberate campaign to sell the vaccine. One physician even suggested the vaccine to be more dangerous than the virus: "We would have more deaths and illness from the vaccine than we have with the flu."[35] The critics were wrong; Asian flu killed an estimated 69,800 in the United States and about 2 million globally.

Ultimately the epidemic dropped off as quickly as it had soared. By November the number of new cases of Asian influenza was in steep decline all across the United States—ironically at the very moment when manufacturers had been able to catch up with the demand for vaccine. The drop-off in new cases, coupled with a lingering distrust of the necessity for the whole campaign, led to a glut of vaccines on the market. By 15 November 1957, 53 million doses of influenza vaccine had been released, but now there were few takers. Some manufacturers were able to sell some of the excess abroad, but

most were saddled with huge stocks of unwanted vaccine. Later, Maurice
Hilleman would estimate that about "half" the 60 million does produced were
returned unsold.[36]

The 1957 vaccination campaign did have some notable successes. For example, the vaccine manufacturers had exceeded their target and had produced
a safe and effective vaccine. Ultimately, however, the vaccination campaign
must be judged a failure, one that provides instructive lessons not only for the
United States but for the global community. Above all else, this campaign
failed because the pandemic spread far more quickly than manufacturers and
others could prepare and distribute a protective vaccine. The new flu strain
was not discovered until it was spreading epidemically, and by that time it
was too late for 1950s technology to prepare vaccine in bulk. This problem
of a speedy virus was exacerbated by a public health system both ill prepared
and disinclined to undertake a large-scale vaccination campaign. The result
displeased everyone involved. Members of the public could not gain access to
vaccine when they needed it, public health officials were unable to protect their
charges, and manufacturers were forced to absorb the cost of a large number of
unsold vaccines. Although no one could know when the next influenza pandemic would occur, all parties needed to be better prepared.

Hong Kong Flu, 1968

As it happened, the next pandemic appeared eleven years later, and in many
ways the 1968 Hong Kong pandemic mirrored that of 1957, even down to its
initial discovery. The response by the WHO and national health programs was
quicker, but vaccination campaigns failed for the same reasons they had failed
in 1957: the virus moved too quickly.

On 12 July 1968 the *Times* of London reported that a widespread outbreak
of respiratory disease was raging in southeastern China.[37] The newspaper article came to the attention of Charles Cockburn. Like Hilleman before him,
Cockburn was no disinterested newspaper reader; rather, he was the chief
medical officer for virus diseases at the World Health Organization, and he
immediately recognized the importance of the report. Five days later the city
of Hong Kong suffered a rapid rise of influenza-like illness. The WHO's representative in Hong Kong, Dr. Chang, forwarded virus samples to the World Influenza Centre in London. When testing there determined that the new strain
differed from the drifted 1957 strain then prevalent, the WIC issued a warning
on 16 August 1968 that a new pandemic was possible.[38]

The appearance of a potential pandemic strain was especially ill timed for
residents of the Northern Hemisphere. For one thing, the new virus emerged
in midsummer, when manufacturers in this hemisphere had already produced

influenza vaccines for the following season and would have little lead time to create a new one before that season began. In addition, the vast majority of roosters had long since been sold off from the brood stock, limiting the egg production vital to the vaccine-production process. Despite these limitations, manufacturers geared up for a crash effort to produce vaccine. Incorporating the experience of 1957, manufacturers sped up the steps necessary to craft a vaccine for the threatening strain and begin production. Within fifteen days manufacturers had settled the technical requirements (potency, dose strength, and purity), a full forty days quicker than in 1957. The first batch was released by day 66, almost a month sooner than had been accomplished in 1957. And by day 83 the manufacturers had produced and released five million doses, again, a little over a month more quickly than had been managed in 1957.[39]

It did not matter. Mirroring the Asian flu infection, the epidemic peaked before the majority of the vaccine was released for use. In North America the pandemic peaked in early January 1969. As had happened in 1957, a sizable percentage of the manufacturer's vaccine went unsold. In Europe the situation was much the same. Vaccine production lagged behind the pandemic, and few citizens received benefits from a protective vaccine. This lag in European production occurred even though the initial wave of Hong Kong flu was less deadly than the second wave, which emerged in the fall of 1969. Only the Soviet Union claimed any success in protecting its citizens from the pandemic through unnamed (and unverified) "prophylactic and anti-epidemic measure[s] performed by the public health services."[40]

In the final accounting, once the numbers of extra dead were calculated, the 1968 Hong Kong flu was less deadly than the 1957 Asian flu had been. About a million people died from the flu globally, with 33,800 of those victims in the United States. Some influenza experts speculate that the Hong Kong pandemic was less deadly because the viral strain was novel only in a shift in the hemagglutinin, and the similar neuraminidase provided partial immunity or lessened the course of infection (Asian flu was designated H2N2; Hong Kong flu, H3N2).

Public health researchers and influenza scientists learned much in the two pandemics, and influenza vaccine manufacturers had mounted tremendous efforts to produce vaccines. But both vaccine efforts failed. Surveillance programs missed the new strains until they had become regional epidemics, public health agencies failed in equitably distributing the vaccine (spectacularly in 1957, less so in 1968), and vaccine manufacturers had been forced to absorb the cost of unsold vaccine. In the years following the Hong Kong pandemic, influenza experts from around the world gathered to discuss how to address these failures and to speed up the vaccine production process so that it could pro-

vide real protection from pandemic influenza. Technical solutions still dominated influenza pandemic response planning, despite the reintegration of the
socialist states of Eastern Europe and the influx of many new nations into the
United Nations. Strong winds of change were beginning to buffet the WHO's
technical focus in the early 1970s, but the relatively small circle of influenza
experts on whom the WHO drew maintained a focus and faith in technical
solutions. The experts decided that prior preparation was the key, and over the
next few years influenza experts sought to consolidate what they had learned
from 1957 and 1968 with an eye to applying these hard-earned lessons to the
next pandemic.

The key elements to successfully limiting the impact of pandemic influenza remained the same as always: surveillance and vaccine production. At the
tail end of the Hong Kong pandemic, an influenza researcher had developed a
new technology for manufacturing vaccines that promised greater quantities
and faster methods of vaccine production. Influenza scientists also developed
two theories that might predict when a new pandemic strain would appear
and what kind of viral type it would be. All these elements would loom large
in 1976. The years 1957 and 1968 provided crucial information about methods
for responding to pandemic influenza, and the results of these failed vaccination campaigns played a large role in the development of the 1976 Swine Flu
Program, when the response to the emerging influenza pandemic was a massive national vaccination effort. But the fallout from this program contributed
to an abandonment of influenza pandemic preparation, and when public health
organizations again began to draw up new pandemic plans, the limitations of
nation-centered approaches remained uppermost in their minds. Still, the vaccination programs of 1957, 1968, and 1976 have shaped public health responses
to novel influenza viruses up to the present day.

CHAPTER 5

The Forecast Calls for Pandemics

Influenza and other pandemic diseases are by definition border-defying agents. The highly transmissive nature of this respiratory disease and the world's tight interconnections ensure that every nation has been susceptible to new strains of influenza. Moreover, the speed with which the virus circulates has accelerated with the pace of transportation advances. Beginning with Russian flu, influenza researchers have avidly tracked the relationship between transportation and the epicenters of outbreaks. Following the 1957 Asian flu pandemic, researchers began to identify a new pattern associated with the widely used new form of transportation: the jet airplane.[1] Health officials of this era believed that the next influenza pandemic would move faster than had any others in human history. Because the 1957 and 1968 vaccination efforts had failed at many levels, preparation and organization for the next pandemic shift was undertaken at levels stretching from the local all the way up to the international. Any program that sought to protect against pandemic influenza would require close coordination among public health organizations. Building on efforts begun in the 1950s, these organizations sought to coordinate in terms of research, surveillance, manufacturing, and organization. A new influenza pandemic would brook no delays.

Protecting against an influenza pandemic was seen as a technical problem, one that could be solved. New predictive pandemic models and faster, more productive manufacturing processes were seen as crucial for blunting or even preventing pandemic spread in the nation. Public health officials anticipated that any successful new approaches to protecting against influenza epidemics would stem from increased research on the virus and its behavior. These advances in preventing the virus would be part of a global effort to control pandemic outbreaks.

The increased knowledge about influenza achieved in the 1930s and 1940s, the ability to grow large quantities of virus cheaply, and the identification of an inexpensive animal model (laboratory mice) enabled many more researchers to study the influenza virus. Although other diseases, including polio, continued to attract more research funding, by the 1950s increasing numbers of people were working on the virus. This wider interest made it clear that some sort of coordination of effort was needed to prevent wasteful duplication in research. Again, such global coordination seemed a natural fit for the World Health Organization. By the early 1950s the expert committee on influenza—which already met regularly to decide on yearly vaccine recommendations—began the task of informally organizing research agendas on topics related to influenza.

Expert committees have a curious relationship with the WHO. Consisting of individuals recognized as experts in the various fields in which the WHO is involved, they are called together to consult on a topic of interest to the organization. The reports or recommendations they issue are provided to the director general of the WHO but are neither binding on the organization nor necessarily accepted as its official policy. Only the directors of the WHO's executive board or the amendments passed by the World Health Assembly officially speak for the organization. In practice, however, the expert committees' recommendations carry enormous clout with the WHO, especially in the case of influenza and the relevant committee's twice-yearly vaccine recommendations. For committees working on matters of technical sophistication, senior WHO leaders are relatively unlikely to intervene in their recommendations. Significantly, the group of experts dealing with the influenza surveillance system has been—and remains—one of the more technically oriented of the WHO's committees.

In many ways the influenza committee's role in the WHO mirrors the WHO's role in global health. The WHO can craft reports and studies and issue proclamations and suggestions, but it cannot really compel acceptance of its goals. In fact, the WHO has few resources of its own, relying almost totally on national health programs to do its work and achieve its goals. The organization maintains a small staff at its headquarters in Geneva and in regional divisions, but it mostly uses people and resources "loaned" to it. Nonetheless, the WHO can bring enormous coercive public pressure to bear on individual nation-states, pushing them to adhere to its prescriptions and to work with the organization in various ways.[2]

The influenza expert committee meetings have tended to be informal affairs, with gatherings considered a meeting of equals. Although the number of researchers working on the influenza virus was growing throughout the later 1950s, the circle of experts then was still quite small, with many scientists having collaborated with their peers or at least visited their laboratories. This clubby atmosphere continued into the 1980s,[3] making it easy for researchers to coordinate their efforts and to remain aware of their colleagues' projects. In addition, the WHO sought to become a clearinghouse for promising research being conducted in the field.

Research interest on the influenza virus exploded with the sudden appearance and spread of Asian flu in 1957. Much of the research, naturally, focused on issues of vaccination and vaccine production, but researchers also recognized that the emerging pandemic presented a unique opportunity to study the virus itself. Some of these studies focused on transmission patterns, viral mutation, and infection in various populations. The WHO's influenza experts sought to carve out a research niche of their own by focusing on the virus's origin—specifically, determining whether an animal reservoir for the virus exists. Influenza scientists were by now well aware of the reports that swine caught influenza during the Spanish flu epidemic. At an informal influenza committee meeting held in Geneva during July 1957, Dr. Kaplan of the WHO suggested to the forty assembled experts that "steps should be taken to collect animal sera so as to be able to determine whether domestic animals played any part in the epidemiology of influenza."[4] Kaplan's suggestion ultimately established a research agenda funded by the WHO that in the ensuing years would contribute to uncovering both the reservoir of influenza strains in the avian population and the role of animals in transmitting the virus to the human population.

Recycling Theory

Spurred by the Asian flu pandemic, scientists tested some of their theories about the virus and how it behaves in times of a pandemic. These experiments confirmed some suspicions but also provided some unexpected results. One observation of Asian flu's infection pattern and antibody production in various populations gave rise to a predictive theory known as the recycling theory.[5]

One type of study useful for charting the impact of this new flu strain relied on determining antibody reaction to the new strain in various populations. Establishing this baseline of reaction rates in different age groups helped researchers to determine how effectively vaccines protected individuals and to retrospectively estimate the morbidity rate of infection in a population. Maurice Hilleman had run such studies in May 1957, which allowed him to determine that the Asian flu virus was a novel strain for the population and thus likely to spread pandemically. The Dutch influenza researcher J. Mulder received some unexpected results from his antibody surveys. Mulder's findings showed that a surprising number in the elderly population (between seventy and eighty-four years of age) produced antibodies to the new influenza strain. He immediately recognized the import of this observation. The human body (generally) produces antibodies only to infections it has already encountered. If the elderly were producing antibodies to this new strain, they must have previously encountered it or something quite similar. Anyone seventy years old in 1957 would have been born in 1887, which suggests that the 1957 Asian flu was either the same as or very similar to the pandemic Russian flu of 1889.[6]

Mulder understood that his observations were suggestive and that they would have to be confirmed at other laboratories. He also recognized that the window of opportunity to get this corroborating evidence was small. Many people would be exposed when the highly transmissive Asian flu reached a community, with some victims experiencing symptoms so mild that they would not even realize they were infected. It would be difficult to obtain a clean and clear antibody comparison in a population already subject to the pandemic. Therefore, Mulder encouraged other laboratories to conduct similar antibody studies prior to the arrival of the pandemic. Mulder sped his preliminary results to the WHO and urged it to broadcast his observations and request further assays. Dr. A. M.-M. Payne complied and on 21 June 1957 sent a memorandum to all influenza centers and observers outlining Mulder's results.[7]

Initially, personnel at other laboratories were unable to duplicate Mulder's observations, casting doubt on the validity of his results, but by the latter part of the summer, researchers in Australia and the United States reported a similar unusual antibody pattern. The most prominent booster of Mulder's evidence relating age to antibodies was Fred Davenport, who had succeeded Tommy Francis as the head of the U.S. military's commission on influenza. Davenport subsequently published the results of his experiments, which agreed with, and added to, Mulder's report.[8]

In the years following the Asian flu pandemic, it became generally accepted that this disease was closely related to the Russian flu of 1889. Mulder's hypothesis that the virus had recirculated into the human population was an interesting observation but of limited practicality. It would take additional information to turn Mulder's hypothesis into something useful for vaccine production. The Hong Kong pandemic of 1968 would provide that additional information.

The sudden appearance and spread of a new influenza strain—dubbed Hong Kong flu for its original isolation—sent researchers scrambling to study the emerging pandemic. As was the case in 1957, one common method for studying the disease was to measure antibody production to the new strain in various populations. In an echo of Mulder's observations, researchers around the globe found that the older population produced abnormally high levels of antibodies in response to the new Hong Kong strain. These studies drew both on Mulder's and Davenport's work in 1957 and on Tommy Francis's theory of "original antigenic sin."[9] Francis had theorized that the first influenza type to which a person is exposed results in a powerful and persistent antibody response. Subsequent infections with different influenza types also result in antibody formation, but not of the volume produced by the first strain's infection. Therefore, high antibody levels produced in response to a virus strain suggest that the strain is similar or identical to the first influenza infection the person had; because influenza is a highly transmissible infection, most people initially encounter it at an early age.

In 1968 observations of high antibody response rates to the Hong Kong flu among the elderly population were discovered in the United States, the Netherlands, and Japan.[10] Simple subtraction suggested that the elderly population of 1968 was first exposed to a similar virus in the year 1900. Although 1900 was not considered to have been a pandemic year, researchers examining medical records and statistics from the time now noticed that an elevated number of influenza outbreaks had occurred then and suggested that it should be considered an epidemic or perhaps mild pandemic year.

Contributing to the validity of the recycling theory—as the observation of antibody patterns suggested—was the new method for naming influenza viruses. When the Hong Kong virus first began to spread, members of the scientific community debated whether it was a new strain.[11] In some tests, the Hong Kong strain produced results radically different from those produced by the prevailing strain (the Asian flu drifted descendant), indicating that the former should be designated as a new strain, A3. In other tests, however, the virus appeared to be similar to the prevailing strain, suggesting it to be part of the Asian flu family (A2). In response, influenza researchers developed (and the WHO adopted) a new naming system that grouped influenza viruses by their surface components (hemagglutinin and neuraminidase). The types of the two components were grouped into "families" that shared similar characteristics. The Hong Kong influenza strain (and its drifted descendants) was designated H3N2, meaning that the hemagglutinin belonged to family H3, and the neuraminidase, to family N2. The 1957 Asian flu was designated H2N2. Spanish flu (typed from Shope's pig samples from 1931) was designated H1N1. The more accurate naming process solved the puzzling test results on the Hong Kong influenza strain. The hemagglutinin was a viral shift, from an H2 to an H3, but the neuraminidase (N2) did not change; tests that measured the neuraminidase thus showed no viral shift.

The recycling theory thus postulated that the 1957 Asian flu was a recycling of the influenza strain that had caused the 1889 Russian flu. Both viruses included hemagglutinin from the H2 family. The 1968 Hong Kong flu, however, was a recycling of the unnamed 1900 flu strain, with the two viruses sharing hemagglutinin from the H3 family. The logic of the recycling theory draws on the "original antigenic sin" reaction of the human immune system. Over time, the strong and persistent viral antibody reaction from the individual's first exposure to influenza is sharpened by repeated exposure to drifted descendants of the original strain. Eventually, the majority of a population builds up resistance to a family of influenza disease. This population resistance to infection makes it increasingly difficult for the influenza virus to maintain its chain of infection in the human population. As a result, the virus dies out or retreats to low levels of infection and is then supplanted by a new family of influenza virus. As time passes, an increasing share of the population comprises members born since the last time that family of influenza virus circulated widely. This enables the population to be primed for the pandemic spread of that family of influenza.[12]

In 1957 those people who carried a strong resistance to the H2 family from their first exposure were more resistant to Asian flu than were the rest of the population. But those aged seventy and above were only a small proportion of the planet's population. Since the vast majority of the world's population had no resistance to the H2 family, Asian flu was able to spread widely and rapidly. In 1968 the H3 Hong Kong virus spread pandemically because those who had strong immune response to the H3 family (the unnamed 1900 flu) constituted only a small fraction of the population. The H3 family had apparently been supplanted by the H1 Spanish flu family in 1918.

The recycling theory not only explained events and observations retrospectively but could be applied predictively. The 1957 Asian flu was a recycling of the H2 family of viruses from the 1889 Russian flu pandemic. The 1968 Hong Kong Flu was a pandemic recycling of the 1900 H3 family of viruses. The next pandemic strain was the 1918 Spanish flu. Therefore, the next strain to appear and spread pandemically should be a member of the H1 family. Also, this new appearance of an H1 type should occur in the near future because the individuals immune to H1 were becoming a smaller share of the planet's population day by day.

The Eleven-Year-Cycle Theory

Observations of flu pandemics in the later nineteenth and twentieth centuries gave rise to another theory about pandemic influenza. The eleven-year-cycle theory was developed and promoted by the prominent influenza researcher Edwin Kilbourne. Kilbourne noted that the gaps between the presumed pandemic years of 1889, 1900, and 1918 were eleven and eighteen years, respectively. He noted that the gap between 1957 and 1968 was eleven years. Moreover, Kilbourne vividly recalled the influenza epidemic year of 1947 (the strain had first appeared in late 1946) because as a young lieutenant he had treated patients stacked up in hallways; moreover, the prevailing vaccine had failed that year because the virus had dramatically changed its appearance. Putting 1946 into the equation marks eleven years before 1957. Kilbourne detected a pattern in influenza pandemics, and if there was a pattern, there must be some method to describe that pattern. If a pattern can be described, subsequent events fitting it can be predicted.[13]

Before Kilbourne could present a hypothesis to describe influenza's infection pattern, he had to be certain that the pattern existed. The major obstacle to his hypothesis was the large gap between the 1918 Spanish flu and the 1957 Asian flu. Kilbourne had partially solved that issue by proposing 1946 as a year of viral shift, but that still left a break from 1918 to 1946. In reviewing medical statistics kept by the United States, the United Kingdom and the League of Nations, Kilbourne discovered a rise in influenza cases in 1929 that he postulated was due to a shift in the virus. Others suggested 1933, the year of Andrewes and Smith's sneezing ferrets. Both years roughly fit the proposed pattern. According to the eleven-year-cycle theory, the years 1889, 1900, 1918, 1929 (1933), 1946, 1957, and 1968 were years of pandemic shift in the influenza virus.[14]

The explanation for this cycle can also be found in "original antigenic sin."[15] When a new strain is introduced into a population that has no immunity to it, the virus spreads easily, with the number of cases or infections quickly soaring to an epidemic peak. Subsequent years have lower numbers of cases because an increasing share of the population had been exposed to the pandemic type. Genetic drift prompts new epidemic peaks, but they are never as high as the one associated with the initial introduction of the new virus, because exposure to the family of influenza results in greater levels of resistance to a similar strain. Over time the population's repeated exposure to versions of the pandemic type increases resistance to that virus family, making it harder for the virus to circulate. By the end of the cycle—about eleven years, in Kilbourne's theory—the population is highly resistant to the grouping of the initial pandemic strain. But this resistance does not extend to other types of influenza virus. When a new or shifted virus appears, it spreads pandemically, and this drives out the prevailing virus, supplanting it with a new family of influenza virus, and the cycle begins anew.

Kilbourne's hypothesis was widely accepted. And why not? The theory provided a logical explanation (with diagrams!) to an apparently observed pattern. Like the recycling theory, if the retrospective theory of the influenza pattern was correct, then it could conceivably be used predictively. If the last pandemic year was 1968, then the next pandemic should arrive somewhere around 1979. Combining the two theories suggested that a new pandemic strain would appear around 1979 and be a recycling of the H1 strain, or Spanish flu. No public health official needed reminding of what had happened in 1918.

Recombination and Vaccine Production

The recycling and eleven-year-cycle theories offered the potential to make surveillance more efficient. Surveillance had failed to detect pandemic strains of influenza until they were spreading epidemically in 1957 and 1968. If the surveillance system had some sort of advance warning, then perhaps it could help identify a pandemic before it took off. But the inability to detect a new strain early only partly explained why vaccination efforts failed in 1957 and 1968. Manufacturers had been unable to produce the vaccine quickly enough to blunt the impact of the pandemics, in part because they had struggled to develop vaccine strains that matched the novel flu type and to produce the material at high levels. In 1957 early strains of Asian flu killed the chicken eggs used to grow vaccine; in 1968 it was difficult to increase the yield of vaccine per egg. At the tail end of the vaccination effort in 1968, however, a new production technique promised to increase both speed and yield. Once again, it was the intrepid Edwin Kilbourne who offered the solution.

Kilbourne's new production technique relied on the influenza virus's proclivity to swap genetic components. When it occurs in the wild, recombination is responsible for the creation of a new, reassembled virus, a process known as viral shift. Kilbourne sought to harness this tendency so as to aid the human population rather than threaten it.[16] His method involved combining a fast-growth, high-yield strain with the strain targeted with vaccination. Kilbourne did this by injecting the Hong Kong strain into a fertilized chicken egg infected with a laboratory influenza virus (then known as Ao/PR/8) and primed with a serum that inhibited the growth of the latter. The combined viruses then swapped genetic components, producing an array of mixed versions. Through titration, Kilbourne selected out those faster-growing mutants that combined the high growth potential of the laboratory donor (Ao/PR/8) with the immunizing characteristics of the Hong Kong influenza strain. Kilbourne repeatedly diluted the solution and incubated it into other fertilized chicken eggs seeking to find the most quickly growing and highly yielding strains. Eventually he selected one he dubbed X-31. The X-31 strain, a Hong Kong flu virus hybrid, produced significantly more virus particles than did the current vaccine seed stock, thereby providing the potential for significantly greater vaccine production.

Kilbourne's X-31 was not developed until mid-October (his laboratory had received samples of the Hong Kong strain only in late September), and the lateness of the hour and the fact that the original virus had been passed through a mammal cell line (monkey kidney) prompted vaccine manufacturers to decline using the new prototype.[17] But the fact that Kilbourne was able to quickly produce a vaccine that offered both excellent protection against the newly shifted virus and high production value had extraordinary relevance for public health. Simply put, Kilbourne's recombination technique would allow manufacturers to make a lot more vaccine in a shorter period of time.

Organization

Surveillance and manufacturing were crucial components of the 1957 and 1968 vaccination campaigns, and their limitations and failures contributed significantly to rendering those campaigns ineffective. But as I have shown, both campaigns lacked adequate coordination and planning. The lessons from the 1957 and 1968 pandemics would need to be applied on both the national and international levels if subsequent vaccination campaigns were to be more efficient. The key to developing an effective vaccination effort relied on prior preparation.

United States Public Health Service officials keenly appreciated that the decision not to designate a central authority for the vaccination campaigns had greatly contributed to the uneven distribution of the vaccine in 1957 and 1968. The demand for vaccine had overwhelmed the supply at the outset of the pandemic, quickly leading officials to abandon priority distribution. Those considered high-priority recipients—whether for public health reasons (they worked in health care or emergency services) or for medical reasons (they were deemed to be at high risk for complications from influenza)—had not received the vaccine first. The overall impact of misdistribution of vaccine stocks served to heighten the public's distrust of the campaign, frustrated public health officials, and ultimately blunted the efforts to mitigate the pandemic's impact on the populace.

Beginning in the late 1960s and continuing into early 1970s, government programs to attack large-scale problems gained popularity. President Lyndon Baines Johnson had declared a "war on poverty," and President Richard Nixon had matched this ambitious announcement with his own call for a "war on cancer." Both "wars" were lavishly funded efforts to attack intransigent problems; both comprised programs run by government bureaucracies. The management of large-scale operations directed by a cadre of government experts was a model perfectly suited for the sensibilities of the Centers for Disease Control. Although not directly controlling the antipoverty or anticancer program, the CDC did manage to carve out a role in both. The CDC flourished in an era when government-managed solutions seemed best. In arenas directly under the CDC's authority, the organization favored large-scale projects, including massive vaccination programs—both domestic and international—such as the smallpox eradication program. But the CDC attempted to run these programs as lean as possible, which for the CDC meant using as few layers of bureaucratic oversight as possible. Even though the organization favored large-scale programs, it delegated authority to officials "on the ground" and kept reporting lines short and directly connected to the CDC hierarchy. This structure was a function of both necessity and proclivity. Funds for public health programs are often in short supply, so providing resources and staff is difficult. Using fewer layers of oversight allowed the CDC management to control the program tightly and served the organization's desire to keep the programs in house.[18]

The decentralized mode of the failed vaccination campaigns greatly affected manufacturing in another, less well-known way. Vaccine manufacturers had twice undertaken large-scale efforts to produce protective vaccines. In 1957 and again in 1968, manufacturers were unable to get vaccine to market before the peak of the epidemic. When producers finally delivered the material in bulk, they found few takers and so were saddled with unsold and unsellable vaccine stocks. Manufacturers signaled they were unwilling to risk the potential costs of unsold vaccines again.

To ramp up production for a crash immunization program, manufacturers would need improved facilities and infrastructure, but maintaining such a productive infrastructure made financial sense only if they had a steady market for influenza vaccine from year to year. The federal government recognized the need to ensure manufacturing capacity for influenza vaccine and had taken steps to increase the number of people who received those vaccines. Beginning in 1960, the USPHS recommended that those in "high-risk" categories—anyone sixty-five or more years old and those with chronic lung ailments—get a yearly flu vaccine. The effort had boosted the influenza vaccine market, benefiting recipients and manufacturers.[19] The overall effect was minimal, however, because as one public health expert put it, "Adults, by and large, just don't like to get vaccinated."[20] Fortunately for those who wanted to bolster manufacturing capacity, manufacturers based in the United States supplied a number of overseas markets as well.

By the early 1970s the USPHS concluded that any large-scale vaccination campaign would need to be centrally organized and administered by the federal government. In addition, recombination technology offered the possibility of producing large quantities of vaccine. Nevertheless, the government would have to do more than merely publicize the need for the vaccine to protect the nation's citizens. The publicity campaigns in 1957 and 1968 had worked; many people knew about the vaccine and wanted to be inoculated, but the doses were unavailable when needed. If the federal government purchased the vaccine, then the manufacturers would be assured of a market, and the USPHS would be able to control its distribution. Increasingly, those in the field of public health began to push for just such an expanded federal role.[21]

Other nations also recognized that they needed to bolster their abilities to respond to the sudden appearance of a pandemic strain of influenza. For nations other than the United States, the major problem had been the lack of vaccine production. The 1957 Asian flu epidemic prompted many other national health programs to make vaccine, but the production rate remained low because much of the vaccine was made "at the bench." Some pharmaceutical firms began to produce influenza vaccine—for example, in France both the Pasteur Institute and Merieux began producing vaccine following the 1957 pandemic—but the market for it was small.[22] No other nation besides the United States had promoted yearly vaccine for those deemed to be at high risk, and in general, influenza was considered a minor seasonal annoyance, of no more importance than the common cold.

The 1968 pandemic began changing this attitude about influenza in European public health circles. Studies stimulated by the Hong Kong epidemic began to reveal the burden of influenza—in terms of the economy, mortality, and symptom-related suffering—suffered every year and not just in pandemic years. Also, the WHO's new system for naming influenza strains clearly demonstrated the virus's shifting nature, which made it necessary to update the vaccine constantly. In the years following the Hong Kong pandemic, France and several other nations began to assess their abilities to respond to a pandemic, as well as the less spectacular yet central issue of the influenza virus's yearly impact. Beginning in the early 1970s, French public health officials sought to increase production of influenza vaccines by promoting wider use of a yearly protective vaccine.

Vaccine manufacturing in the United Kingdom followed a similar path.[23] In the early 1970s the major influenza vaccine producer in the United Kingdom, a Glaxo Pharmaceuticals subsidiary named Evans Medical, was producing approximately 1.2 million doses a year. This figure had increased in the years following the Hong Kong pandemic flu strain, but the U.K. market for influenza vaccine was still quite low. Influenza vaccine was only a part of Evans Medical's portfolio of vaccines. The company found greater demand for, and thus more profit in, veterinary vaccines. Production capacity on influenza vaccine would increase only if there was an increased demand for the shots. Despite some large institutional purchases—for example, British postal workers were offered free influenza vaccines—demand for influenza vaccination remained light in the United Kingdom.[24]

The United Kingdom also had a very vocal antivaccination league active in the community in the 1960s and 1970s. J. Donald Millar, the coordinator of the WHO smallpox eradication effort in West Africa, recalls that health officials did not respond aggressively when smallpox was inadvertently introduced into the United Kingdom from Pakistan in the early 1960s. In some cases, asserted Millar, the illness had progressed "five or six generations before they got it under control."[25] Millar believes that vocal critics of vaccination in the United Kingdom restrained the National Health Service from aggressively inoculating possible contacts with those infected with smallpox and overall dampened people's willingness to receive any type of vaccine.

In one nation, however, the government and the public health system succeeded in greatly increasing vaccine production and use following the Hong Kong flu pandemic. The Japanese government began annually inoculating children in primary and middle schools both because the 1968 pandemic had wrought significant harm and because schoolchildren play a disproportionately large role in spreading influenza (seen most notably in the 1957 pandemic). This Japanese vaccination policy fostered a robust market for influenza vaccine (20 million doses just for schoolchildren in 1973), which stimulated influenza vaccine manufacturers to increase their production capacity.[26] But Japanese efforts to expand the use of influenza vaccines appear to have been the exception rather than the norm. Despite efforts to increase production, most other national pharmaceutical firms lagged behind the major U.S. manufacturers in terms of production capacity.

In addition to acknowledging the need for greater production and increased coordination within each nation, public health officials recognized the necessity to foster greater intergovernmental and international organization.

The years 1957 and 1968 clearly demonstrated the global nature of influenza; in each case, the pandemic virus that arose in one location had rapidly circled the globe. Freely exchanging information about the virus would benefit all nations. To foster international exchange of the most recent knowledge of the influenza virus, the National Institutes of Health, in the United States, sponsored a series of meetings designed to address topics of the influenza virus and strategies to protect the public from the disease. Lists of attendees to meetings read like a global who's who of influenza research, and the presentations and discussions were republished in the *Journal of Infectious Diseases* for wider dissemination.[27] The workshops presented state of the art knowledge among influenza researchers, including the practical application of techniques to detect and protect against the influenza virus.

The circle of researchers and administrators who collaborated on influenza research comes close to the model of functionalism promoted by international relations theorists. Unlike earlier scientists, whose often nationalist competitions for medical discoveries served as proxies for empire conflicts of the times, influenza researchers now saw themselves as members of an elite club of experts. They attended the same conferences, collaborated on research projects, and visited each others' laboratories to share knowledge and learn techniques. There were, to be sure, still some elements of national identity, but these were subsumed under the larger dictates of science. As Walter Dowdle pointed out, the WHO's meetings of influenza experts promoted an atmosphere in which it "would have been absolutely unacceptable" to "carry the national policy onto the international scene" (he added that it had "always" been this way and always would be); he too asserted that the researchers' principal allegiance was to science.[28] The group was open to new members, both as a matter of collegiality and for the practical reason that new members made the surveillance net wider and more effective, but membership hinged on mastery of the technical issues and language of biomedical influenza research.

Besides the NIH-sponsored gatherings, meetings and workshops held by other groups discussed all manner of topics related to pandemic influenza, including how to improve vaccination campaigns when facing a new pandemic strain. In a workshop held in Switzerland in January 1976, public health influenza experts met to discuss strategies for responding to an influenza pandemic and to assess the current state of the world's ability to uncover a viral shift and mount a large-scale vaccination program. The results were hardly reassuring.[29]

The delegates at the Swiss conference agreed that surveillance was steadily improving.[30] The number of laboratories involved in the WHO influenza surveillance network was increasing, and thanks to WHO-led training efforts, the laboratories' surveillance was becoming more reliable. But, the delegates noted with concern, significant gaps existed in the surveillance net, especially in "developing" countries. Most worrisome was the fact that the previous two pandemic strains were believed to have originated in China, which remained cut off from the outside world because of Chairman Mao's policies. Mindful of the 1957 and 1968 examples, the assembled public health experts agreed that a major shift in either of the influenza virus's surface components (hemagglutinin and neuraminidase) offered pandemic potential. The experts agreed that evidence of this type of shift constituted sufficient evidence to issue an early global alert. It was clear that although surveillance was improving, it was still far from optimal to provide early detection of an emerging pandemic, and early detection is vital if governments are to wage a protective vaccination campaign.

Manufacturing capacity, too, had improved since the 1968 Hong Kong pandemic. Kilbourne's recombination technique greatly accelerated the quantity of vaccine that could be produced. By the mid-1970s, most manufacturers had become familiar with the technology, and several researchers were using it. But even as the technology improved, production facilities (outside the United States) had not greatly expanded. The British influenza expert Joseph Smith estimated that an emergency vaccination campaign, creating only monovalent vaccine, could produce enough to protect no more than 30 percent of the United Kingdom's population.[31] The situation in Britain was roughly comparable to that of other "developed" nations. The existing production capacities within the developed countries could certainly be expanded to the point of providing sufficient vaccine to protect all their populations; no technical constraint precluded achieving that goal. But the expansion of production required significant expenditures of government financing, and during the 1970s economic realities made such funding appear doubtful.

Indeed, financing for public health was in scarce supply at this time. The recession sparked by the oil crisis of 1973 had bitten deep into government coffers. Public health programs labored under constricting budgets. Some research programs had to be abandoned altogether, and there was even concern that the day-to-day operations of research laboratories would be affected.[32] Like surveillance, manufacturing capacity had improved in the years since the Hong Kong pandemic emerged, but vaccine production was far from optimal.

By the end of 1975 all those in the influenza research community agreed that an influenza epidemic was imminent. Many scientists were influenced by the two previously mentioned predictive theories, one of which suggested that a viral shift was due eleven years after the 1968 Hong Kong pandemic and the other, that it was likely to be similar to the 1918 Spanish flu (H1N1). Other influenza experts thought they detected a pattern of instability in the prevailing strains of influenza, a pattern that resembled events prior to the pandemic shifts of 1957 and 1968.[33] The views of these scientists were not merely their personal convictions; because these experts worked in various organizations, their observations became the views of those agencies. For example, the National Institute of Allergy and Infectious Diseases, in the United States, flatly stated that "every 10–12 years a major modification takes place rendering whole populations susceptible to the new strain" and that "the next such pandemic [was] predicted for the late 1970s."[34]

The expectation of an imminent pandemic was a truly international belief within influenza research circles, but it held a special attraction in the United States. Many public health experts there believed that, if they were lucky, the United States had sufficient manufacturing capacity to protect its citizens, a belief in productive capacity shared by the manufacturers. Maurice Hilleman, now the director of virus and cell biology research at the Merck Institute for Therapeutic Research, wrote John Seal, the acting deputy director of the National Institute of Allergy and Infectious Diseases, warning, "Pandemic 1978, or thereabouts, is a real thing that can likely be substantially controlled by application of killed vaccine *provided* there is advance preparation . . . [and] central coordination and planning must reside somewhere in the government."[35] Hilleman should know; he had been in charge of vaccine development at Merck since he left the Walter Reed Army Institute of Research after the 1957 pandemic.

In many ways, the early 1970s were heady times in the field of public health. Newly developed vaccines were making a serious dent in preventing illness in the industrial world, new and more powerful antibiotics seemed to control many rampant and deadly bacterial infections, and it seemed that the biggest challenge remaining lay in figuring out how best to export these medical advances to the developing world. The sentiment of imminent mastery over infectious diseases is visible in a statement from the late 1960s frequently attributed to U.S. Surgeon General William Stewart, who is claimed to have said that it was "time to close the book on infectious diseases."[36] This feeling of optimism was not without basis, for humanity's greatest killer of all time, smallpox, had been driven to a handful of locales and seemed poised for extinction. Smallpox's imminent eradication was purposely planned and prosecuted by humankind, making these exciting times indeed.

There were, to be sure, critics who noted the expensive failure to eradicate malaria, the stubborn persistence and resurgence of measles, and the spotty vaccination coverage in the poverty-stricken pockets of the United States.[37] But the difficulties of wider access to successful prophylactic methods were seen as challenges to overcome rather than insuperable obstacles. Public health officials spoke of eradicating diseases, not just limiting their impact. Nowhere was this sentiment more pervasive than at the CDC. Galvanized by the arduous but successful programs of eradicating malaria in the United States and smallpox across the Americas, and their leading role in eradicating smallpox worldwide, CDC experts began to consider what other diseases might be candidates for eradication. This optimistic spirit permeated the organization, and on the eve of the Swine Flu Program, epidemiologists could write joking notes saying things such as, "My condolences on your recent bout with the flu; flu is the next disease we will eradicate!"[38]

The CDC had steadily increased in power and prestige throughout the 1960s, and its laboratory acumen and epidemiological expertise made it a recognized leader in issues of health.[39] Building on the strong base created by Alexander Langmuir, CDC director David Sencer successfully reorganized the agency's operations to give them a more international focus. The CDC inherited the foreign quarantine program in 1966, the year Sencer was elevated to the directorship, and Sencer authorized shifting surveillance efforts abroad, reasoning that fighting diseases overseas prevented them from being imported into the United States. Sencer called this "nice budget logic," but it allowed the CDC to operate worldwide. Along with participating in international epidemiological efforts modeled on Langmuir's EIS program and smallpox and malaria eradication operations, the organization became involved in a number of other international projects under the flags of both the United States and the WHO.[40]

The CDC was not the only or even the major beneficiary of renewed funding and organization in medical research. The 1950s and 1960s are seen as the "golden years" for the National Institutes of Health, whose budget increased from $29 million in 1948 to $1.4 billion in 1967. Congressional leaders continually pushed to increase funding for research in general and for pet research projects in particular. American economic might was being turned into American scientific might. Dramatic increases in the number and effectiveness of diagnoses, treatments, techniques, drugs, and vaccines followed this research investment bonanza. This research pattern reinforced the technical biomedical approach to health prevalent in the United States.[41]

Following the 1957 pandemic, researchers and public health officials carefully studied pandemic outbreaks, their impacts, and failed vaccination efforts with an eye both theoretical and practical. The influenza experts wanted to understand the virus and control any subsequent pandemics.[42] Those groups interested in controlling potential pandemics (public health practitioners, influenza researchers, and vaccine manufacturers) prepared for the next epidemic of influenza. Protecting the public against such a pandemic was seen as a technical problem, but only a handful of national health programs possessed the capability and infrastructure to respond quickly. The constraints of a vaccination campaign—the need to identify a new strain, create a vaccine prototype, produce it in large quantities, and set up a distribution system to rapidly and fairly deliver the vaccine—meant that time was of the essence. If a new strain appeared, the experiences of 1957 and 1968 indicated it would move quickly. As Dr. Michael Gregg, a CDC epidemiologist put it, "For several years, . . . epidemiologists at CDC had played the 'what if' game: What if a new strain of influenza came along and there was a pandemic?"[43] In February 1976 it appeared as though the "if" had had arrived.

CHAPTER 6

"Chance Favors the Prepared Mind"

In January 1976 influenza researchers and public health officials around the globe coordinated their efforts to speed up their responses to pandemic influenza. At Rougemont, Switzerland, public health experts met to evaluate the current status of influenza surveillance and vaccine manufacturing and to discuss methods of improving both. The predictive eleven-year-cycle and recycling theories added impetus to influenza research, providing an almost audible ticking sound to preparations for the next pandemic. When Martin Goldfield, an epidemiologist for New Jersey, sent his unidentified influenza samples to the CDC headquarters in Atlanta, he had no idea that he was initiating the first step in a decision chain that would end in the creation of the National Influenza Immunization Program (or Swine Flu Program). The novel influenza samples were received by an organization that had been preparing—in both national and international terms—for the next pandemic strain.[1]

January 1976 was cold in south-central New Jersey, and the crowded conditions and stress of training made the base at Fort Dix an ideal amplifier of respiratory diseases.[2] As influenza researchers and public health experts were meeting in places such as the National Institutes of Health offices outside Washington, D.C. (on 12 Jan. 1976), and at the Swiss resort town of Rougemont (26–28 Jan.), a minor epidemic of respiratory disease was circulating at

Fort Dix. The epidemic resulted in an unexpectedly high hospitalization rate, predominantly among recent trainees. On Thursday, 29 January 1976, the post's medical officer, Colonel Bartley, sent eight samples to Dr. Goldfield's laboratory to settle their friendly wager. Lab technicians at Goldfield's laboratory injected the material into fertilized chicken eggs and left them to incubate over the weekend. On Monday, 2 February, Goldfield harvested the material and tested it to determine whether the specimens contained influenza virus. Goldfield quickly typed four of the eight samples as A/Victoria, an H3N2 Hong-Kong-drifted descendant recently detected in Hawaii. Two of the other viral packages responded to tests indicating they were influenza strains but did not react to any of the reagents that Goldfield had on hand. Colonel Bartley later shipped an additional eleven samples, which turned up two more unidentified influenza strains. Of the nineteen units tested by Goldfield's laboratory, seven were typed A/Victoria and four revealed unidentified influenza strains. Goldfield dutifully shipped these mystery items to the CDC in Atlanta for typing on 6 February.

When Goldfield's samples arrived in Atlanta, they were delivered to the laboratory where two virologists—Gary Noble and Alan Kendal—were charged with identifying influenza. Unlike Goldfield's lab in New Jersey, which possessed only a limited number of reagents, the CDC laboratory contained freeze-dried reagents extending all the way back to 1931 (the 1931 sample, coincidentally, was collected by Shope from midwestern pigs). Goldfield's jest that the strains were probably swine aside, the unidentified subjects were likely to be some drifted relative of Hong Kong flu that Goldfield's laboratory had been unable to detect; growing influenza virus can be a fickle business. But swine influenza was on the minds of the two virologists. Gary Noble had identified two mystery strains that other researchers had been unable to type just a few weeks before. One strain came from a sixteen-year-old boy afflicted with Hodgkin's disease who had died in September 1974; the other came from an eight-year-old Wisconsin boy who had recovered from a severe illness in October 1975. The identity of the material was unknown until Noble thought to try samples against swine flu reagents. Both results came back positive. But those two cases were seen as anomalies. Both children had been in contact with pigs on their farms, and there was no evidence of spread beyond those two isolated cases. In addition, it was presumed that the sixteen-year-old's fatality was hastened by his immunocompromised state due to Hodgkin's disease. The Fort Dix samples were viewed like any other unidentified test result: interesting, but not of immediate concern. This blasé view was about to change.

On Wednesday, 4 February 1976, Private Lewis began his doomed final day of training at Fort Dix, collapsing and dying on the return march that evening. On autopsy, tracheal swabs were collected from the corpse. The preliminary cause of death was called bronchitis or bronchial pneumonia because Lewis's lungs were filled with bloody fluid. On 9 February Goldfield's laboratory had identified the mystery strain in the cultures taken from Lewis, and Goldfield shipped this specimen to the CDC, where it arrived on 11 February 1976. At the time, Kendal was harvesting viral samples from the first batches from Goldfield, for he needed additional material to run his tests. With the new quantity of viral material, Kendal conducted his tests with a greater sense of urgency. The mystery virus had been part of a miniepidemic at Fort Dix and had killed an apparently healthy young man. Examining the material with an electron microscope suggested the samples were an influenza virus, and by the next morning tests determined that the virus was from the influenza A family. Kendal tested the strains against a number of reagents, including ones for swine influenza. By that evening he had his results: the samples reacted only to the swine influenza reagents. The virus was swine, specifically, HiswN1.

Kendal and Noble immediately conveyed their results to Walter Dowdle, who directed a virology laboratory that worked for both the CDC and the WHO. Dowdle called CDC head David Sencer, in Washington, at nine o'clock that evening.[3] The identity of the virus had officially become more than a subject of friendly wagering. The next morning Sencer called the National Institutes of Health, the Bureau of Biologics, the U.S. military, and the New Jersey Public Health Department to set up a meeting to discuss the results; it was scheduled for Saturday, 14 February.[4]

A Mystery Unveiled

The 14 February 1976 meeting at the CDC was a small affair, including only the major figures involved in the immediate detection. Dr. Goldfield was there in his role as the director of New Jersey's public health lab, and he had brought samples from the initial cases for retesting in a "clean" laboratory (one that had not done influenza testing) so as to rule out contamination as a cause of the swine flu identification. Fort Dix was a military base, and Colonels Philip Russell and Franklin Top represented the armed forces and their continuing interest in influenza vaccination. John Seal was the acting director of the National Institute of Allergy and Infectious Diseases, which had a long-running focus on influenza research. Dr. Harry Meyer headed the U.S. Food and Drug Administration's Bureau of Biologics,[5] and he also represented the interests of the FDA itself, which was charged with testing and certifying the safety and efficacy of influenza vaccines. The CDC was represented not only by Sencer, who chaired the meeting, but also by Walter Dowdle, who discussed the process of determining the identity of the new virus, and by members of the CDC staff. On the way into the meeting Dr. Goldfield had again joked to Gary Noble that the strain was probably swine. Noble did not fully confirm Goldfield's guess, merely replying, "Maybe you're closer than you think."[6]

All the attendees at the meeting suspected that the Fort Dix cases had important implications, hence the emergency meeting, but only the CDC staff knew the identity of the mystery virus. When Walter Dowdle reported the virus was typed as swine, there was a moment of stunned silence. Reportedly, Colonel Russell's head jerked up and his jaw dropped open, "the picture of astonishment," according to one meeting participant.[7] All the participants understood the potential public health implications of this identification. Dowdle and the CDC staff also discussed the swine flu cases of the preceding two years from Minnesota and Wisconsin. Perhaps Fort Dix was part of a chain of events in which the swine influenza virus was becoming better adapted for human transmission.

While the assembled experts at the 14 February meeting recognized the implications of the Fort Dix discovery, they also understood the need for further work to confirm the initial results. The first step was to verify the identification. The CDC had already begun this process by retesting samples from Dr. Goldfield's laboratory. The second course of action was to determine the contours of the outbreak at Fort Dix and look for any spread outside the camp or around the world. The military had already agreed to do a "quick and dirty epi" under the direction of Colonel Top to determine whether the infection continued to be transmitted at the camp and how widespread it had been.[8] Dr. Goldfield pledged to survey the communities around the base and ensure that various samples thought to show influenza infection, which physicians around the state routinely submitted, would be typed. The CDC committed itself to searching for cases nationally and to encourage the WHO influenza surveillance system to be vigilant globally. The CDC would also make and distribute reagents so that surveillance laboratories could positively identify the new strain. The group agreed that the typing of the strain merited rapid but sober publicizing, so they decided that once retesting confirmed the strain's identity, the information should be published immediately in the CDC-produced *Morbidity and Mortality Weekly Report (MMWR)*, a publication for anyone interested in epidemiology and medicine around the world; the report published a brief paragraph on the results in its 20 February 1976 issue.[9] The scientists agreed not to inform the popular press.

In addition to taking these steps to ramp up surveillance, the experts wanted to get a jump on manufacturing requirements. Having already considered these issues, Dr. Goldfield had sent a sample of the virus to Edwin Kilbourne's laboratory. Goldfield hoped that Kilbourne, who had harnessed the virus's recombination for vaccine production, could create a high-growth, high-yield recombinant for the A/New Jersey strain. In addition, the CDC itself would try to create such recombinants using a sample from the Wisconsin swine flu of 1975.

Despite the immediate attempts to create a vaccine strain of the new virus, the assembled experts were cautious about getting ahead of themselves. John Seal's memorandum submitted for the meeting's record stated the consensus of the group regarding the matter: "It is too early to speculate about the meaning [of the new virus] in terms of pandemic potential or other significance of the situation although this was a part of the discussion." But the pandemic potential of the novel influenza strain could not be ignored, as Seal noted under the heading of "Problem" in the memorandum. Seal stated, "The real question is—is this the beginning of the next pandemic?—will we expect widespread outbreaks of Swine Influenza in the U.S. next fall?" The answer to these questions could not definitively be determined from the evidence at hand at the 14 February meeting, but prudently, Dr. Meyer, as head of the BoB and liaison to the vaccine manufacturing community, intended to get recombinant strains into the hands of vaccine manufacturers as soon as possible.[10]

The discovery of the new virus at Fort Dix was fortuitous to those interested in manufacturing influenza vaccines. Unlike the pandemic years of 1957 and 1968, where the new virus was identified in late spring and mid-summer, respectively, after influenza vaccine manufacturers in the Northern Hemisphere had shut down their production lines, the February identification of the new virus occurred at the peak of influenza vaccine production. In the United States, the group charged with recommending the recipe for the yearly influenza inoculation—the Advisory Committee on Immunization Practices (ACIP)—had recently met and agreed on the strains to be covered by the protective vaccine, A/Victoria and B/Hong Kong. Anticipating this recommendation, manufacturers had been producing A/Victoria and B/Hong Kong virus in bulk.[11] Vaccine manufacturers in the Northern Hemisphere were making vaccine at a high rate, but they were approaching the ends of their production targets. Meyer recognized that the manufacturers could easily continue production with a new seed stock of vaccine, but they would need to know "within the next 30 days or so." The assembled experts at the 14 February meeting hoped that influenza surveillance would demonstrate definitive evidence about the new swine flu's pandemic potential. Seal summarized the problem: "This [vaccination] decision would be very difficult if the only evidence is that of a small localized outbreak at Fort Dix."[12]

The three levels of surveillance—on the camp, throughout the state, and across the nation or globe—were likely to have differing levels of accuracy and confidence in detecting the new virus. Because of the smaller population at Fort Dix and the relative control over its personnel, officials anticipated that the military would be able to determine quickly and accurately how many troops had been infected with the new strain there.[13] The public health experts hoped that enhanced surveillance in New Jersey would detect any infections outside the camp. These experts realized they would need some luck to detect whether swine flu virus was circulating at low levels nationally or internationally.

Swine flu's appearance was fortunate for the timing of vaccine production, but the same could not be said about the timing for surveillance. February and March signal the end of influenza season across the Northern Hemisphere. Fewer and fewer cases of influenza infection were detected as the weather warmed. If the surveillance system was going to monitor swine flu, public health officials needed the system's members searching for the novel virus immediately. Accordingly, Walter Dowdle alerted the WHO sentinel system to immediately ship unidentified influenza strains to his laboratory in Atlanta, and he sent reagents to the new swine flu strain to over 200 laboratories globally.[14] David Sencer wanted to ensure that state health officers clearly understood the importance of enhanced vigilance for influenza. On 18 February 1976 he sent a telegram to all such authorities, stating that four "Type A Viruses with antigenic characteristics of swine influenza [had] been isolated"; he added that the CDC was "aware of 2 human influenza cases in the U.S. caused by swine virus" (i.e., the Minnesota and Wisconsin cases in 1974 and 1975). He announced that the discovery of the new virus had prompted an "intensive investigation at Ft. Dix and in New Jersey into origin strains and possible spread" but admitted the limits of the current knowledge: "[It is] not yet known if this strain is circulating elsewhere in the United States. Laboratories are urged to submit to CDC isolates differing substantially from current Port Chalmers/Victoria strains."[15]

The Sencer telegram is certainly not alarmist, but it does convey a sense of urgency through the use of such phrases as "intensive investigation," "possible spread," and "laboratories are urged to submit . . . isolates." Considering the intended audience—state public health officials—and the source of the telegram (the director of the CDC), there is little doubt that the message of a potentially dangerous new flu strain was conveyed. State health officials would be acutely aware that the influenza season was nearing its end, taking with it the hope of determining whether the strain was circulating. Also, the inclusion of two earlier and geographically dispersed cases of swine flu infection would reinforce the need for vigilance everywhere. The new virus just might be lurking anywhere.

With the expanding circle of people informed about the discovery of novel influenza strains at Fort Dix, the national media began to make inquiries. To forestall uninformed or misguided reporting, the CDC decided to hold a press conference on 19 February 1976. In later interviews, members of the public health community complained about press coverage surrounding the Swine Flu Program, especially the press's linking of A/New Jersey (the strain's official designation) to the Spanish flu of 1918. While charges of poor or misguided reporting have validity in some aspects, charging the press with emphasizing swine flu's connection to Spanish flu is unfair, for the CDC itself made that connection in its first press conference.

A Mystery Announced

H. Bruce Dull, assistant director of the CDC, stood before the press on 19 February 1976.[16] Dull laid out the facts of the moderate influenza outbreak at Fort Dix. The predominant strain recovered at the camp was A/Victoria, the Hong Kong drift, but the other strain recovered had "antigenic characteristics of swine influenza virus. These latter viruses were from four cases of influenza, one fatal." Dull reported that this was the first time that swine flu viruses had been associated with an outbreak in the human population, but cautioned, "Whether this is significant or merely a curiosity is unknown at this time." Dull also informed the assembled press that although A/Victoria was causing elevated influenza cases at the moment, the virus did not appear to be sufficiently different from the Hong Kong strain to cause a pandemic. Dull declared that while influenza viruses were not isolated until the 1930s, it had "been speculated that viruses of the 1920s and perhaps before were similar [to swine flu]. The 1918–19 pandemic [had] been a special topic of conjecture because of its high mortality and unusual characteristics," but there was "no way to be sure whether the swine-type virus was associated with that event." Dull went on to discuss the heightened surveillance efforts then being conducted and closed with a bland statement of uncertainty: "Whether a swine-type influenza virus may become the predominant strain in the United States and elsewhere cannot be answered at this time."

Predictably, the national media emphasized the alarming aspects of Dull's press conference. The *New York Times* had a first-page story headlined "U.S. Calls Flu Alert on Possible Return of Epidemic's Virus," whose author, Harold Schmeck, suggested that the "virus that caused the greatest world epidemic of influenza in modern history—the pandemic of 1918–19—may have returned."[17] The *Wall Street Journal,* the *Atlanta Constitution,* and *Newsweek* made similar connections between the Fort Dix strain and Spanish flu.[18] All three nightly television network newscasts (ABC, CBS, and NBC) ran stories high-lighting the relationship between swine flu and the 1918 pandemic.[19] The template for this press coverage was set by the CDC itself, which established that the swine strains might be connected to the 1918 pandemic; that four cases had been detected, one of them fatal; and that the strain might become the predominant strain next year.

Exacerbating the problems of information flow between the press and the scientific community was the two groups' use of an essentially different language. The scientists used carefully calibrated phrases such as "antigenically similar" and allowed only that swine flu strains could become the predominant strain. But the press translated these comments into an alarming warning: the old virus had returned and could cause a pandemic. In a later review of the media's coverage of the Swine Flu Program written for the *Columbia Journalism Review,* David Rubin noted that "the single most important variable in the quality of coverage was the background of the reporters." Rubin found that the *New York Times, Washington Post,* and *Los Angeles Times* generally handled the story well, but by and large, "reporters . . . were not equipped to ask basic scientific questions about the vaccine, its administration, its composition, and the inoculation program as a whole."[20]

To be fair to the journalists, however, their job was complicated by the fact that the science community did not speak with one voice on the relationship between swine flu and Spanish flu. While many reputable researchers sought to downplay the connection between swine flu and the 1918 pandemic, others equally reputable sought to emphasize this relationship because the strains isolated at New Jersey could indeed be the harbinger of another pandemic, perhaps as deadly as the one in 1918. These scientific disputes over the relationship between A/New Jersey and the Spanish flu pandemic were publicly displayed at a later ACIP meeting, in May 1976, where Edwin Kilbourne stated, "The only thing we can say is that only two A-genes of the [Fort Dix] virus resemble the 1918 virus," adding, "It is unfair and probably unwise to keep using this [1918 virus link] as a justification for the vaccination program[;] . . . to trade in these fears is something that will come back to haunt us." Dr. Reuel Stallones, dean of the University of Texas School of Public Health, disagreed, stating, "If it were not for 1918 we would not be sitting here trying to immunize all these people. That's the reason we're doing it. . . . I feel quite strongly about this."[21] Confusion about scientific terminology, disputes within the scientific community, and a tendency to emphasize the worst-case outcome in reporting are not limited to 1976. If anything, the trend has accelerated with the proliferation of news and other media outlets.

The Circle Expands

Less than one week after determining that a novel influenza strain was circulating at Fort Dix, the cat was out of the bag. The press had already widely reported the discovery and intense investigation for more cases and was openly speculating on the possibility of a pandemic, perhaps even the return of the deadly Spanish flu. The day after the press conference, 20 February 1976, a larger meeting of influenza experts—including representatives of vaccine manufacturers—met to review the evidence thus far and begin to consider responses to the appearance of the new virus.

This larger meeting, held at the National Institutes of Health's campus in Bethesda, Maryland, was jointly chaired by the NIH (represented by John Seal), the CDC (represented by David Sencer), and the BoB (represented by Harry Meyer).[22] All the attendees knew about the Fort Dix swine flu strains, and the meeting included a large number of scientists involved in research, production, and manufacturing of the influenza virus and influenza vaccines plus members of the press.[23] The meeting introduced little new evidence, but open discussion of the appropriate response to the new strain took center stage.[24] If addressing this new virus required a massive vaccination effort (and the scientists were careful to emphasize the conditionality), success in the venture would take a tremendous effort on the part of everyone, including scientists, manufacturers, and public health officials. But the scientists generally concluded that it could be done. And the difficulty of mounting a large vaccination effort was no doubt exciting, an aspect clearly illustrated by Harry Meyer, who admitted that much of what he did daily was "not terribly interesting," even calling such activities "real chores," but expressed a certain eagerness in the face of a potential pandemic: "To have a challenge of something that is a real public health interest is really stimulating."[25]

Meyer was not the only scientist stimulated by the Fort Dix cases. Walter Dowdle, chief of virology at the CDC, reported on the evidence from previous human infections with a swine influenza strain. This transmission evidence suggested that Fort Dix might be part of a pattern, with the virus increasingly moving across species, from pigs to humans. But the cases at Fort Dix were qualitatively different: "This [is] as far as we know the first of what would appear to be human to human transmission of swine virus. . . . That's why it alarmed us."[26] Dowdle's concern with the implications of the new virus's person-to-person transmission was seconded by Edwin Kilbourne, who theorized how this new virus might have come about and referenced the experience of the previous pandemic years. The hard-earned lessons of influenza research and pandemics were not in vain, however, as Kilbourne reminded his auditors: "I really think that if ever [there] were a time for concerted action and united action on the flu front, it is right now because we have in the wings excellent vaccine candidates with new vaccine approaches, live virus vaccines . . . and other approaches have been tried."[27]

Maurice Hilleman, now with Merck pharmaceuticals, echoed Kilbourne by drawing on the previous pandemic years as instructive for vaccine manufacturing, but he advised against the use of live-virus vaccines as still having too many problems.[28] In any event, he argued, live-virus vaccines were not needed, because a tremendous effort on the part of industry, the government, and the public would suffice to produce 200 million doses. For that to happen, however, "there would have to be some very heroic decision-making very soon." Manufacturers would have to know shortly, certainly before 1 April 1976, whether they were going to produce a monovalent swine influenza vaccine.[29] Harry Meyer agreed with Hilleman's estimation and timetable but also suggested that a new distribution system would be a key element of any vaccination program, for if the pandemic arrived early in the next flu season (October or November), the efforts would come too late: "It is entirely possible that very little of that [200 million doses of] vaccine in the existing system would actually have gotten to people, in which case you have lost your primary opportunity to have an effect upon mortality and morbidity in the flu."[30]

By the end of the meeting, the assembled experts had generally concluded that protecting the public from a swine flu pandemic required speedy preparations for a vaccination effort. Manufacturers were encouraged to accelerate recombination experiments in the hopes of creating a quickly growing high-yield vaccine strain. The momentum for a massive program began to build.

In the days following this meeting, work on surveillance and manufacturing continued on parallel tracks. Influenza researchers continued the laborious process of collecting, incubating, and testing viral samples at the levels of the camp, the state of New Jersey, the nation, and around the globe, hoping to detect further swine influenza cases. Manufacturers continued to work on developing a recombination strain for creating a vaccine that protected against swine influenza and was suitable for mass production. Scientists from vaccine manufacturing firms had left the meeting with samples of the virus collected from Fort Dix and a much earlier swine influenza strain gathered by Richard Shope in 1931. The latter strain had the advantage of having already been used as a vaccine seed stock by the military from 1955 to 1969. In another remarkable coincidence in the events surrounding the discovery of A/New Jersey at Fort Dix, Shope's strain had been labeled A/Swine/1976/31, where the "1976" referred to an animal from which the sample had been harvested.[31]

Walter Dowdle had recognized the advantages of using a previous vaccine strain as early as 18 February 1976, when he suggested to Fred Davenport—who had worked with the strain when he chaired the army's board on epidemiological diseases in the 1950s and 1960s—that Davenport should discuss his experiences using the vaccine at the forthcoming 20 February meeting.[32] By 27 February all manufacturers were declaring that the production capacity of the Shope-derived material was "good."[33]

Nonetheless, production capacity of the virus was only part of the key to an effective vaccine strain. Any vaccine candidate would need to be a good match with the wild strain circulating. The Shope vaccine offered some protection, but the antigenic differences between the 1931 Shope virus and the 1976 A/New Jersey strain were sufficiently large that antibodies to the former did not offer complete immunity protection to the latter. On 5 March 1976 Dowdle reported that A/Swine/1976/31 offered only partial immunity to the new strain and so should not be used to produce vaccine. In contrast, the A/New Jersey/8/76 virus itself grew very slowly when placed into eggs, thus making it unsatisfactory as a vaccine production seed stock. Fortunately, Edwin Kilbourne's recombination experiments were beginning to bear fruit. On 27 February 1976 Kilbourne was able to report that he had isolated a high-growth-rate, high-yield recombinant of A/New Jersey.[34] This recombinant strain, which Kilbourne dubbed X-53, was selected for vaccine production and was used in the extensive safety and potency testing to develop the dose level and safety of the vaccine.[35] Kilbourne wedded the quickly growing high-yield laboratory strain A/Puerto Rico/8/34 with the A/New Jersey/8/76 type to create a hybrid that produced high levels of protective immunity and high quantities of viral material.

Kilbourne's laboratory was one of only a handful with expertise in the recombination technique. The use of recombinant strains in commercial vaccine production dated back only to 1971, but spurred by the Fort Dix cases, it seemed more laboratories were pushed to try it.[36] The looming prospect of more laboratories dabbling in recombinant experiments concerned Kilbourne, who realized that he and other vaccine researchers did not completely understand exactly what packets of genes were being swapped when they combined two viruses. The opaque nature of the recombination process might result in some unforeseen dangers. As Kilbourne described the method at a later influenza meeting, on 25 March 1976, "I think we have to appreciate that this remains a bit of a black [box] at the moment because we don't know the genes that are transferring. The evidence suggests that it is more than one gene. Whether it is three polymerases or two polymerases or whatever, we are not clear on."[37]

After the 20 February meeting at Bethesda, several influenza researchers and pharmaceutical manufacturers took samples of the A/New Jersey strain so that they could work on recombinants for vaccination. Kilbourne wanted to ensure that the scientists were cautious when using the technique. Shortly after the meeting, he sent a letter to Seal, Krouse, Meyer, and Dowdle expressing his concerns.

> Although in the past I am on record as minimizing the dangers of recombination experiments with influenza viruses, I have never taken the position that these are without hazard and I am concerned about the fact that a number of us are now undertaking such experiments without peer review of our protocols. . . . No one wants constraints on his research less than I do . . . [but] it does appear to me that we could be subject to serious criticism by the rest of the scientific community if we continue to "wing it" as we have been doing under the pressure of the present crisis.[38]

Kilbourne's solution was to suggest creating a coordinating commission to oversee surveillance and manufacturing efforts; however, no such separate commission was created.

Kilbourne was worried that researchers working with recombinants might inadvertently develop a strain more dangerous than the strain against which the scientists were seeking to create a vaccine. For example, the Fort Dix strain, A/New Jersey (H1swN1), grew slowly and was therefore not especially transmissible. The cocirculating strain at Fort Dix, A/Victoria (H3N2), proved to be a highly transmissible and thus quickly spreading virus. Experiments combining the two might inadvertently create a highly transmissible novel strain of influenza, with the worst aspects of a new type (to which few had immunity) merged with highly efficient spread. Also, lethality could not be measured in the laboratory. Perhaps combining some relatively benign samples would create a deadly strain that might then escape the laboratory setting. As I will show, such concerns were not unfounded. Of course, nothing could be done about combination events happening in the wild.

Lacking formal oversight of the murky recombinant research, the scientists had adopted cautious rules of thumb. Even though the "Mayo Clinic" swine influenza strain showed the highest yield and growth rate of the recent swine influenza types, scientists declined to use it as a donor for vaccine research because it had come from the fatal case of the sixteen-year-old boy with Hodgkin's disease. When the decision to not use the Mayo Clinic virus as a vaccine candidate was announced at a large influenza workshop held on 25 March 1976, there was a period of silence from the assembled experts. One attendee, Dr. Jordan, appeared to speak for the group when he said, "To put a strain from a Hodgkin's patient into 200 million Americans, although you think it absolutely safe, would be a risk you wouldn't want to take." Walter Dowdle observed that as an informal policy, the CDC never distributed samples from fatal cases as subjects for research.[39]

By the first weeks of March 1976, the elements for large-scale production of swine influenza vaccine were falling into place. An effective and efficient strain for vaccines (X-53) had been produced and distributed; manufacturers were at work creating seed stocks; and production was beginning to wind down on the A/Victoria and B/Hong Kong strains already recommended for the next year's vaccine. The manufacturers were only waiting for public health experts to decide what to do about A/New Jersey.

In retrospect, it is surprising that the initial epidemiological work and pandemic forecasting was so narrowly focused on a purely national response. The disjuncture of crafting national health policy decisions to combat a global pandemic threat is jarring when considered in the light of the international preparation and evaluation in which influenza scientists had engaged following the failed 1957 and 1968 exercises. The United States certainly fulfilled its reporting duties for the influenza surveillance system, and officials there hoped that global surveillance might detect other epidemic foci, but the initial discussion and plans about responding to the new virus did not consider other nations or international organizations. As events unfolded and a vaccination campaign became a real possibility, the USPHS did invite health officials from other nations and observers from the WHO, but the responses they considered remained focused on the nation.

Several factors explain this resolutely national vaccination decision. The first lies in the inherent weakness of the WHO structure. The WHO advocates for health globally, but it relies almost entirely on the resources of national health programs. Therefore, the first framework for health decisions is always a national one. Second, because the WHO has few independent resources, the influenza system has focused on surveillance rather than action. The organization's headquarters served as a clearinghouse for information rather than a center for action against influenza outbreaks. Third, influenza pandemics were seen as problems that required rapidly deployed and highly technical solutions. Finally, the USPHS believed—probably with good justification—that only the United States possessed the resources and infrastructure to carry out such a large-scale campaign. And whether even the United States could do so remained an open question. Thus the template for responding to an imminent influenza pandemic was a nation-centered program, and this was what U.S. health officials considered from the outset.

The decision to recommend some type of vaccination effort hinged on findings from the various levels of surveillance. In the weeks following the 14 February 1976 meeting outlining the discovery of swine influenza at Fort Dix, the WHO influenza surveillance system scrutinized field reports for evidence of swine influenza outbreaks. Although outbreaks of influenza and influenza-like diseases continued steadily through the end of February and into March, none of the infections were typed as swine influenza.[40] Surveillance at the national level yielded the same results. To some degree this surveillance outcome was expected. The tiny proportion of influenza samples typed versus the large number of identified and unidentified cases made detecting the swine flu virus unlikely; either the virus would have to spread at a high level or the researchers would have to get lucky. Searching for swine influenza cases was made even more difficult by the fact that the A/Victoria strain was causing a sharply elevated epidemic, the highest rate since the pandemic arrival of its ancestor Hong Kong flu in 1968.[41] If swine flu was seeding itself at low levels, it would be difficult to detect against the backdrop of an A/Victoria epidemic.

The public health experts had higher expectations for the surveillance effort throughout New Jersey. Martin Goldfield had greatly increased the number of samples his laboratory would type, and he placed a special emphasis on the population surrounding the base at Fort Dix.[42] Goldfield's laboratory had tested 17 samples in the week ending 13 February 1976. After the Fort Dix material was identified as swine flu virus on the following day, Goldfield's laboratory ramped up its typing work. In the week ending 20 February 1976, the laboratory tested 204 samples, typing 61 as A/Victoria. The following week they tested 301 samples, fingering 71 cases as A/Victoria. Goldfield's laboratory found no additional cases of swine influenza strain outside the camp. Although the lab had greatly expanded the identification of influenza cases, the number of samples tested still represented only a small percentage of the number of people who contracted influenza in New Jersey during that time. Still, Goldfield and the CDC were confident in stating that the epidemic of influenza enveloping the state was caused by A/Victoria, not the swine flu virus.

The public health experts concerned with tracking the swine influenza strain were certain that the U.S. Army's epidemiological investigation of Fort Dix would provide the most complete picture of the new strain. To assess the spread of swine flu there quickly, Colonel Top decided to do a 10 percent random sampling of the camp's population from 17 to 27 February and to test the blood of all recruits who had been hospitalized during the January outbreak.[43] Colonel Top was relying on seroarchaeology to provide the outline of swine influenza at the camp.

As was discussed previously, the human immune system produces antibodies designed to neutralize an invader after infection. Recent or violent infections produce a more rapid and voluminous antibody response to a subsequent infection by the same pathogen. Over a lifetime, the body produces a library of antibodies to all the invaders the immune system has neutralized, and this library can be read with the right tools. But the data from seroarchaeology must be read carefully. Some individuals infected with one type of influenza strain develop a cross-immune response to others. Also, since the antibody response reveals the possible lifetime exposure to an infectious agent, previous exposure to any swine strain of influenza might trigger an antibody response to a different but related swine strain. In the case of swine flu at Fort Dix, Colonel Top had to keep some sets of information in mind. The cross-reaction or background rate of antibody rise in response to the swine influenza strain, even if the individual was not previously exposed, was determined to be approximately 5 percent. Recruits at Fort Dix were inoculated with a trivalent influenza vaccine on induction, so Colonel Top suspected that these recent injections might elevate cross-reaction rates a percentage or two. Also, since swinelike H1N1 strains were the predominant family until 1930, those born before that date would also show elevated antibody responses. Later testing showed a 90 percent antibody reaction to swine influenza strains among this older population.

The CDC had identified four cases of swine flu from the camp population. Dr. Goldfield had subsequently identified a fifth recruit who produced antibodies to the swine influenza strain. Colonel Top's testing of the blood of recruits who were hospitalized during the abbreviated influenza epidemic uncovered an additional eleven cases. The evidence for a sustained swine influenza chain of infection was beginning to emerge.

The second part of the epidemiological survey—Colonel Top's 10 percent sampling of the camp's population—revealed the larger pattern of swine influenza activity at the camp. As I have shown, incoming recruits to Fort Dix arrived at the reception center, where they spent the next three days doing the bureaucratic tasks of filling out forms and being allocated supplies. In this stay at the reception center, they also received a number of inoculations, including the trivalent influenza vaccine. The larger group of approximately 800 men was subdivided into units of 50 and further separated into 8-man sleeping quarters. The whole group was reconstituted for some training exercises and for mess. During their basic training, the troops were restricted to the base for the first month, a practice still current. These facets of camp life for the new recruits made it likely that a respiratory virus would readily spread between the trainees.

Blood tests performed on the two cohorts of recruits inducted into the camp in the weeks beginning 5 January 1976 and 12 January 1976 exhibited a 20 percent elevated antibody reaction rate to swine flu. The 19 January inductees had a 12 percent reaction rate, and subsequent cohorts never exceeded 7 percent (roughly comparable to the anticipated 5 percent background rate). Platoons in which one member had been hospitalized during the influenza epidemic had the highest reaction rates, ranging from 15 to 63 percent.[44] All the units with high reaction rates had begun training in January or early February. For close contacts of confirmed cases, 37 of 110 (or 34 percent) produced antibodies to A/New Jersey, while only 6 percent of those with no direct contact produced swine influenza antibodies. From his random sampling, Colonel Top concluded that A/New Jersey had circulated through the camp in January and early February, ultimately infecting approximately 500 men there. Human-to-human transmission was confirmed, and a chain of infection lasting several weeks was suggested. These were two key elements of an influenza pandemic. On 24 February 1976 Walter Dowdle wrote in his laboratory notebook, "Screen pre marital sera–now know did *spread*."[45]

Colonel Top's epidemiological investigation revealed that positive swine influenza antibody response was disproportionately associated with incoming recruits who had spent their first couple of days in Fort Dix's reception center, making it likely that a new recruit had brought the infection there, prompting the outbreak. Colonel Top polled these recruits to see how many had been in contact with pigs shortly prior to their induction. He turned this list of twenty-two names over to the CDC to check the recruits' household contacts.[46] The CDC tested 172 blood samples drawn from close contacts of these twenty-two recruits; 19 of these samples produced a high reaction of antibodies to swine influenza. Discarding those over the age of fifty, whose antibody response was clouded by the prevalence of H1N1 strains in their youth, the CDC zeroed in on the eleven household contacts of a recruit from "Fayettesville," Pennsylvania.[47] Four of the household members (aged eleven, twelve, twenty, and twenty-five) produced high antibody reactions to A/New Jersey. None but the recruit had direct contact with swine, and several of the household—including three of the four swine-positive members—also tested positive for infection with A/Victoria. Many of the household contacts distinctly recalled two separate flulike illnesses running through the family. Testing of the wider community, including forty-one of the eleven- and twelve-year-olds' classmates, did not uncover additional high antibody rates. Apparently the recruit became infected with swine influenza from contact with pigs and transmitted the infection to his family, but the infection had spread no further in the community.

Officials at the CDC concluded that the Fayetteville recruit was the likely index case for A/New Jersey. Public health officials were especially concerned about the dual infection in the recruit's family. A/Victoria was proving to be a highly transmissive influenza infection, and researchers were beginning to understand the role of animals, especially pigs, in serving as "mixing vessels" for different influenza viruses; furthermore, their own experiments in recombination demonstrated the array of viruses formed when two strains combined.[48] Perhaps the strain of influenza from the pig had picked up enhanced human transmissibility by combining with A/Victoria in a household member who had a dual infection. A/Victoria had been cocirculating at Fort Dix with A/New Jersey and was even now climbing above the epidemic threshold in dozens of states. If the two viruses had combined once, they might do so again.

The CDC had confirmed that A/New Jersey was a novel strain of influenza. Colonel Top's epidemiological investigation of Fort Dix had demonstrated that the virus had passed from human to human for several generations. H. Bruce Dull's press conference on 19 February 1976 had been careful to state that it was not clear whether the Fort Dix cases were "significant or merely a curiosity." Basing their opinions on the surveillance data gathered by Colonel Top, more of the public health officials working on the Fort Dix case were becoming convinced that the swine flu strain was significant rather than curiosity.

The pressing demands of manufacturers and the vaccination experiences of 1957 and 1968 weighed heavily on the minds of public health experts. But the evidence collected was contradictory. A/New Jersey was novel and had spread from person to person, but the epidemic had stopped, and no additional cases were found outside the camp. A novel flu strain that spread through humans made a pandemic possible, but quantifying that possibility was a hopeless task. A later survey of experts involved in assessing swine flu's pandemic potential for the next year produced a range of probabilities, from a 2 to a 49 percent chance of a pandemic occurring in the fall of 1976.[49] Additional outbreaks would make deciding to mount a vaccination campaign easier, but it increasingly appeared that additional outbreaks would not soon be uncovered. The difficult decision to undertake a vaccination campaign would need to be made based on the evidence at hand.

The challenges these health officials faced in predicting the course of events from such scarce data is emblematic of problems such officials must continually confront. The behavior of biological organisms always contains an element of chance, and the influenza virus more so than many others. As had their predecessors in 1976, public health officials in 2009 faced an influenza virus whose course of infection remained maddeningly unpredictable. But crafting public policy does not rely solely on the scientific assessment of the possible outcomes of biological events. The scientists can determine a range of what can happen, but it is up to public health and elected officials to determine what should be done, though what *should* be done is always limited by what *can* be done. In the event, the answers to these questions must be determined quickly, or the passage of time removes the possibility of doing anything at all. In the weeks following the identification of the new strain of influenza at Fort Dix, public health officials began to consider a large-scale vaccination campaign to protect the public against an influenza strain they dubbed swine flu.

CHAPTER 7

An Act of Will

In the world of a bureaucratic organization, any action that seeks to change the usual course of affairs must overcome a high level of inertia, not only because the new option counteracts established and entrenched protocols, but also because the proposed activity must be considered and accepted at a number of levels. Making a decision outside the norm is not a onetime event; rather, it is something that must be reargued and carefully stewarded through the various levels of the organization. Successfully navigating this process requires an influential person to champion the cause and continue to promote it as it moves up the hierarchy. In the case of the Swine Flu Program, that person was CDC director David Sencer. Sencer held his post for ten years, and under his leadership the organization greatly expanded in reach and prestige. After extensively interviewing others in the CDC, Neustadt and Fineberg termed the staff there as being "devoted" to him. Arthur Silverstein, drawing on his experience as a congressional science fellow attached to the Senate Health Subcommittee, described Sencer as a "tough, competent bureaucrat" who ran "a very tight ship at the Center[s] for Disease Control" and who had "large ambitions for himself, large ambitions for his agency, and a deep commitment to its mission—preventive medicine."[1]

Once the influenza scientists became convinced that a pandemic was possible, Sencer knew that some sort of a vaccination decision had to be made. Sencer was greatly impressed by the predictive aspect of Edwin Kilbourne's theory that influenza pandemics follow an eleven-year cycle, and he was reminded of the hypothesis again when, coincidentally, Kilbourne contributed an op-ed piece to the *New York Times* detailing his theory and recommending preparations for a possible pandemic. Remarkably, the piece appeared on 13 February 1976, the day before the CDC told a few experts about the novel strain at Fort Dix.[2] Based upon his direct experience in 1968 and what he knew about 1957, Sencer realized that any vaccination campaign would have to operate differently from previous attempts if there was to be any hope of protecting a large percentage of the public. Sencer found that Meyer at the BoB and Seal at NIAID agreed with him, but he knew that he would have to convince many others. No authorization of such a program could be made at the higher levels until the lower levels had signed on, and the first level in the decision-making chain for vaccination consisted of the Advisory Committee on Immunization Practices. Sencer called for an emergency meeting to be held on 10 March 1976.

Sencer had been instrumental in the creation of the ACIP, which he initiated shortly after becoming director of the CDC in 1966.[3] Prior to the creation of the ACIP, developing a vaccine and offering it to children always required the creation of a new, ad-hoc "public health advisory committee." These individual committees would work closely with the American Academy of Pediatrics to issue recommendations and guidelines to individual physicians. Sencer and others in the CDC thought it better to approach immunization "as a policy" rather than create "a separate entity for each disease." The ACIP was designed to bring together public health experts from various backgrounds—the American Academy of Pediatrics, state health departments, academia, the BoB, and others—to issue recommendations for the use of various vaccines. The committee issued guidelines to help administer money allocated to state and local health departments under the Vaccine Assistance Act of 1962, which was earmarked for children five and under. One of the ACIP's tasks was to recommend the recipe for the next year's flu vaccine, and in 1976 the group had met on 5–6 February to determine which strains to target in the next flu season. Sencer called the 10 March 1976 meeting to assess whether the public required protection from A/New Jersey as well in the forthcoming year.

Although the ACIP had been created under the auspices of the CDC, which generally provided the epidemiological and virological data that the committee used in making its recommendations, the ACIP was no rubber stamp of the director's goals. Instead, it was staffed by prominent members of the public health community who took their roles seriously. The ACIP also tended to be deliberative, with the evidence and facts involved in a decision known beforehand. But as Sencer realized, the time pressures on this decision were extreme, and he himself had become convinced that a large-scale vaccination effort was necessary. A staff meeting at the CDC on 27 February highlighted concerns about the slow pace of the ACIP and a belief in the need for a large-scale immunization program.[4]

Gaining the recommendation of the ACIP was absolutely critical for mounting any large-scale vaccination campaign. Because the committee was seen as a deliberative body of experts drawn from outside government service, their concurrence on the potential danger of the new viral strain was likely to be a powerful tool in gaining supplemental funding. Even if the circumstances were unusual, Congress would insist on following proper procedures. No vaccination program would be forthcoming without the imprimatur of the ACIP. Sencer was determined to get the committee on board.

The 27 February CDC staff meeting, held a few days after Colonel Top had collected the evidence for human-to-human transmission at Fort Dix, included representatives from the BoB, CDC, NIH, and the U.S. Army. In a discussion led by David Sencer and Harry Meyer, the group summed up its points. First, the individuals assembled recognized that they could not make a decision "independent of ACIP." Second, merely issuing the recommendation that swine flu be added to the current recommendation of 20 million doses of trivalent vaccine for high-risk patients was a "cop-out non-decision." Finally, even though the ACIP was meeting two days before the Armed Forces Epidemiological Board (AFEB) meeting scheduled 12 March 1976,[5] it was likely that the military's board would make its decision first. The fact that the assembled group considered the addition of A/New Jersey to the 20 million doses for high-risk patients to be a "cop-out" suggests that Sencer and the group were strongly considering a more expansive vaccination campaign. Any delay by the ACIP in issuing its guidance would threaten the possibility of making such an effort. If the group waited too long, the limitations of the vaccine production process would make any program moot. The ACIP must make its determination quickly.

The United States Public Health Service was not the only group whose attention became drawn to influenza. Gar Kaganowich, a congressional staffer for the Senate Committee on Appropriations, sent a note inquiring what the Department of Health, Education, and Welfare was doing about the potential epidemic. The letter wound its way through the department, eventually landing on Sencer's desk on 3 March. His reply on 5 March suggests the type of response Sencer favored. After briefly sketching the discovery of the virus and the initial responses undertaken by the USPHS, Sencer reported that the

ACIP would be meeting on 10 March with "the U.S. Armed Forces, Bureau of Biologics, National Institutes of Health, State of New Jersey and the World Health Organization" to consider the need for a possible immunization campaign "to control swine virus-like influenza." He stated that thus far, the CDC efforts had cost $33,000: "The need for additional funds will become known next week after our review of the epidemiologic findings and an assessment of the vaccination program required."[6]

In this letter to Kaganowich, Sencer signaled his intentions to the Senate Appropriations Committee: the events at Fort Dix were serious enough to command the attention of civilian and military health experts in the United States and the WHO, a program to "control" this new influenza strain might be necessary, and the vaccination program was likely to be large enough to require special appropriations. Since ACIP recommendations were already covered under the budget in the Vaccine Assistance Act, Sencer was alerting Congress that swine flu might be an extraordinary circumstance that would require an extraordinary response.

On the eve of the 10 March 1976 ACIP meeting, Sencer met with several of his top advisers to discuss their views about the epidemiological and vaccination issues to be discussed the next day.[7] He and the advisers concluded that the epidemiological evidence supported the possibility of a pandemic and that some sort of vaccination effort would be required to protect the public. One group of the CDC staffers argued that the logic of the new virus required a universal campaign to deliver vaccination to all citizens. Some of the more cautious members suggested that large quantities of vaccine be manufactured but that inoculation not begin unless a pandemic had clearly emerged. The strong proponents of nationwide vaccination pointed out that distributing the vaccine from central locations would require several weeks, and even after inoculation, the immune system requires two more weeks before it produces protective levels of antibodies. The highly infectious virus combined with the high rate of spread enabled by modern air travel meant that an emerging pandemic would likely outstrip any hurried distribution scheme, which would rapidly become extremely chaotic as individuals and organizations clamored for the vaccine. Sencer apparently kept his own counsel, for several of the participants later reported they were not sure which way he was leaning after the meeting.

The ACIP Meets

The 10 March ACIP meeting was called to order by the committee's chair, David Sencer, at 9:00 a.m. Underscoring the importance of this meeting, the room was packed with a host of interested observers. In addition to five

ACIP members, the member ex officio Harry Meyer, and the liaison with the American Academy of Pediatrics, the invited included three observers from the WHO; Colonel Russell, from Walter Reed; Edwin Kilbourne, from the Mount Sinai School of Medicine; Goldfield and Altman, from New Jersey; sixteen CDC staff members; and a journalist.[8] The proceedings followed an unusual format. Normally, the ACIP meets for two days, during the first of which the CDC presents epidemiological information and then proposes its recommended course of action. The committee members discuss and debate the evidence and then overnight draft their proposal. The second day includes reworking the draft until the committee members concur on their recommendation. David Sencer reports that at this meeting, the CDC did not suggest a course of action, wanting the group to reach its own conclusion.[9] After the morning session, when the epidemiological evidence gathered at Fort Dix was presented, Sencer presided over a free-ranging debate on the proper course of action. This debate involved everyone at the meeting, not just the official committee members.

John Seal was vindicated in his prediction that crafting a vaccination decision based on only the Fort Dix outbreak would be difficult. Attendees at the meeting lamented the costs of the program and the upheavals the vaccination effort would cause in other public health programs and in people's lives.[10] Others retorted that the expense of the campaign was "peanuts" compared to the estimated $4 billion an outbreak would cost.[11] Some questioned whether manufacturers would be able to produce sufficient quantities of vaccine, to which Harry Meyer reported that if given the order, manufacturers could have 100 million doses by September, with more to follow if needed. Other members suggested waiting for a second outbreak, perhaps delaying the decision to as late as June. Russell Alexander adopted a cautious attitude, agreeing that manufacturing a vaccine might be needed but insisting that some thought should be put into deciding when to inject the vaccine. Reuel Stallones forcefully argued for a large-scale campaign, stating, "Flu vaccine has not yet done anything—we bombed out in 1957—we need a *large* effort."[12]

The minutes for the meeting show a congruence of opinion on several points concerning the Fort Dix outbreak.[13] The group agreed that person-to-person spread was well documented at Fort Dix and that outbreaks of A/New Jersey swine influenza were possible the following winter. Accordingly, production of vaccine should continue, and a plan for administration be developed. The committee might consider recommending two vaccines: a bivalent vaccine containing A/Victoria and A/New Jersey for high-risk individuals and a monovalent A/New Jersey for the rest of the population.[14] If such a program was developed, federal authorities should both purchase the vaccine and deliver it to the public.

As was predicted at the 27 February CDC staff meeting, by the end of the day the ACIP had been unable to agree on a recommended course of action. It had not even made the "cop-out" decision of proposing A/New Jersey's inclusion in the next year's recipe of influenza vaccine for the high-risk population. The delay in deciding on a course of action discouraged some of the influenza experts there. Walter Dowdle noted, "Final decision has not been made—*in spite of paper.*"[15] But other officials concluded that the ACIP was ultimately going to recommend a large-scale effort. Donald Berreth noted, "It is apparent to me that it is only a matter of time before a decision to go all out on vaccine production will be made."[16] Sencer himself was confident that the ACIP was going to suggest a massive vaccination effort, and he had the means and the desire to push the committee to that decision quickly.

The ACIP had deferred suggesting a government response based on the Fort Dix evidence, and its members longed for a second outbreak, which would make their decision easier. But they recognized that if they delayed too long, time would take the decision out of their hands. By the end of the meeting, they agreed to think about the evidence and await polling by telephone for their assessments. Sencer, who would be in charge of the individual phone calls, was strongly convinced of the need for a large-scale effort to protect the public from a pandemic. He recalled that prior to the 10 March meeting, he viewed A/New Jersey as a real threat: "It had been ten, twelve years and it had been quite cyclical. And so, it looked as though we had the possibility of an introduction of a new strain[;] . . . we felt that we should not capitalize on 1918, but on the fact that influenza was a recurring pandemic disease, and that we had indication that there might be a pandemic and we had measures that we could do to stop it in this country."[17] Clearly both the eleven-year and recycling theories weighed heavily on his mind. Sencer came out of the ACIP meeting with two objectives: to get the ACIP to recommend a total vaccination effort and to convince his superiors to institute such a program.

Sencer began selling the idea to his superiors the next day. In a remarkable document dated 11 March 1976 and titled "FY 1977 Influenza Immunization Initiative," he laid out the logic for a massive vaccination campaign.[18] The objective of the document was "to assure the development of an effective national influenza immunization program aimed at providing protection to the total U.S. population of 213 million during the influenza pandemic forecasted for the Winter of 1977 [corrected to 1976 by an unknown party]." The objective was followed by seven points designed to achieve this goal, including steps concerning manufacturing, distribution, and surveillance, and to study the program's effectiveness. The second page of the two-page document listed ten assumptions that bolstered the need for such a large vaccination effort. Several of the assumptions echoed statements endorsed by the ACIP, but some went beyond what the ACIP had been willing to conclude just the day before. Sencer and the other drafters of the document assumed that "additional outbreaks [could] be predicted," judged "present evidence and past experience indicating the possibility of widespread influenza in 1977" to be "substantive," and urged that "programs of immunization should begin immediately."

The language used in this document is clear, declarative, and decisive. It is not the hedging language of the science community, with phrases such as "it may be possible," "it is likely," and "it is unknown"; to the contrary, the language is concrete: an influenza pandemic is "forecast," additional outbreaks are "predicted," the evidence is "substantive," and immunization programs should begin "immediately." This document was drafted for decision makers, not scientists.

Adding impetus to the view that Fort Dix represented a potentially dangerous warning of an impending pandemic was the armed forces' decision to inoculate all troops against the new viral strain. Meeting two days after the ACIP and evaluating the same evidence, the military medical experts quickly agreed to purchase swine flu vaccine for all active-duty personnel. In addition, they called for the use of recombinants to produce the vaccine, clearly anticipating that their shots would be part of a larger vaccine order.[19]

Action Memos and Phone Calls

The day after the armed forces' decision, 13 March 1976, David Sencer began drafting a memorandum outlining the vaccination options for the Department of Health, Education, and Welfare.[20] The memo begins with an outline of the facts surrounding the discovery of A/New Jersey; couching the matter in scientifically cautious phrases, Sencer wrote that the new virus was "antigenically related" to the Spanish flu virus and that though feasible, producing protective vaccine would take an "extraordinary effort" on the part of manufacturers. He then listed the core assumptions involved in crafting the recommendation. Here Sencer abandoned the cautious language of scientists for the action language of decision makers: "Present evidence and past experience indicate a *strong* possibility . . . of widespread influenza activity." He characterized the situation as requiring a "go or no go" decision, one that had to be made immediately, adding, "It is assumed to be socially and politically unacceptable to *plan* for less than 100 percent coverage of the nation's 213 million citizens."[21]

The memo then detailed four possible courses of action—together with their pros and cons—to address the situation entailed by this alarming set of facts and assumptions. The first option called for no action by the federal government. On the positive side, the government would not waste money if the pandemic did not arrive. On the negative side, the government would be castigated for not responding if it did, and as Sencer pointed out, the "administration can tolerate unnecessary health expenditures better than unnecessary deaths and illness." He did not and needed not mention that 1976 was a presidential election year, and if the pandemic came, it would likely occur at the height of the campaign season. The second course, labeled "minimum response," called for a vocal federal response urging vaccine manufacturers to make vaccine and for citizens to purchase it, but little other federal involvement. On the upside, the federal government would have high visibility in reacting to the new flu strain but face little financial costs. On the downside, the government would have no guarantee that vaccine manufacturers would increase their supply of vaccine or any control over its distribution. This second option thus recapitulated the course of action that had failed in 1957 and 1968. The third option, "government program," called for complete federal control of the process from start to finish. The federal government would guarantee purchase of up to 200 million doses of vaccine from manufacturers, and the vaccine would be distributed by the public health network. This option would guarantee sufficient vaccine production for all and fair delivery of the shots, but at a substantial cost; it would also shut out the private system of distribution through physicians and their offices. The fourth and final option, "the combined approach," sought to take advantage of the strengths of both the public and private medical systems. To ensure adequate production and equitable distribution of vaccine, the government would guarantee purchase and delivery of the material. Public health departments would hold mass vaccination campaigns, but the injections would also be distributed to private physicians, who could administer inoculations in their offices. This system would avoid unnecessary duplication of services while maintaining supply and distribution control. The "combined approach" was cheaper than a full-blown government program and likely to be the most efficient. This fourth option was the course of action recommended to HEW secretary Mathews.

This "action memo" was designed to enact the ACIP's decision that a potential pandemic of swine flu in 1976 required a massive immunization campaign to protect every citizen of the United States. There was only one problem: the ACIP had not yet made its decision. Months after the Swine Flu Program was initiated, David Sencer suggested to Neustadt and Fineberg that he had written this memo in response to the ACIP's recommendation of a universal national vaccination program, suggesting it to have been the consensus of the committee: "I asked the Committee to sleep on it and let us phone them the next day to make sure they still felt the same way, which we did—and they did."[22] In addition, at a meeting of the National Commission for the Protection of Human Subjects of Biomedical and Behavioral Research held on 17 August 1976, Sencer reported that the members of the ACIP had been "polled again by telephone on the 12th" and he "prepared a proposal at that time."[23]

Sencer's later recollections on the order of the phone calls and the drafting of the "action memo" are incorrect. Several draft timelines created in the earliest days of the program list the phone calls to the ACIP members as occurring on 17 or 18 March 1976. Sencer himself provided the 19 March date in a calendar of events distributed at meeting of the Association of State and Territory Health Organizations held on 2 April.[24] Whichever date is correct, the memo was clearly created before the ACIP had voted on its recommendation. Indeed, if the 18 March or 19 March date is correct, the memo was delivered to the secretary of HEW before the ACIP had decided. Sencer had not drafted the recommendation for a massive vaccination campaign in response to the decision of the ACIP; rather, he had already drafted and perhaps even submitted it before he contacted the committee for its decision.

The timing of the events surrounding the "action memo" and Sencer's phone calls to committee members may well arouse curiosity as to what was said in the phone calls. Unfortunately, no transcript or notes from them exist. But the structure of the polling itself was geared to ensure a positive vote for a massive vaccination campaign. Here was the powerful CDC director, who was a strong proponent of a large-scale campaign, phoning each member individually to record his or her recommendation. The ACIP members would have no opportunity to gauge whether others had doubts; instead, they would be forced to rely on Sencer for an account of the other members' opinions and preferences. And in fact, some suggest that Sencer was willing to be duplicitous in gaining ACIP support. According to Neustadt and Fineberg, one member of the committee recalls being informed that "an all-out program was required for Congressional approval, [and] another that the White House was insisting on immunization."[25] There is also some suggestion that Sencer did not reach all the members. Sencer himself cannot positively recall reaching all the members by phone, stating, "I think I did[;] I don't know. But I think I did. I know I reached a good majority of them, if not all of them."[26] However the decision came about, the ACIP recommended a national vaccination campaign to inoculate every citizen.

Escalation

With the ACIP on board, or at least with Sencer having anticipated its being on board, the next step in the decision chain was the secretary of HEW, David Mathews. Sencer, who asked for a meeting with the secretary on 15 March 1976, had been in contact with Theodore Cooper, Secretary Mathews's deputy (and a physician), preparing him for the topics Sencer intended to discuss. Cooper was out of the country, but his deputy, James Dickson (also a physician), was authorized to stand in for Cooper in the meeting. Although Cooper and Dickson had scientific backgrounds, Sencer would be pursuing his case with the political appointee Mathews and through him the Ford administration. He intended to express the urgency as clearly and decisively as he could.

Sencer had begun this process of underscoring the potential danger of A/New Jersey in the action memo he had drafted, which was in the hands of Mathews's inner circle prior to the 15 March meeting. He had bolstered the hedging scientific evaluation of the Fort Dix swine flu strain as a "possible" pandemic strain by calling the possibility "strong." The intensifying qualification suggested that a pandemic was more likely than not, a clear escalation of the threat A/New Jersey posed.[27] The problem was that no one could predict the new strain's effects. It could be no more than a scientific curiosity, or it could be worse than Spanish flu. Sencer's language suggested that the matter lay toward the latter end of that scale; it certainly depicted the pandemic as more likely to occur than not.

Sencer intended to push his recommendation in the meeting with Mathews because of rumors that the secretary was "unwilling to make a decision." Any delay would make a vaccination decision moot, and Sencer was convinced that a big effort was required. When Mathews asked about vaccine manufacturing time pressure, Sencer replied, "There are many things that force a decision, but this is the first time that a rooster has ever made you make a decision."[28]

In retrospect, Sencer need not have pressed his case so hard at this meeting, for Mathews and his advisers were already convinced.[29] In a departmental meeting held prior to meeting with Sencer, Mathews solicited thoughts on the business of the day from his staff. When Dickson summarized the action memo from Sencer, the discussion dissolved into stories about 1918. In *Epidemic and Peace, 1918* Alfred Crosby points out that the American people had forgotten Spanish flu to a remarkable extent, and this is certainly true for institutional and public memory.[30] But in anecdotal and folk memory, the Spanish flu pandemic retained powerful force. If the influenza experts had been reluctant to make connections between A/New Jersey and Spanish flu, the same could not be said about the HEW hierarchy and the Ford administration. As one participant at the staff meeting reported to Neustadt and Fineberg, "We understood that it might not happen . . . but lots of us had tales to tell about what it might be like if it did."

Going into the meeting with Sencer, Mathews had the worst-case scenario of swine flu uppermost in his mind. Mathews was a political appointee, so he recognized the political as well as the public health implications of A/New Jersey. When he pressed Sencer on the probability of a pandemic of swine flu, Sencer replied "unknown." For Mathews, then, a vaccination decision was inevitable. As he stated it to Neustadt and Fineberg:

> The moment I heard Sencer and Dickson, I *knew* the "political system" would *have* to offer some response. No way out, unless they were far out from the center of scientific consensus . . . [and] they weren't. . . . As for the *possibility* of another 1918 . . . one had to assume the *probability* greater than zero. If they say "unknown" that's the least they can mean. Well, that's enough for action if you know in time. You can't face the electorate later, if it eventuates, and say well, the probability was so low we decided not try, just two or five percent, you know, so why spend the money. The "political system" should, perhaps, but *won't* react that way . . . so again it's inevitable.

Mathews was on board, and he would be taking the recommendation to the next level: the White House.

In fact, Mathews was so convinced that he sent a memorandum to James T. Lynn, director of the Office of Management and Budget (OMB), saying that the HEW department would be preparing a recommendation for a vaccine campaign that would require special appropriations.[31] In the memorandum, Mathews further escalated the likelihood of a swine flu pandemic, stating that "a major flu epidemic" would arrive with the coming fall; that the nation would "see a return of the 1918 flu virus," which is "the most virulent form of flu"; and that this virus would "kill one million Americans in 1976." Unbeknownst to Sencer, this alarmist memorandum was circulating in the Ford White House, and it or some other unknown document spawned grave misperceptions about the strain that were being discussed by President Ford's top advisers.

Remarkably, in only five days the questions about swine flu were replaced with certainties. On 10 March 1976 the ACIP had been so unsure of a potential pandemic of influenza that it had not even agreed on the "cop-out" decision of merely recommending vaccination to high-risk patients. By 15 March

Secretary Mathews was boldly predicting a pandemic that would kill a million Americans. To be fair to Mathews, however, he did only what Sencer had done. Sencer reset the likelihood that A/New Jersey would prompt a pandemic from a bare possibility to a strong possibility; Mathews further reset it to a certainty. Sencer had carefully stated that A/New Jersey was "antigenically related" to the 1918 virus. Mathews declared it was the same virus. In a few days the decision to craft a massive vaccination campaign had picked up tremendous momentum. Stopping it now would be far more difficult than allowing it to continue. Only one more decision needed to be made to launch the program. And that decision would be the president's.

No one person can be an expert in everything, not even the president. So presidents must rely on close and trusted advisers to help them make decisions. Even though a president can call on any number of experts to discuss his or her options, it ultimately comes down to the president and those advisers. Sencer escalated the potential dangers of a swine flu pandemic to convince his boss, HEW secretary Matthews; Matthews had escalated the threat to convince the president. Both these men understood the basics of the virus and had deputies who were well versed in pandemic behavior. But President Ford's close advisers did not have such mastery of medical issues, and a distorted view of swine flu's threat emerged in this circle.

A 22 March 1976 memorandum from her deputy, Randall L. Woods, informed a midlevel executive branch staffer named Margarita White that scientists were predicting the "'probability' of a large outbreak." Highlighting his source as Deputy Assistant Secretary for Public Affairs (HEW) Ed McVeigh, Woods stated that swine flu was "highly contagious" and had "an incredibly high mortality rate" for the uninoculated.[32]

On their own, misperceptions of swine flu's dangers among midlevel staffers are not too concerning. But such evaluations of the threat were also held by the president's senior advisers. In a "sensitive/eyes only" memorandum for the president's inner circle of Bill Baroody, Jim Cannon, Dick Cheney, and Jim Connor, Jack Marsh reported that swine influenza was a "particularly virulent strain of virus which[,] if contacted [sic] by humans, is likely to result in a fatality"; Marsh reported that projections of fatalities placed them as high as "one million."[33] Such alarming projections were at odds with the consensus of the influenza scientists.

Presidential decisions also have individual impacts, for they sometimes involve questions of life or death. The personal nature of swine flu's dangers were brought home to President Ford in a sweet handwritten letter from the parents of David Lewis. They thanked the president for his swine flu vaccination decision, saying that in making it he had "showed real concern" and spared other parents from grief: "[It] can't bring us back our son, [but] we have assurance that it will help protect other sons and daughters."[34]

President Ford was at the time locked in a hotly contested primary battle with Ronald Reagan for the Republican nomination. If an influenza pandemic appeared, it would likely come at the height of the campaign for the fall election. The juxtaposition of the vaccination and presidential campaigns has prompted some critics to charge the entire plan was a scheme to bolster Ford's election efforts.[35] But on examination, it appears that any political aspects of the decision were of secondary concern.[36]

Ford was alerted to the possibility of a massive vaccination campaign request by his staff on the afternoon of 15 March 1976. Ford's staff—OMB director James Lynn, his deputy Paul O'Neill, and staff member James Cavanaugh—met with Ford to briefly describe the Fort Dix outbreak and the HEW memorandum. Cooper had discussed the contents of Sencer's memo with Cavanaugh. Ford agreed to schedule a meeting for the following week, 22 March 1976. At the meeting, Ford quizzed his advisers on the likelihood of a pandemic, the cost, and whether there would be enough fertilized chicken eggs to support manufacturers' production needs (he was assured on that point by the secretary of agriculture, who said, "The roosters of America are ready to do their duty"). Ford was convinced of the potential threat of the new strain, but he was troubled by the scientific uncertainty behind the decision. To his credit, Ford reached outside his circle of advisers and announced that he wanted to hear the consensus of the scientific community directly. To do so, he requested a separate meeting with the nation's leading influenza research scientists, plus a handful of prominent scientists not affiliated with the research. This separate meeting would allow the president unfiltered access to their thoughts on the program and a useful scientific consensus to score as a publicity opportunity for the decision. The meeting was set for the afternoon of 24 March 1976.

After the president requested this meeting with scientists, HEW officials, Meyer, Seal, and Sencer scrambled to come up with a list of invitees. They quickly compiled a list of fifty people that was trimmed to thirty for the prosaic reason that only thirty chairs fit into the cabinet room.[37] Some critics charged that the room was stacked with supporters of the vaccination plan, but the people in attendance seem to have been chosen because they were the most prominent researchers. The attendees included the senior influenza researchers Kilbourne, Hilleman, and Davenport and, in a crowning touch, both polio heroes Albert Sabin and Jonas Salk. The event was the only time the two bitter rivals graced the same stage in support of a medical discussion.

The President Decides

At 3:30 p.m., 24 March 1976, President Ford addressed the hastily assembled group.[38] Sencer led off the meeting by summarizing the Fort Dix outbreak and explaining the recommended course of action. Ford turned to Salk, who strongly endorsed the recommendation. He then turned to Sabin, who also strongly endorsed the vaccination plan. Ford went around the table soliciting the views of the assembled scientists, even asking for a show of hands in support at one point. All agreed with the recommendation. Ford specifically asked for dissenting opinions, but none was offered. He even retired to a side room with the invitation to speak with him in private; no one took him up on his offer. Finally, Ford returned to the cabinet room and asked Salk and Sabin to join him as he addressed the nation.

From the description of the special meeting with the president, it certainly appears that Ford was serious about soliciting the views of the assembled scientists and providing the opportunity to register complaints about the decision. It should be pointed out, however, that as Ford was meeting with the scientists, his press officer was releasing a background fact sheet to the assembled media about the decision the president was about to make. Also, at least one meeting attendee thought the consultation was all for show, stating that while he and the others waited for the meeting to start, "President Ford left the Oval Office and passed the open door by the Cabinet room. He was wearing a white shirt. When he reappeared minutes later, his shirt was T. V. blue."[39]

Ford had made his decision, pro forma or not. Flanked by Salk and Sabin, Ford addressed the nation:

> One month ago, a strain of influenza sometimes known as swine flu was discovered and isolated among Army recruits at Fort Dix, New Jersey. The appearance of this strain has caused concern within the medical community, because this virus is very similar to one that caused a widespread and very deadly flu epidemic late in the First World War. Some older Americans today will remember that 548,000 people died in this country during that tragic period. . . . I have been advised that there is a very real possibility that unless we take effective counteractions, there could be an epidemic of this dangerous disease next fall and winter here in the United States. Let me state clearly at this time, no one knows exactly how serious this threat could be. . . . The facts that have been presented to me in the last few days have come from many of the best medical minds in this country. These facts do not suggest there is any cause for alarm. . . . The facts do suggest, however, that there is a need for action now—action by the Government, action by industry and the medical community and, most importantly, action by all of our citizens.[40]

After the announcement, Salk and Sabin joined Sencer, Cooper, and Mathews at the press conference to field questions from the media.

The language Ford used in his speech was mild, calculated to suggest potential danger without prompting panic. Ford accurately reflected the uncertainty of a pandemic through the use of phrases such as "a very real possibility," "could be an epidemic," and "no one knows how serious this threat could be." But Ford's portrayal of the likelihood of a pandemic was undercut by the dire and dramatic fact sheet distributed to the press.[41] The fact sheet stated, "This flu strain, which had been dormant for almost half a century, was the cause of an epidemic in 1918–19 that killed an estimated 548,000 Americans. . . . Present evidence and past experience indicate a strong possibility that this country could experience widespread swine influenza in 1976–77. . . . These are the ingredients for a severe epidemic or pandemic. Pandemics of influenza occur at approximately 10-year intervals." It also announced, "The President believes that it is important to take effective counter-measures to avoid an outbreak similar to the one in 1918."

The White House fact sheet served as the end point of the process to escalate the threat of A/New Jersey. In this depiction, the virus from Fort Dix was the same as the dreaded 1918 killer, merely laying "dormant" for half a century. There was a "strong possibility" of a pandemic of this deadly flu, and President Ford's actions had been taken to forestall an "outbreak similar to 1918." These portrayals of the dangers of A/New Jersey shaped the media's description of the vaccination decision far more than the president's speech did. When the American public turned on the television or picked up the newspaper, they saw the return of Spanish flu to be the justification for the vaccine program. Whether or not they intended this view—and it is abundantly clear that the experts rejected this simplistic relation between A/New Jersey and Spanish flu—it was what the scientific advisory panel endorsed and what the heroes of polio validated.

In two short weeks, A/New Jersey had gone from a possible pandemic strain to a near certain return of Spanish flu, and the process had occurred without the introduction of any new evidence. The process of escalating the potential threat of the new strain accelerated in the hierarchy of the HEW department and the Ford administration, but it had begun with David Sencer.

The next day the CDC, the BoB, and NIAID cosponsored a massive meeting—over sixty influenza researchers, scientists, and manufacturers were listed, plus representatives of the media—to explain the president's decision and discuss vaccine formulation recipes and research issues associated with the program.[42] A heated discussion ensued over whether influenza B vaccine should be included in the doses offered to the high-risk population. Not a single scientist questioned the validity of the swine flu decision. During the discussion, both the 1918 Spanish flu pandemic and the failed examples of 1957 and 1968 were raised to justify how the program had taken shape.[43] The tone of the meeting can be summarized as resolute excitement. The task before these public health experts was going to be difficult, but, the assembled scientists agreed, the job was one that not only *should* be done but *could* be done. The National Influenza Immunization Program was under way.

Several elements came together to hasten the move from discovery of the novel virus on 13 February 1976 to the president's announcement on 24 March. First, the failed vaccination campaigns of 1957 and 1968 demonstrated that early detection and rapid decision making were crucial for any successful protective inoculation effort. In the years following the Hong Kong flu of 1968, the public health, research, and manufacturing communities had worked closely to prepare for the next influenza pandemic. The two predictive theories also helped accelerate the decision process. A/New Jersey fit both the recycling theory and the eleven-year-cycle theories for the next pandemic strain. The fact that the virus was novel was the most important element leading scientists to conclude that a vaccine program was necessary; the virus's relationship to Spanish flu was the crucial element for the political administration. The subtle and not-so-subtle amplification of the likelihood of a pandemic also helped speed the decision along. Finally, the nature of the challenge at hand was exciting for the public health community. Harry Meyer, the BoB's chair, discussed how A/New Jersey posed a set of challenges different from the "chores" he usually faced; ACIP member Reuel Stallones emphasized how a vaccination campaign provided him a way to "give back" to society. This "can-do" ethos permeated the program. J. Donald Millar, director of the Bureau of State Services at the CDC and hand-picked by David Sencer to coordinate the campaign, encapsulated this mind-set in a memorandum he sent to the members of his team six days before Ford's decision. Millar wrote, "The Federal Government has adopted the position that all 213 million Americans should be immunized against swine influenza by December 31, 1976 (that's 282 days from now)." Figuring out how to do this monumental task would be the team's job. Millar closed by stating, "The decision to conduct a national influenza immunization program presents the biggest challenge in preventative medicine since polio vaccination in the late '50s. This should be an exciting time, and we ought to be able to have some fun with it. I look forward to working with you."[44]

The escalation of swine flu's danger played an important role in the U.S. vaccination decision. In explaining and seeking to convince nonscientists of the program's necessity, the spokespeople at various levels of the scientific community (especially Sencer and Mathews) simplified the uncertainty and emphasized the likelihood of the threat. This well-meaning attempt to highlight the potential dangers of the virus created a distorted vision of the new virus. In the echo chamber of the nonscientist circle of presidential advisers, the less dangerous potential outcomes of Fort Dix disappeared, and only the most dire vision of a Swine flu pandemic remained. This failure of translation from the science to the lay community remains a stumbling block in all wise decision making on matters of science and medicine in the public policy arena.[45]

The overwhelmingly technical approach to the problem nicely illustrates the dominant mind-set in the USPHS hierarchy. The vaccination program would be a big job, but a big job the USPHS, and especially the CDC, believed it was prepared to handle. Thinking big in matters of health was the CDC's religion. Such daunting tasks were seen as exciting opportunities to do some real public health. The leadership of the CDC believed it was ready, willing, and able to get protective vaccines into the arms of the American public before a swine flu pandemic could hit.

The desire to meet the challenge of A/New Jersey was not replicated elsewhere around the world. Over the next couple of weeks, the portrayal of the pandemic potential offered by the new strain was minimized. The World Health Organization developed a much more benign interpretation of the potential threat of A/New Jersey, and this milder assessment of the novel virus undergirded the vaccination decisions of other nations. But just as nonscientific factors shaped the perception of swine flu's pandemic potential in the United States, practical concerns about vaccine production shaped the assessment of a pandemic in the forum of the WHO. Concerns over potentially dangerous live-virus research and production limitations played a large though unacknowledged role in crafting the WHO's wait-and-see response. The WHO's concern over what could be done shaped its interpretation of what should be done.

CHAPTER 8

A Different Interpretation
Emerges

The World Health Organization is forced to straddle a sometimes uncomfortable divide between the global and the local. The organization is resolutely broad in outlook, an attitude exemplified by the first principle of its constitution, which states, "Health is a state of complete physical, mental, and social well-being and not merely the absence of disease or infirmity."[1] To achieve the lofty goal of ensuring such health globally, however, the WHO must rely almost entirely on national health organizations in implementing its various tasks, and these national health organizations differ enormously in terms of resources and capabilities. Quite simply, many nation-states are in such desperate economic straits that they lack either the resources to contribute to global health issues or the equipment and training to implement the technologically driven programs the WHO has tended to favor. Those nations able to help fund the organization and to provide equipment and personnel to global health programs have an outsized role in driving the WHO's agenda. In 1976, by far the loudest voice in the WHO was the United States, which was the largest contributor both of funds ($40 million in fiscal year 1977, a full 25 percent of the WHO's budget) and of scientific experts to run WHO projects, most notably the effort to eradicate smallpox.[2] This benefactor had just initiated an expedited immunization program to safeguard its citizens from a possible swine flu pandemic; what would the WHO recommend to its other member states?

The United States played a similarly outsized role in shaping the WHO's technical focus. Scientists from that country predominated on a number of expert advisory boards. Moreover, U.S. money often underlay U.S.-style technical programs for disease control or health improvement. The scientific experts from the United States were part of a technical elite largely drawn from a small number of "developed" nations. Although increasing numbers of WHO member states were arguing for new approaches to health, these new demands had little impact on the more technical programs in the 1970s. The WHO surveillance system is a prime example of the technical elite approach to health.

By 1976 the WHO's expanding influenza surveillance system encompassed ninety-seven centers in sixty-seven countries, all actively engaged in shipping influenza samples to WHO collaborating centers.[3] As in 1947, the collected influenza samples were sent either to the United Kingdom (Mill Hill, in London) or to the United States (Atlanta), where the sophisticated work of strain identification was carried out. The CDC served a dual role, acting as the expert source for influenza virus identification for both the United States Public Health Service and the WHO. In practical terms, the WHO thus received precisely the same information that the USPHS did. Walter Dowdle, the director of the CDC's virology division, quickly passed along relevant information about the Fort Dix outbreak to Charles Cockburn, the director of the WHO's division of communicable diseases. Cockburn and Dowdle worked closely on responses to the new influenza strain, agreeing on the official name for the reference strain (A/NJ/8/76) and, with D. A. Henderson, coordinating simultaneous press conferences to publicize the discovery of the virus.[4]

The structure of the WHO influenza surveillance system called for close coordination between the two collaborating reference centers. As was mentioned earlier, tensions between the heads of these two centers had hindered efficient cooperation in the late 1940s and early 1950s. By 1976, however, the tensions had long since dissipated, and the two laboratories worked in a close harmony facilitated by the fact that their longtime heads, Geoffrey Schild and Walter Dowdle, were good friends. In fact, the scientists at the highest levels of influenza research were all well acquainted with one another, often visiting each other's laboratories to observe techniques and research.[5] The tightness of communication among WHO headquarters in Geneva, London, and Atlanta, however, did not extend throughout the entire WHO influenza surveillance system, and communication problems would become public after President Ford's 24 March 1976 announcement of the U.S. vaccination program.

The discovery of a new influenza virus at Fort Dix provoked trepidation among scientists at the top levels of the WHO. These scientists had been looking out for just such an event since 1968. Like the USPHS, the WHO was concerned by the U.S. Army's epidemiological evidence of person-to-person transfer at the camp. When the CDC invited representatives from the WHO to the 10 March 1976 meeting of the Advisory Committee on Immunization Practices, the WHO sent three prominent influenza experts: Geoffrey Schild, a former head of the World Influenza Centre at Mill Hill who had recently moved over to the National Institute of Biological Standards and Control (the United Kingdom's counterpart to the U.S. Bureau of Biologics); John Skehel, Schild's replacement at Mill Hill and codirector of the World Influenza Centre; and Paul S. Bres, chief medical officer for the WHO's virus division. These influenza experts did not just passively observe the meeting but instead participated in the debate over the course of action the ACIP should endorse, with Bres being recorded as declaring that it would be "safest to go [with] vacc."[6]

Bres and Schild summarized the discussions in an official report for the WHO, and the evidence of a potential swine flu pandemic presented at the meeting clearly impressed the WHO representatives.[7] The report provided the highlights of the epidemiological evidence concerning Fort Dix, and the authors agreed that the evidence of "man-to-man transmission of the virus was amply demonstrated." Bres and Schild also summarized the options for vaccination being debated—bivalent or trivalent for individuals at high risk, monovalent for the entire nation (over 200 million people), or both. The report roughly parallels the notes of attendees and the official minutes of the meeting later produced by David Sencer.

At the end of the report, Bres and Schild added comments on the meeting that they grouped into five points, and what they say and do not say indicates their impressions of the evidence. Bres and Schild reported, without comment, that this novel virus was transmitted from person to person. Therefore, surveillance should be stepped up, especially in the Southern Hemisphere, where influenza season was just beginning. They also suggested that the surveillance efforts enlist veterinarians to survey pig populations. Serological surveys should be conducted to determine baseline reaction rates in various populations, and the WHO should supply reagents so that more laboratories could be brought into the search for swine influenza strains. The two influenza experts also cautioned that "National Influenza Centers should not introduce live swine influenza-like viruses into their laboratories at the present time," a recurring theme for the WHO in the mid-1970s. Their final observation is the key for appreciating their conclusions about the evidence generated by Fort

Dix: "A meeting might be convened with the producers of vaccines in Europe at a date pending the deliberation of the Bureau of Biologics which will be known very soon."

The two WHO experts had just sat through a meeting in which various levels of vaccination campaigns were being discussed, including a massive nationwide immunization program to rapidly produce, deliver, and inject over 200 million protective shots. Bres and Schild did not challenge this conclusion; rather, they suggested that European manufacturers might need to get started working, too. They also suggested that other nations should use the recommendation of the Bureau of Biologics as a starting point in making their own decisions. Bres and Schild apparently found the evidence presented at ACIP meeting concerning.

In addition to attending the meeting and coauthoring a report for the WHO, Geoffrey Schild sought to coordinate research between his laboratory, in London, and Walter Dowdle's, in Atlanta. He informed Dowdle of the three types of research his workers would be doing.[8] First, they would seek to produce a high-growth-rate, high-yield recombinant strain, an effort that would mirror Edwin Kilbourne's work and studies then under way at the CDC. Second, they would conduct dose-response surveys of inactivated vaccines to determine the optimal vaccine schedule for various populations. Third, they would attempt to develop a safe and effective live-virus vaccine. These live-virus vaccine experiments would be undertaken in strict isolation conditions at the Medical Research Council's Common Cold Unit, a governmental research facility in Salisbury. Ultimately this research never produced any live-virus vaccines, but as I will discuss, this type of study appears to have been the genesis of a controversial experiment that some WHO experts later cited to justify not recommending a large-scale vaccination campaign.

From the initial discovery of the novel virus on 14 February 1976 up through the 10 March ACIP meeting, the WHO had marched in lockstep with the USPHS. But as the USPHS began to accelerate momentum toward endorsing a universal vaccination campaign, the WHO began to develop a different interpretation of the pandemic potential of A/New Jersey. This gulf of interpretation regarding swine flu widened considerably following President Ford's announcement, on 24 March, of a massive vaccine campaign; when the WHO convened a special meeting on influenza on 7–8 April 1976, the policy it endorsed could best be described as "watchful waiting." In much the same way that the USPHS had gone from confusion to certainty in only a few short weeks, the WHO went from concern to ambivalence. As I have shown, factors beyond those of "science" had been involved in generating the U.S. decision; "nonscience" factors would shape the WHO recommendation also.

Changing Interpretations

In the days following the 10 March ACIP meeting, the USPHS and the Department of Health, Education, and Welfare began to settle on a massive vaccination campaign as the response to the Fort Dix outbreak. Those involved in the process, and outsiders who worked closely with the organizations involved, discerned the increasing momentum for a vaccination program of some sort. For those outside the system, however, especially those who had relied on the *Weekly Epidemiological Record* and the *Morbidity and Mortality Weekly Report,* Gerald Ford's announcement must have come as a surprise. Both these public health bulletins had provided little indication that the Fort Dix cases required such a dramatic response.

Contributing to the surprise other public health experts had at the announcement of the U.S. vaccination decision were the relatively poor communications throughout the WHO surveillance system. There were exceptions; as was noted before, communication between WHO headquarters in Geneva and the two reference laboratories in London and Atlanta were tight. Charles Cockburn learned of the probable U.S. programmatic response not just from the detailed report of the ACIP meeting but also by a phone call from Walter Dowdle on 19 March.[9] But the free flow of information did not extend throughout the WHO system. Claude Hannoun, head of the WHO's collaborating center for respiratory viruses in France, stated that his center's communication with the surveillance system was generally limited to "receiving letters" about upcoming meetings. In the weeks after announcing their vaccination program, USPHS officials received inquiries from around the world about the epidemiological evidence used to make the decision, including one from the prominent polio researcher Herdis von Magnus, who was the director for the WHO collaborating center for virus reference and research in Copenhagen. It is surprising that someone of her stature in the WHO was not kept informed of the evidence related to the new influenza virus, and this lapse is emblematic of the inadequate communication throughout the entire surveillance system.[10]

In the weeks following President Ford's announcement, the USPHS worked to distribute the epidemiological justification of the decision as widely as possible. Questions about the facts supporting the U.S. vaccination decision were a sign of poor communication within the WHO surveillance system but not a direct challenge to the scientific logic of the program. Nonetheless, the United States responded quickly to those who marshaled the epidemiological research to question the validity of the decision, for these types of criticisms did not signal mere confusion about the evidence but rather challenged the scientific interpretation drawn from the data. Embarrassingly for the United States, that first criticism came from a WHO official.

Media coverage of Ford's announcement was accompanied by a comment from an unnamed WHO official who was "surprised by the American plan for vaccine" and said that "no other countries [had] plans for mass vaccination."[11] This immediate expression of surprise by a WHO official was a blow to the credibility of the U.S. decision, for the USPHS had continually emphasized its close coordination with the WHO in responding to the events at Fort Dix. Officials in the United States immediately pressured the WHO to officially support the U.S. decision, and that pressure appears to have succeeded, because the next day the media reported that the WHO endorsed President Ford's plan for inoculation.[12] Officials at the USPHS declared that the WHO official quoted had simply been uninformed of the data supporting the planned vaccination program. Those officials fully informed of the collected evidence were able to clarify the logic of the decision and thus were in a position to speak authoritatively of the program.[13] Such assertions may be correct, but the damage had been done. The stigma of WHO criticism of the U.S. program would stick.

The WHO issued a press release to demonstrate its support for the U.S. decision, but a close examination of the document suggests that the WHO was beginning to distance itself from the U.S. vaccine plan. Some WHO officials were skeptical of A/New Jersey's pandemic potential as early as 24 February 1976, but the process of developing a response different from the U.S. plan was first articulated in the press release.[14]

The press release repeats much of the epidemiological information that the USPHS used to justify its recommendation for a large-scale vaccination campaign but draws a less alarming set of conclusions from it. For example, the press release states that "altogether 500 recruits were infected by a new strain," a depiction that minimizes the fact that the miniepidemic encompassed human-to-human transfer of the new virus for several generations. It acknowledges that "the new strain satisfies some of the criteria associated with pandemic strains" but then soothingly downplays the transmissibility risk: "It is known that some strains spread rapidly and others do not." In addition, the release emphasizes that recruits at the camp infected with swine flu had undergone a course of infection no more serious than that of other influenza infections.

The press release's milder depiction was factually correct; it lay within the continuum of outcomes stretching from "scientific curiosity" to "worse than Spanish flu." But the WHO was emphasizing a future course for A/New Jersey that was closer to the former than to the latter. In addition to depicting the discovery of the new strain of influenza in a less alarming light, the press release suggests an underlying strategy for the vaccination campaign never claimed by the United States and one decidedly unlikely to work.

The WHO press release agreed that, if the new strain could produce an epidemic, there would be sufficient time to mass-produce a protective vaccine, a historical first. And U.S. authorities did include this justification in making their decision. The spokesperson, however, included an additional reason, one not cited by the United States: "Widespread rapid vaccination in the country where the strain has first appeared could greatly reduce the risk for the rest of the world." Here the WHO was beginning to develop a rationale for not recommending that its member states mount a large-scale campaign by mischaracterizing the goal of the U.S. vaccination plan. The vaccination program announced by President Ford was designed not to prevent the emergence of a pandemic but to protect U.S. citizens from the pandemic anticipated to appear. Officials at the USPHS seriously doubted that they had uncovered the first cases of the new influenza strain, and they feared that the new virus was seeding itself around the world at low levels beyond surveillance detection.[15] A vaccination effort to inoculate every citizen from Maine to Hawaii (indeed, any U.S. citizen around the world), set to kick off in the fall, would not offer protection to people in Mexico or Canada, or for that matter, Geneva or Tokyo. Here, in a statement designed to support the U.S. plan for a massive vaccination campaign as a way to forestall a possible pandemic, we can see the WHO beginning to take steps toward developing a more benign interpretation of the new flu strain.

Although this WHO press release mischaracterizes one of the goals of the U.S. vaccination plan, it does not directly challenge the scientific validity of the claims underlying it. The expression of surprise aside, the WHO had scrupulously avoided directly criticizing the U.S. response, and in the earliest days following the identification of the new flu strain at Fort Dix, it had closely coordinated its comments with U.S. influenza researchers. The policy of not challenging the U.S. decision was about to change, and the source of that challenge was a dismaying one for the USPHS.

The events at Fort Dix and the U.S. immunization plan pressed the WHO to advise its member states on the potential threat of the new virus and provide a range of responses that individual national health programs should consider adopting. The WHO called for an emergency meeting where its influenza experts would craft an official recommendation for such responses. The scientists and public health experts were invited to attend a two-day meeting in Geneva on 7–8 April 1976. Committees and meetings of scientific experts are a staple of the WHO's modus operandi, and Walter Dowdle, who was often involved in these conclaves, described the meetings as informal affairs, with the attendees acting as consultants.[16] Nonetheless, while these committees do not necessarily dictate the policies of the WHO (a point not always clearly understood by the invited experts), their prescriptions and reports carry enormous clout in directing WHO policy. In the field of influenza research, the expert meetings were generally practical affairs, where the subject at hand involved coordinating and disseminating research information, discussing new strains, or evaluating prophylactic and treatment options. The most important task of the influenza experts' meeting was to decide on the WHO's biannual recommendation for the upcoming influenza season. After the experts agreed on the recipe, the WHO would distribute seed stock to vaccine manufacturers around the world. In the give-and-take of these meetings, the experts hash out the recommendation that the WHO hierarchy then generally passes along, for it lacks the expertise and technical background to alter the report's conclusions.

All the experts attending the meeting of influenza were given ample opportunity to discuss and debate various points, but it bears underscoring that the structure of WHO influenza surveillance was strictly hierarchical, with samples traveling to one of two coequal strain identification laboratories. While the invited WHO experts generally all had experience working with the influenza virus, the two directors of the laboratories that did the typing of unknown influenza viruses had the greatest experience working with a variety of strains. And both Dowdle and Schild were well respected by their peers. It is natural, then, to presume that the opinions of these two men carried more weight than did those of the directors of national laboratories, if only because the work of identifying and studying novel influenza viruses was done in their labs. On the eve of the 7–8 April 1976 experts meeting in Geneva, the former director of the World Influenza Centre in London, Geoffrey Schild, offered a pointed critique of the U.S. vaccination plan. In an interview that appeared in the 5 April 1976 *San Francisco Chronicle*, Schild characterized the U.S. decision as a "'somewhat immoderate' response to the Ft. Dix phenomenon."[17] Schild then went on to detail the United Kingdom's vaccination plan to incorporate swine flu into the mix of vaccines offered to high-risk patients but not to attempt to reach other members of the population. This program was a decidedly low-key response that stood in stark contrast to the massive effort proposed by the United States.

At first glance, calling the response "somewhat immoderate" does not seem unduly harsh, but the critique should be seen in context. Schild not only had been the director of the World Influenza Centre laboratory until just a few months earlier but also had moved into another prominent position in the field of influenza research and vaccination: director of the National Institute of Biological Standards and Control. Schild's comments can be read as suggesting that the U.S. decision was rash and hasty or perhaps influenced by factors beyond the science of the new virus. In fact, the newspaper article quotes two anonymous "well-known government experts in communicable diseases" who asserted that the vaccination decision reflected political considerations ("this is a Presidential election year"), a charge that Schild's critique supports. The article would not be the last place such accusations about the program were leveled.

WHO Influenza Experts Meeting, 7–8 April 1976

The April 7–8 WHO meeting brought together influenza experts from thirteen nations in addition to health officials from the WHO, United States, and United Kingdom.[18] As was stated before, the purpose of the meeting was to assess the potential impact of the virus uncovered at Fort Dix, New Jersey, and to craft a recommended response to this new virus that the WHO could issue to its member states.

The WHO had no power to initiate its own responses to the new virus. Any program would have to be carried out at a national level. The WHO could provide its best determination of what the Fort Dix cases represented, but it had little ability or infrastructure to aid in a vaccination campaign. Just as in 1957 and 1968, national protective programs were the only available response to an international pandemic threat, and such programs would necessarily be limited to the few states that had the technical capabilities to undertake such efforts. Which states had the means to conduct an emergency program remained an open question.

The meeting was opened by Dr. L. Bernard, the WHO's assistant director general, who thanked the delegates for coming on such short notice.[19] The purpose of the meeting, according to Bernard, was to provide the organization's member states expert advice about the new influenza virus. This new strain was a concern, he said, because of its "man-to-man" spread and "its antigenic relationship to the swine influenza–like virus which caused the 1918 pandemic." Bernard thanked the CDC for rapidly providing the epidemiological evidence it had gathered and for quickly shipping reagents to nodes in the influenza surveillance network to help them detect the new virus. These contributions were crucial to aid the WHO influenza program in fulfilling its primary aim, which according to Bernard was to detect new viral strains and to make vaccine seed stock available to manufacturers as quickly as possible.

Bernard's opening address was forthright about the purpose of the meeting and laid out the scientific questions at hand in relation to the events at Fort

Dix. The virus was new, had been transmitted from person to person, and might (or might not) be related to Spanish flu. The experts were to analyze these points with an eye to recommending whether the new virus should be allocated to vaccine manufacturers. These issues were all scientific questions. At the close of his speech, however, Bernard issued a curious caution, one not related to the science of the new virus. Bernard advised the assembled experts not to overlook the fact "that countries in the developing world would have no facilities for vaccine production." The limits of vaccine production were not a scientific problem but a political one.

Bernard's comments were emblematic of new winds beginning to blow in the WHO.[20] In the later 1960s and the 1970s, the technical, biomedical approach that had dominated WHO programs began meeting increasing dissatisfaction for several reasons. First, WHO membership was swelling with newly founded "developing" nations emerging from decolonization. These states constituted 70 percent of WHO's membership by 1970, and they often found the technical solutions offered by the WHO to be impractical given their material and technological situations.[21] Some states also resented the vertical, or "stovepipe," approach of focusing exclusively on the eradication of a single disease. Proponents of this model could point to the dramatic success of the smallpox elimination campaign, while critics could counter with the colossal failure of malaria eradication. At its height, between 1959 to 1966, the malaria program consumed 27 percent of the WHO budget.[22]

Delegates of developing states called for greater WHO support for the cultivation of basic health-care services and pointed to the Chinese model of "barefoot doctors" as the best use of WHO funds. This mode of moderately trained medical personnel drawing on local or indigenous health practices to care for their charges stood as a polar opposite to the technical biomedical approach adopted by WHO experts. Champions of this stress on basic health care included the newly elected director general, Halfden Mahler (1973–1988), and the movement culminated in the 1978 Primary Health Care Conference at Alma-Ata (now Almaty), in the Soviet Union, whose resolution issued a call for "health care for all" by the year 2000.

This new social focus in health care, which emphasized broader, society-wide improvements, echoed a strand of thought popular in the 1930s under the League of Nations Health Organization. Although this resurgent interest in social mediation for health problems would roil the WHO membership and affect budgets in the 1980s and 1990s, it had little direct impact on the experts of the influenza committee, who resolutely maintained a focus on technical approaches to influenza pandemics.

Combating influenza pandemics thus remained a technical concern, and until this sophisticated, nation-centered approach was discredited, national health programs took the lead in protecting individual nations' populations from infections. Although programs to forestall influenza pandemics would adopt new models, influenza surveillance continued to rely on complicated and expensive machinery and processes.

After Bernard's welcoming speech, and with his caution about uneven vaccine production ability in their minds, the delegates gathered to discuss the new virus. The first order of business was electing a chair for the meeting and two individuals who would record the proceedings. V. M. Zhdanov, from the Soviet Union, was elected chairman, with Walter Dowdle and H. Bijkerk (from the Netherlands) elected reporters. According to Dowdle, these informal meetings did not require votes or parliamentary procedures. Instead, the appointed reporters were responsible for writing up the meeting's conclusion with input from the chair and the secretariat of the WHO. The draft conclusions and recommendations were presented to all the participants, and modifications of the document were solicited from the floor. The final product was then approved by the reporters and the chair.[23]

After the election of the board, the meeting turned to epidemiological evidence concerning the current influenza season. Several nations were experiencing elevated influenza morbidity rates that they attributed to the A/ Victoria strain (the Hong Kong drifted descendant). No nation had uncovered swine flu strains circulating in its population. The discussion then turned to the events at Fort Dix. Two representatives were there to discuss the science of the new virus and the program on which the United States had settled. Walter Dowdle discussed the discovery of the virus and its characteristics and summarized the epidemiological evidence associated with the localized epidemic. Dowdle was, of course, a regular attendee at these expert meetings and was well known to the scientists from the other nations. The second U.S. representative, however, was unfamiliar to most of the influenza experts. This man, J. Donald Millar, was tasked with explaining the structure of the National Influenza Immunization Program and how it intended to vaccinate every U.S. citizen.

Millar was not an influenza expert but considered himself an "immunization program implementer."[24] He had joined the CDC in 1961 and was soon enmeshed in organizing large-scale vaccination campaigns. He had been an administrator of the dramatically successful program to eradicate smallpox and control measles in West Africa. This program served as a template for efforts to eradicate smallpox globally, and its massive measles vaccination campaign quickly inoculated over a 120 million people in West Africa. As Millar recalled, this was over 80 percent of the population, who were inoculated by mobile teams using jet-injector guns. After Millar had helped manage successful programs abroad, CDC director David Sencer brought him back to the United States to organize public health programs with various state representatives. His experience organizing mass vaccination campaigns made him a natural choice to administer the vaccine program under development in 1976, and so Sencer tapped Millar as the man to actuate the president's decision within the CDC. Millar saw his role at the Geneva meeting merely as one of explaining the program the USPHS intended to undertake. He was not seeking counsel from the influenza experts there, and he did not feel the need to lobby for or justify the decision the United States had made.

The presence of Millar, whose expertise lay outside influenza, and the role he envisioned for himself seemed to have rubbed some people at the meeting the wrong way. Claude Hannoun, who had been attending influenza experts' meetings in Geneva since 1970, found Millar's presentation to not fit the venue well.[25] As Hannoun recalled, conversations at these meetings usually revolved around technical issues, such as "the antigenic relationship in the hemagglutinin inhibition test between strain so and so and the strain so and so." Millar's presentation was stiff and formal, and according to Hannoun, Millar responded to questions from the experts by saying, "the President of the United States does not want to gamble with the life of the American citizens," which Hannoun characterized as "very unusual for [these] meetings!"[26] Hannoun recalled that he and other delegates were a little frustrated about the discussion of the U.S. decision, for he did not think the answers provided were scientific, the sort other nations would need to make their decisions properly.

Millar's role as spokesperson for the U.S. vaccination campaign disrupted the politically neutral scientific discussions that dominated these expert conclaves. These technically oriented influenza experts saw themselves as dispassionate evaluators of the scientific merit of the confusing mix of information. Millar, however, sought only to implement a decision already made and so was uninterested in the scientific debate. Be that as it may, the distinction between impartial scientist and political operative is not nearly as clear-cut as the experts assembled in Geneva might have liked to believe. Many of the influenza experts appearing on the international stage of the meeting would return to play national roles back home. They surely would know their nations' capabilities for vaccination programs, and it is hard to imagine that such knowledge did not play some role in their evaluations at the meeting's broader level.

Regardless, the meeting broke for lunch with the attendees pondering the fact that U.S. health officials had thought the epidemiological evidence of the novel strain's human-to-human transmissibility sufficient to justify a program to inoculate all their citizens. This massive program would stretch U.S. vaccine manufacturers to their limits, which meant that it was unlikely that much, if any, of the doses produced in the United States would be available to other markets. Vaccine for other nations would have to come from domestic sources, and the capabilities of these national producers were a matter of concern. Up to this point in the meeting, other national health programs had not directly challenged the U.S. program. That all changed at the afternoon session with the initial suggestions of a markedly different approach to the Fort Dix virus, and it was the WHO that would provide the justification of this new approach.

CHAPTER 9

WHO Decides

In the morning session of the 7–8 April 1976 influenza experts meeting at Geneva, the two representatives from the United States, Walter Dowdle and J. Donald Millar, had carefully laid out the epidemiological evidence uncovered at Fort Dix and the rationale behind and method of the U.S. vaccination campaign. None of the influenza scientists challenged the science behind the vaccination decision or directly disputed the logic of the U.S. program. As the afternoon session of the meeting began, however, it became clear that representatives from other national health programs did not draw the same alarming conclusions from the epidemiological evidence as the United States Public Health Service had and were disinclined or unable to mount large-scale vaccination programs. Some of the assembled influenza researchers were concerned about the use of live-virus vaccines, which they considered overly dangerous. Wanting to downplay the potential dangers of the new virus and, at least in some cases, to elevate the results of a controversial experiment, many influenza experts at the meeting favored a milder projection of A/New Jersey's pandemic potential. The resulting World Health Organization report evolved from an alarming depiction of the new virus to one far more calming. The recommendations that the WHO ultimately forwarded to its member states emphasized a policy of watchful waiting rather than immediate action.

The experts returned from lunch and began the afternoon session with an overview of other national health programs' planned responses.[1] Doctor Marguerite Pereira, codirector of the World Influenza Centre, summarized the U.K. National Health Service's plans. As previously indicated by Geoffrey Schild, U.K. health officials had developed a low-key response, merely incorporating A/New Jersey into the existing vaccine recipe (offering protection against A/Victoria and B/Hong Kong) to make a trivalent vaccine. This trivalent vaccine would be produced at the usual levels. As Pereira described it, this vaccination decision was based on the fact that undertaking a mass vaccination campaign presented two major problems. First, acquiring the funds needed to support such a program was difficult in the current economic climate. Second, British health officials had neither the experience nor support infrastructure to produce, distribute, and inoculate a significant portion of their population in rapid order.

Immediately following Pereira's discussion of the United Kingdom's limited response, Geoffrey Schild detailed the results of an experiment conducted at the Common Cold Unit, in Salisbury. Two researchers—A. S. Beare and J. W. Craig—had infected six volunteers with the A/New Jersey strain. The resulting infections were generally mild: one moderate course of influenza, two mild cases, and three subclinical cases.[2] This study thus indicated the infection caused by A/New Jersey to be not especially severe, and certainly not like Spanish flu.

Retrospectively, the intentional infection of six human volunteers with a novel influenza virus is seen as remarkably dangerous, both to the subjects and to the public at large. There was no way of knowing whether the infection would prompt a violent reaction in the subjects, and passing the sample through a human host could help the virus adapt for more efficient human transmission. Thus, infecting the human subjects might have inadvertently sparked a pandemic if the strain had escaped the laboratory. Sir John Skehel recalls that the Beare and Craig experiment was discussed at later influenza meetings, and the general attitude was that the experiment should never have been done because of the risks associated with it.[3]

Beyond the potential dangers of deliberately infecting human volunteers with a novel virus, there were serious questions about the value of the evidence generated from the experiment. An infection produced in a laboratory setting cannot mimic a natural infection. Serial passage through human hosts adapts the virus for greater transmission between humans, and laboratory infections cannot replicate that process. As Walter Dowdle later stated, "It just simply isn't the same as if you have millions of people infected with the same agent."[4] Also, as the experimenters acknowledged, the virus used in the study had been passed through chicken eggs six times in preparation for infecting the subjects. This process (injecting, incubating, and harvesting the viral material) weakened the strain and in fact mirrored an old method used to prepare influenza viruses for use in a vaccine. Edwin Kilbourne, whose laboratory at the New York Medical College had created over thirty vaccines or vaccine-candidate reassortant strains, commented that being "passed through an alien host [chicken eggs] like that" weakens the virus. Strains employed to create vaccines used to be "based on the simple act of . . . serial passage in the egg. They weren't temperature sensitive, they weren't cold adapted [other methods to develop vaccine strains] or anything. They were just passages. . . . If you passed it a few times you couldn't infect anyone."[5]

In sum, then, the deliberate infection of human volunteers at the Common Cold Unit was reckless both because it could have prompted a dangerous course of infection in a volunteer and because the virus could have escaped the laboratory to serially transmit in the surrounding population. At the same time, the experiment was of dubious value, because the process of preparing the virus for inoculation weakened the wild strain, making any severity information suspect. Dowdle did not find Schild's presentation of the study particularly helpful, and he doubted that other scientists at the meeting found the information compelling for the issues at hand. Nevertheless, he said, some of the U.K. representatives really pushed the results of the experiment at the conclave.[6]

Dowdle's assessment of the Common Cold Unit experiment is clear, but those of other influenza experts are less so. Assuming that the experiment did have relevance to issues of swine flu, the results did bolster the argument that A/New Jersey prompted a mild course of infection. The test spoke to the crucial issue looming over the experts' discussion: was swine flu going to be similar to Spanish flu? The relatively innocuous course of infection in the six volunteers suggested it would not. In addition, Dowdle's notes do not show any of the experts questioning the value of the experiment at the meeting, and Schild's summary of the outcome of the experiment was one of only two pieces of evidence—the epidemiological evidence at Fort Dix was the other—included in the experts' report to the WHO's director general. The Common Cold Unit study would be cited not only by critics of the U.S. vaccination decision but also by proponents of the Swine Flu Program, who focused on a different set of data generated by the experiment to bolster their decision. The results of the study would be a part of the discussion about the A/New Jersey strain for the next several weeks.

After Schild presented his report, the representatives of various states discussed their nations' planned responses. At the low end, Japan's contingent admitted that their country had not yet started any sort of planning. Though somewhat further along, France announced that it had made no decision as to whether a monovalent vaccine should be produced and, if produced, whether it should be stored or injected immediately. And the Soviet Union declared its intention to prepare and stockpile 20–50 million doses of killed vaccine for emergency use. The problem for these WHO experts was the one facing the USPHS experts: there just was not enough information to predict what the new virus would do. As the WHO virologist Martin Kaplan pointed out, although the data from Fort Dix offered the "first proof of human to human spread," the lack of evidence for such transmission elsewhere might be due solely to the "poor surveillance system." He added, "Only a handful of people are looking—[we] need more *information*."[7] Much like the ACIP, the WHO influenza experts lamented the paucity of information on which they would be forced to reach a decision.

Similarly unclear was the public's likely response if the WHO recommended the sort of large-scale inoculation program that the United States had proposed. Claude Hannoun suggested that responses to a mass vaccination campaign could range from "panic" to a "lack of interest." Neither outcome would be desirable, but panic was certainly something to be avoided. And of course, officials would have to be careful about alarming the public if they did not have some sort of remedy to address citizens' concerns.

As the representatives from various nations summarized the status of their countries' plans, Charles Cockburn, director of the WHO's communicable diseases division, solicited the Chinese experts for information about their government's intentions. The Chinese had only recently begun to engage in international cooperative organizations following a long period of isolation driven by the Cultural Revolution. The two Chinese scientists were not well known to the other influenza experts, and the influenza community at large knew little about China's expertise in vaccine production and the scientific aspects of the virus. The Chinese influenza expert stated that researchers in his nation did not have much experience in creating killed vaccines and found them "difficult to make." They therefore recognized that they could "not produce killed [vaccines] for all millions."[8]

If the Chinese and other nations could not protect their citizens with killed vaccines, perhaps the solution lay with live-virus vaccines. These vaccines are easier and cheaper to make (because the virus does not need to be inactivated and purified), easier to deliver (because the dose is inhaled rather than injected), and easier to produce in large quantities (because, since the amount of material needed to inoculate someone is smaller than an injected dose, the per-egg yield is higher). In theory, live-virus vaccines are greatly weakened strains that generate courses of infection so mild that recipients barely notice they are ill. Nevertheless, the weakened virus is sufficiently robust to prompt a powerful, long-lasting immune system response. Because the virus mimics the natural course of infection, some experts thought the immunity produced by the live-virus vaccine would be superior to injected killed-virus vaccines. In the 1970s weakened live-virus strains were shaped to replicate only at low temperatures, thereby limiting their ability to reproduce in the warmer human body. Such cold-adapted viruses minimize replication in the individual (making the infection even shorter and milder) and prevent further transmission to others (because the virus does not reproduce effectively in the inoculated, it produces fewer copies to infect others). These attenuated, cold-adapted live-virus vaccines promised much greater vaccine coverage and protection.

In practice, however, the unstable nature of the influenza virus undermined the use of live-virus vaccines. Its high mutation rate during replication increases the probability that the virus will revert to a higher virulence, transmissibility, or both. The National Institutes of Health in the United States had been working on creating attenuated live-virus vaccines for years, but their laboratory efforts had been bedeviled by the attenuated strains' reversion to greater transmissibility and virulence. The NIH had sponsored a meeting of influenza researchers to discuss and assess preparations for a future influenza pandemic, with a focus on the status of attenuated live-virus vaccines. The meeting, held on 12 January 1976 (remarkably, another group of influenza experts who were meeting as swine flu was circulating at Fort Dix), brought together the major U.S. researchers working on live-virus vaccines. The consensus of the group was that the technique showed great promise for accelerating vaccine production levels and shortening the time of production but that live-virus vaccines remained in the "research phase." In two letters subsequent to the meeting, Maurice Hilleman, director of the Merck Institute for Therapeutic Research, suggested that the current limitations on live-virus vaccines be explicitly spelled out in the final report of the meeting. Hilleman stated, "The recombinant live vaccine approach carries potential scientific, political, and economic liabilities of substantial magnitude" and warned that there "should be proof of safety from the standpoint of reversion . . . [and] reasonable assurance that recombinants with virulent virus [would] not occur in the field and so cause a worse pandemic than might otherwise have occurred."[9] Hilleman expressed his concerns that such assurances were not in place for the live-virus vaccines then being developed in the United States.

The WHO's concerns, however, extended beyond those about the tendency of strains used in live-virus vaccines to revert back to greater transmissibility or virulence. The eastern bloc nations, spearheaded by the Soviet Union, had been using attenuated live-virus vaccines at least since the 1957 Asian flu, and they asserted that live-virus vaccines were "the best flu prophylactic."[10] But the Soviets had never provided detailed data on the vaccine strains they created or any samples of the attenuated live-virus vaccine to the WHO.[11]

Some influenza experts strongly favored the use of live-virus vaccines and considered them the only "means of mass immunity against new virus subtypes," although they admitted that "the problem of producing them repeatedly and infallibly" had "not . . . been solved."[12] In 1971 the WHO sponsored an "informal consultation" on the state of international collaboration in research on live-virus vaccines. The subsequent report from the meeting summarized the discussion there. In its conclusion, the report called for increased international collaboration on live-virus vaccine studies, but it also noted a troubling facet of live-virus immunization. Point 3 under "Assessment of Attenuation" suggested that attenuated strains possess "no ability to spread from person to person and revert to virulence on passage," but elsewhere the report conceded that there had "been few attempts to study point number 3 and there [were] no agreed methods for measuring spreading ability."[13]

In the early 1970s, Geoffrey Schild began to suspect that the attenuated live-virus vaccines used by the Soviets and other eastern bloc nations were prompting chains of transmission from the inoculated to the uninoculated. In 1974 Schild observed a pattern of persistent lag of viral types in influenza samples sent from the eastern bloc to his laboratory for identification (the Soviets had only recently begun sending the WHO samples of influenza strains circulating in that nation). In a 19 July 1974 letter to Walter Dowdle, Schild remarked that although all the isolates from the Southern Hemisphere were related to A/PC/73, the samples sent from the Soviet Union and Bulgaria resembled A/England/72. The latter strains might have been persisting, but, he observed, these samples could also have been "re-isolations of live vaccines." That same day Schild sent Cockburn a letter, marked "in confidence," in which he conceded that the 1972 variant might have been persisting in Eastern Europe but suggested as an "alternate explanation" that "live attenuated vaccine strains [were] being re-isolated in these areas," adding, "It will not be easy to establish if this is the case."[14] Detecting whether Soviet vaccine strains were the same as the samples collected for typing in London would be especially difficult because the WHO lacked samples of Soviet live-virus vaccines with which to compare the suspect cases.

Circulating live-virus vaccine strains were dangerous partly because of their ability to revert to virulence but primarily because they could combine with the circulating wild strains of influenza. The attenuated live-virus vaccine strains are selected for their ability to infect humans in order to ensure that the vaccine "takes" and produces a strong immune response for protection. If such a virus combined with a novel strain, or a strain with high levels of transmissibility or virulence, the resulting hybrid could be dangerous and even deadly, possessing both novel surface components that allowed it to evade the human immune system and the ability to infect human hosts effectively.

Therefore, when nations discussed using live-virus vaccines to solve their vaccine coverage problems at the 7–8 April 1976 WHO influenza experts meeting, Geoffrey Schild, Walter Dowdle, Charles Cockburn, and other scientists viewed this idea with alarm. When the WHO virologist Kaplan summarized the afternoon discussion to that point by stating, "Some countries (China) must use attenuated vaccine for mass use" and asking, "What sort of statement should come out regarding the use of live attenuated vaccines[?]" Dowdle marked these comments in his notes with two big exclamation points. He was later to state that the final report included the phrase "extreme caution" with respect to using live-virus vaccines specifically because several investigators outside Western Europe intended to develop and test such vaccines.[15]

One of these nations outside Western Europe was China, which had been purportedly producing and using live-virus vaccines at least since 1972. Dr. W. G. Laver, who was associated with the Department of Microbiology at the Australian National University's John Curtin School of Medical Research, in Canberra, sent a report to the WHO summarizing his visit to China. Laver and Dr. Robert Webster were traveling with seventeen other Australian medical professionals (physicians, surgeons, dentists, and others) at the invitation of the Chinese Medical Association. The nearly monthlong trip (from 9 September through 4 October 1972) took the team on a tightly controlled tour of hospitals and research facilities. Laver and Webster spent a full day visiting the National Vaccine and Serum Institute at Peking, where they met a number of doctors and gave a lecture on influenza. The translator and discussion leader for the tour was Dr. C. M. Chu, who informed Laver and Webster that the institute produced live-virus vaccines. At that time they were using a cold mutant variety of the 1968 Hong Kong strain and were producing and distributing 10 million doses a year. How much the Chinese could ramp up this production in 1976 was an open question, but apparently the Chinese had shown the ability and inclination to make and use live-virus vaccines.[16]

By the end of the first day's session at the April 1976 WHO meeting, the individuals who were to draft the ensuing report—Walter Dowdle, H. Bijkerk, V. M. Zhdanov, and a senior representative from the WHO secretariat—were faced with a series of dilemmas. Many nations of the world—including the most populous nation, China—could not produce inactivated vaccine on a large scale. Attenuated live-virus vaccines offered the potential for greater ease of production, larger quantities of material, and simpler inoculation, but they were dangerously unstable. The A/New Jersey virus was new and had clearly passed from human to human at Fort Dix, but the minor epidemic there had stopped, and thus far no additional outbreaks had been detected. Some—though not Dowdle—thought that the small-scale study by the British Common Cold Unit had suggested the A/New Jersey virus might prompt a mild course of infection. Finally, the United States had already committed to a massive vaccination campaign to inoculate all its citizens, an effort that would consume most, if not all, of the production of pharmaceutical firms based there. It was likely that other nations would have to produce their own vaccine if they wanted to inoculate their citizens.

The inactivated influenza vaccine productive capacity outside the United States in 1976 remains a bit of a mystery. The WHO did not conduct a global census of inactivated vaccine production until the twenty-first century, with an accurate count extending back only to the year 2000. This survey, "Global Distribution of Influenza Vaccine," shows that in 2003, at least 95 percent of the almost 292 million doses produced originated in nine nations (Australia, Canada, France, Germany, Italy, Japan, the Netherlands, the United Kingdom, and the United States). The estimated 231 million doses of vaccine produced in 2000 were more than twice the quantity of vaccine produced a decade before.[17] A partial list of vaccine manufacturers in 1976 lists eighteen manufacturers in twelve nations but makes no mention of capacity and omits eastern bloc nations (with the exception of Romania).[18]

In the absence of hard numbers, one is required to base vaccine production estimates on impressionistic recollections of capacity from those involved in vaccine research and public health at the time. Walter Dowdle believed that several Western European nations, Australia, and Japan could pull off large-scale (if not universal) vaccination campaigns, and there is some evidence to bolster this assertion. Japan had been inoculating 20 million schoolchildren a year with influenza vaccine since 1973. Claude Hannoun estimated that French vaccine manufacturers could produce 4–6 million doses in a normal year of vaccine production but could have tripled that output "in case of a very severe situation" by producing a monovalent vaccine. This level of production could have vaccinated 50–60 percent of the French population. In addition, the Italian government had informed the pharmaceutical house SCALVO that it intended to embargo all the firm's swine flu vaccine (estimated at 10 million doses) if a pandemic arrived.[19]

Other public health experts doubted that many nations could mount large-scale campaigns, at least on a crash basis. For David Sencer, the problem was not technical capabilities but infrastructure. Manufacturers in the United States dominated the global market for inactivated influenza vaccines, partly because the CDC had been recommending yearly vaccines for those deemed to be at "high risk" (over the age of sixty-five or with chronic lung ailments) since 1960. "Flu was not a major vaccine anyplace other than in the United States." Producing flu vaccine requires a steady supply of fertilized chicken eggs and a sterile environment. To begin rapidly producing vaccine, "it takes buildings . . . it takes eggs[;] . . . you don't build those overnight."[20]

A similar point about the difficulties of rapidly ramping up vaccine production was made by Ian Furminger, who was head of research and development and a production manager at Evans Medical, the Glaxo subsidiary that manufactured virtually all the influenza vaccine in the United Kingdom in 1976. Evans annually produced just over a million doses of influenza vaccine for the domestic market in the mid-1970s. Furminger estimated that in an emergency, Evans might have been able to increase production to around 3 million doses by producing only a monovalent vaccine and by running the factory around the clock. The lack of facilities prevented any greater level of production. He said, "It's very difficult to rack up your production, mainly because you don't have the incubators in which to put the eggs"; also, you have to purify the egg-produced material, and "you have got to have centrifuges to purify it." Furminger stated that Evans did not have excess unused capacity and believed that other European manufacturers had similar yearly production rates and similar limitations on capacity.[21]

Perhaps the most compelling testimony on vaccine production capacity in 1976 comes from D. A. Henderson, whom the CDC had loaned to the WHO to administer the global eradication of smallpox program. Henderson remained on the CDC payroll and naturally had close contacts with the organization, and he had from the outset been in the loop concerning events related to Fort Dix. He worked closely with Cockburn on the implications of the swine flu discovery, and his senior status in the WHO led to his serving as acting head of the communicable diseases division when Cockburn was absent or unavailable. Either at the 7–8 April 1976 influenza experts meeting in Geneva or at a meeting shortly before, Henderson chaired a discussion group of vaccine manufacturers from around Europe. Henderson recalls that the informal meeting was called to discuss possible manufacturers' responses to the new influenza strain. Henderson stated: "I remember this very well. . . . From what the manufacturers that we were talking to could tell us, there was little production capacity. . . . Influenza vaccine was made in very small quantities, there was little influenza vaccination going on in these areas at all, and the manufacturers were not in a position to greatly expand this capacity." Henderson replied in a colorful fashion when asked whether the experts at the April 1976 WHO meeting had a good sense of the limited production capacity of manufacturers outside the United States: "We got a very good sense and the capacity was zilch."[22]

Drafts and Final Reports

The final report of the meeting, with the experts' recommended responses to the new influenza strain, would be drafted with these limitations in mind. The experts would try to present a set of recommendations falling somewhere between Hannoun's poles of "lack of interest" and "panic." The drafts of the final report reveal the push and pull of these competing prescriptions.

The first draft of the report listed seven recommendations.[23] The first point was both soothing and alarming: "Since it is by no means certain that A/ New Jersey strains have the capacity to cause widespread disease, there is no justification for public alarm. In particular it should not be inferred that the present situation is the same as that which existed at the beginning of the 1918 epidemic. Nevertheless health authorities would be wise to prepare contingency plans for a possible pandemic . . . with the adaptation of existing health services to an exceptional situation." Points 2, 3, and 4 suggested heightened surveillance of human and animal populations and the prompt shipment of unusual strains to the WHO collaborating centers. Point 5 recommended inactivated vaccine production continue with recombinant A/New Jersey strains and that nations pursue one of three possible strategies: create a trivalent vaccine with A/Victoria and B/Hong Kong; immediately use A/New Jersey to create a monovalent vaccine; or store vaccine in bulk as an emergency reserve. The recommendation also suggested that additional information about the virus's pandemic potential would emerge in the ensuing months. The sixth point assured authorities that information about dose levels and schedules would be forthcoming. The final point stated that "extreme caution" was necessary if attenuated live-virus vaccines containing A/Swine strains were used for experimental purposes because of "possible reversion to virulence." Dowdle penciled in an additional notation to this sentence by adding "or recombination with other influenza strains." Dowdle also penciled additional phrases for possible insertion into the text at the bottom of the page, including, "The WHO recognizes that prod. and purchasing may represent a considerable outlay of public health funds," and "Live vaccine should not be used in the absence of further spread at this time."

The recommendations from this first draft would serve to calm any hysteria about the new virus by emphasizing the absence of any certain evidence that a new Spanish flu was looming or that the A/New Jersey strain would cause a pandemic. Influenza experts recognized the special fear that Spanish flu induced and sought to ensure that they downplayed any relationship between this swine flu strain and the horrifying killer from 1918. It was not the first time that WHO authorities had recognized the relationship's potential for producing panic. In July 1965, M. F. Warburton, head of the laboratory at Commonwealth Serum Laboratories in Australia, wrote Charles Cockburn at the WHO to inform him that his laboratory had detected a patient stricken with influenza who tested positive for the A/Swine type. Warburton stated that his laboratory had kept "the isolation and its identification" secret because "disclosures of the type of virus would be likely to cause some panic in the light of its relationship to the 1919 epidemic." Cockburn replied, "Your decision to keep things entirely confidential for the present was very wise and I shall certainly say nothing about it until you tell me that I can do so."[24]

The draft recommendations were forthright about the pandemic potential of A/New Jersey, however, and so suggested that national health programs prepare for an "exceptional situation." The WHO experts wanted to clearly state that these preparations should not include the use of attenuated live-virus vaccines unless the pandemic was indubitably under way and that "extreme caution" should be used in experiments to create such vaccines. The drafters of the document were intensely concerned about the accidental release of A/New Jersey strains.

The second draft of the final report included a summary of the information produced at the meeting and a revised list of recommendations.[25] The document began with a summary of Assistant Director Bernard's address, in which he had stated that concern of A/New Jersey's "man-to-man" spread was one of the reasons for seeking advice from the influenza experts. This important phrase, however, was omitted from the summary of Bernard's speech, which read, "The appearance of a new strain of influenza A at Fort Dix, New Jersey in the United States of America February this year has caused much concern all over the world."[26] The revised statement is factually correct but presents a milder description of the issues at hand. Human-to-human spread is a key component in a pandemic and was one of the primary elements that influenza researchers cited as justification for vaccination campaigns.

The report downplayed the epidemiological evidence from Fort Dix as summarized by Dowdle and Millar. The investigation of the outbreak at the camp clearly demonstrated serial passage of a novel virus for several generations, which are key ingredients for a pandemic. Human transmission is implied but never explicitly stated in the summary of their evidence. For example, in conveying the data that demonstrated the virus to have passed for several generations, infecting approximately 500 recruits, the report stated,

"Approximately 500 swine influenza–like infections may have occurred during the 4–5 week period."

In addition, the report gave greater prominence to evidence that suggested a pandemic was unlikely or that the resulting infections would be mild. Immediately following the summary of information from Fort Dix was a summary of the Common Cold Unit's experimental infection of six volunteers. The study's most striking finding was the mildness of the resulting infections. Although Dowdle (and others) did not think the study relevant to a possible pandemic, it was the only evidence aside from epidemiological data to be included in the report, thus elevating it to a higher level of importance than several of the experts had intended.

The evidence presented in the report had not changed and was factually accurate. But the alarming points in the report had been presented mildly and the elements that suggested A/New Jersey would not prompt a pandemic were given greater prominence. This trend of presenting the information gathered about A/New Jersey mildly was also visible in the "Conclusions and Recommendations" section of the report.

The five recommendations retained much of the first draft's language, but some new elements were added. The first point stated that A/New Jersey had caused outbreaks at Fort Dix, with "approximately 500 men being infected," again soft-pedaling the human-to-human and serial passage of the outbreak. The point went on to emphasize that no further outbreaks had been discovered: "It is entirely possible that this may have been a unique event in a military recruit population and will not lead to wide-spread epidemics." The second and third points suggested that surveillance be increased and further studies of influenza types in human and animal populations be initiated. The fourth point again stated flatly that "countries currently producing influenza vaccine should be encouraged to initiate production of an inactivated vaccine" and listed the three possible strategies: the addition of A/New Jersey to currently recommended vaccines, the administration of a monovalent vaccine, or storage in bulk. The fourth point also suggested that the decision on which course of action to pursue might be based on evidence "obtained in the forthcoming months." The fifth and final recommendation restated the explicit cautions on attenuated live-virus studies and use.

The final report continued the trend of downplaying the alarming aspects of the Fort Dix outbreak and further emphasized a policy of "wait and see" for its recommended response.[27] This emphasis on waiting for additional information before initiating vaccination was most visible in point 4 of the five-point "Conclusions and Recommendations" section of the report, which reordered the three possible strategies for vaccine-producing nations to pursue: storing in bulk, adding A/New Jersey to existing vaccines, or producing monovalent vaccine. The decision on the best course of action to pursue would be obtained "via the surveillance network."

The evolution of the document was now complete. Evidence suggesting a possible dangerous course of events was presented blandly and quickly offset with evidence that suggested a benign outcome to the new virus. The WHO's recommendations were a call not to action but to increased vigilance. If action was needed, the report suggested that the evidence would come from the WHO's influenza surveillance system.

A similar toning-down process was visible in the press release that accompanied the report, though it does express more urgency regarding preparation for a possible pandemic.[28] The first draft of the release highlighted the relevant information of the meeting, and tellingly, it summarizes the epidemiological evidence from Fort Dix but does not mention the Common Cold Unit experimental infection of six human volunteers. The release suggests that health authorities "should prepare contingency plans" for a "potentially exceptional situation." Dowdle included a penciled notation at the bottom of the page to include the phrase "further investigation revealed that as many as 500 men had been infected[,] which demonstrated the capacity of the strain to spread person to person." "Person to person" was crossed out and replaced with "among humans." The release was not alarmist but clearly and directly indicated the elements of the swine flu outbreak that suggested a pandemic.

Like the influenza experts' report, the final press release toned down the possibility of a pandemic by modifying the characterization of the evidence and presenting a milder depiction of the new strain. For example, the release, titled "Experts' Recommendation on New Flu Strain," began, "Despite its potentialities, the new influenza strain isolated in the USA has not yet caused the kind of epidemics seen in 1957 and 1968."[29] But even with this caveat, the release presents the epidemiological evidence more directly than does the report produced by the meeting. The press release characterizes the events at Fort Dix as demonstrating the "capacity of the virus to spread among humans" but does not mention waiting for further information from the surveillance system. The release was more of a call to action for vaccine-producing nations to prepare for "possible epidemics" than a recommendation to wait and see.

As one of the primary authors of the WHO's report on the experts' meeting, Dowdle was involved in drafting both the report and the press release. Speaking about the 7–8 April 1976 meeting years later, Dowdle did not recall there being a "big fuss" over the phrase "person-to-person" and suggests that the report's wording made the term inessential. But Dowdle did agree that the revisions made from to draft to final version were clearly designed to make the document more calming. Ultimately, however, Dowdle stated that the document in Geneva reflected his thinking, too. The science at Fort Dix was clear—it was a novel strain, and there was person-to-person spread—but the next set of data was not there; the virus did not appear to be spreading, either in the area surrounding the camp or anywhere else in the world. As Dowdle said, "No matter how bad your surveillance is, you should have picked up something."[30]

The other U.S. representative at the meeting, J. Donald Millar, had a different impression of the key elements of the meeting and its impact on the report: "[No other nation] wanted to go our route, but nobody thought they could go our route." Only the United States had the vaccine production capacity to mount such a program and the logistical expertise and experience to coordinate the delivery and injections. The United States had carried out the large-scale vaccine campaigns in West Africa and had provided the lion's share of workers to organize and staff the global eradication of smallpox. As Millar stated it, there were a thousand CDC employees out in the various state health departments whose specialty was the implementation of public health programs. Many of the people involved in planning and implementing the Swine Flu Program were old "African hands" who were "eager to get back into some mass campaigning." Millar retained notes he had taken at or shortly after the Geneva meeting. He understood the opinions of influenza experts from other nations to have been categorical: "*NO WAY* vaccine can be made for more than a few developed countries . . . [or] could be delivered [throughout the world] even if available."[31]

Perhaps the person with the best vantage point to get an overview of the influenza experts' meeting was D. A. Henderson. As previously discussed, Henderson had a unique mix of experience; he was not only familiar with influenza and the WHO but had been involved in coordinating activities with both national health services and vaccine manufacturers. He had developed the U.S. system for tracking the 1957 Asian flu pandemic; he headed the WHO-sponsored campaign to eradicate smallpox globally; and he had worked closely with Charles Cockburn specifically regarding swine flu at Fort Dix and more generally at the WHO's communicable diseases division. Again, when filling in for Cockburn as director of that division, Henderson had chaired a meeting of vaccine manufacturers who had expressed their limited capacity for rapid production of influenza vaccines on an expedited basis. In a 1979 letter to Richard Neustadt criticizing Neustadt and Fineberg's interpretation of events in their book *The Swine Flu Affair,* Henderson stated: "We did convene an international group and made available to them all the facts. They had the option of 'viewing with concern' [and] alarming their own population but with limited capacity to respond with vaccine. Or, as they elected to do, highlight the fact that the disease was mild, they would commence to produce vaccine to the extent possible and would 'wait and see.' In retrospect, the decision of the international committee may be viewed as sound and rational when, in fact, I know the decision to have been born of necessity."[32]

In developing its recommendations, the WHO had traveled opposite to the direction the USPHS took in reaching its decision. Whereas the U.S. authorities increasingly emphasized the potential dangers of the new influenza strain, the WHO emphasized the evidence that suggested a mild pandemic spread or none at all. Both decisions were, in their own ways, shaped by non-scientific elements. Many in the United States perceived it necessary to over-emphasize the probability of an influenza pandemic to ensure that the Ford administration would support the inoculation campaign and that Congress would fund it. For the WHO, the relative inability of national health systems to produce inactivated vaccines, the concern over the premature use of un-stable live-virus vaccines, and fears of provoking panic had prompted a toning down of the potential pandemic threat of A/New Jersey.

Whatever the truth about the various member states' vaccine production capabilities, the fragmentary information available implies that influenza experts formed an elite group who concurred on a technical approach to the new viral strain. Significantly, even China, the home of the barefoot doctors, which had only recently rejoined the WHO, was discussing the technical solution of live-virus vaccines. The experts shared the scientific know-how, but it seems that—aside from Japan and maybe Australia and France—the expertise was not backed with productive and government support for large-scale in-oculation programs. Because influenza had not been made a vaccination priority previously, national industries had not invested in vaccine production. Ian Furminger's experience with Glaxo is telling; the firm made more money from animal vaccines than from human vaccines. Without an infrastructure on which to build, it would have been much more difficult—if not impos-sible—to ramp up manufacturing to support a crash immunization program.

The uneven capabilities in the handful of nations represented at the in-fluenza experts' meeting created different thresholds for triggering program-matic response. For various reasons—previous preparation for a campaign, large domestic manufacturing capacity, prior financial support for influenza vaccines, strong commitment to technical solutions—the United States had a greater willingness to respond to a potential pandemic with a large inoculation solution. For other nations, attempting a similar program would have been, if not impossible, at the least much more expensive and disruptive; therefore, they needed much greater surety that a pandemic was in the offing. The WHO was in an impossible position, and it is not surprising that the evidence suggesting a pandemic to be unlikely seemed the most compelling to it.

The break between the United States and the WHO was now clear. Only Canada opted to pursue a vaccination program similar to the one in the United States. But the United States and Canada would face a number of obstacles in carrying out their vaccination programs. When a flu epidemic did come in 1977, moreover, it was not the epidemic anticipated by the influenza experts. Instead, the unusual event served as the second blow in a one-two punch that discredited the interventionist approach to influenza pandemics and dampened enthusiasm for pandemic planning for the next two decades.

CHAPTER 10

A Program Begins and Ends
and an Epidemic Appears

The United States and Canada were alone in planning large-scale vaccination programs, and the two nations would each have to overcome a host of challenges if the campaigns were to succeed. With respect to logistics, they confronted similar problems, but each nation also faced unique obstacles. In the United States, some of these challenges were anticipated, some were anticipated but not properly communicated, and some were completely unexpected. In Canada, obtaining vaccine for the program presented an overwhelming difficulty. Finally, the influenza virus itself remained a wild card. The anticipated influenza epidemic did not arrive in 1976. An unanticipated epidemic did occur the following year, but with a little human help. As a result of these momentous two years, the interventionist approach to influenza pandemic planning was sharply discredited, and preparation for a possible influenza pandemic atrophied over the next two decades, until reawakened by events in 1997.

The Swine Flu Program Begins

In the early spring of 1976, influenza researchers in the United States anticipated a possible pandemic, public health experts proposed a vaccination effort to protect the public, and the president endorsed such an undertaking. Now the difficult task of creating the program began. Authorities would have to solve a number of logistical and organizational issues, and the administrators of the National Influenza Immunization Program got right to work on them.

The United States Public Health Service officials involved did freely state that there might not be a pandemic, but the hard work of creating a mammoth vaccination campaign colored their perceptions of the ambiguous evidence. Nowhere is this shaping of perceptions clearer than in the USPHS experts' response to the Common Cold Unit experiment. As was previously discussed, some members of the WHO expert committee on influenza thought the experiment to have demonstrated that the new virus from Fort Dix, A/New Jersey, prompted a mild infection and thus posed no great danger to the public. Officials at the USPHS keyed on a different aspect of the experiment. For U.S. researchers, the primary evidence generated from the experiment was the virus's transmissibility. For example, J. Donald Millar stated that although the experiment was too small to draw any definitive conclusions, it did indicate that A/New Jersey was "quite infectious." Michael Hattwick, the chair of a unit devoted to "respiratory and special pathogens" at the CDC's Bureau of Epidemiology, labeled the fact that "all 6 people spread virus" to be "unusual" and judged the experiment to have proved that the swine flu virus would be "very infectious." Even Walter Dowdle, who strongly downplayed the relevance of information from the experiment, stated that it "demonstrated" the virus to be "capable of infecting man and spreading."[1]

The wildly divergent conclusions drawn from the Common Cold Unit experiment highlight the difficulties of using scientific information to craft public policy. For the British, who faced serious problems of vaccine production stemming from financial and infrastructural constraints, the experiment demonstrated the mildness of the infection and hence justified a minimal response to the new virus. For the U.S. public health administrators who had already committed to a massive vaccination program, the infectious nature of the virus was the most prominent aspect revealed by the data. Both scientific conclusions were plausibly true, but the relevance of the data was viewed from different perspectives: one nation had opted for a massive response, and one had opted for a minor response.

Whatever their feelings about the likelihood of a swine flu pandemic, U.S. public health officials could not organize the massive program before them with only half-hearted steps. The time pressures and challenges to be overcome were tremendous and required full commitment from all those involved. The first issues to be addressed were technical. Vaccine manufacturers were busily growing seed stock for the vaccine by injecting Kilbourne's recombinant strain X-53 into fertilized chicken eggs, incubating the eggs, and harvesting the viral material. The next step was to package the bulk viral material into doses of specific potency levels for the individual shots; the potency information would come from the USPHS. The CDC and the National Institutes of Health collaborated on a series of pilot studies to determine effective dose levels and reaction rates to the influenza vaccine injections. The results would be announced in June at a special joint meeting.

The resulting study of over 5,200 adults and children was the largest civilian influenza vaccine trial ever undertaken at that point.[2] The results of the tests were announced on 21 June 1976 at a meeting jointly hosted by the CDC, the National Institute of Allergy and Infectious Diseases, the Bureau of Biologics, and the U.S. Department of Defense. High antibody protection levels and low reaction rates were achieved at the 400 cca level of vaccine for those twenty-four years of age and older. Slightly lower protection rates were observed at the 200 cca level. The results were favorable, and the following day the Immunization Practices Advisory Committee (IPAC) issued its recommendation that the vaccination program continue and the 200 cca single-dose vaccines be used for those aged twenty-four and older. Using the 200 cca level instead of the slightly more effective 400 cca level would double the amount of vaccines that could be produced with only a minimal decline in effective antibody response.[3]

The results of the trial were not as favorable for those under twenty-four, however. This group of subjects did produce effective antibody response to single-dose levels of vaccine, but higher levels of viral material and whole virus preparations were associated with higher reaction rates, generally involving fevers or sore arms. Low dose levels did result in a lower level of side effects— fewer and milder—but they did not yield sufficient antibody levels to ensure protection. Preliminary results suggested that younger children required two-dose schedules, where the first dose "primed" the patient for a second dose of the vaccine three to four weeks later. High levels of vaccine protection were achieved with the doses separated in this fashion. Vaccine trials in this younger population required more study, so the IPAC members deferred issuing a vaccine recommendation for this group.[4] As with the adult population, vaccine reaction rates in children gave no indication of the serious neurological complaints that would later be associated with the swine flu injections.

A second, practical goal to be attained was getting official congressional sanction for the program. President Ford's announcement on 24 March had merely stated that such a program was required. Authorization and funding would have to come from the Congress. In a series of hearings before the House Subcommittee on Health and the Environment, chaired by Congressman Paul Rogers, and the Senate Subcommittee on Health, chaired by Senator Ted Kennedy, public health and administrative experts testified on the necessity of the program. The plan emerged intact after Senator Kennedy was dissuaded from piggy-backing other childhood immunization plans onto the program, and the bill authorizing the program was signed into law (Public Law 94-266) by President Ford on 15 April 1976. The manufacturers' production of vaccine was now guaranteed for purchase.[5]

The program was to provide individual states with money and vaccines to implement the injections. Each state and territory had to apply for a grant through the CDC, detailing its plan for vaccine distribution and administration. All sixty-two grant awards had been submitted and fifty-six plans had been reviewed and approved by 15 June 1976.[6]

The authorities thus recognized that the tasks to be completed included determining effective dose levels and reaction rates, getting authorizing legislation, and developing project grants with the states for implementing the program. Another issue involved liability, and although this too was foreseen, it became such an impediment that it threatened to halt the program in its tracks. More specifically, the issue concerned determining ultimate legal responsibility for a vaccine produced and certified by private pharmaceutical firms working under government auspices and purchased and administered by public health agencies.

Liability Issues

The question of liability for vaccines, which had been brewing for years, had roots stretching back to the infamous Cutter incident of 1955.[7] Cutter Laboratories, a California-based pharmaceutical firm, had not mastered Jonas Salk's detailed virus inactivation method for producing killed-virus polio vaccines and so had inadvertently distributed polio vaccines with live virus still in it, leading to artificially produced polio infections. Although the pharmaceutical maker Wyeth and perhaps a few other producers of Salk vaccine experienced similar problems, Cutter's doses were far and away more contaminated with live virus material than were any other production lots. Ultimately Cutter Laboratories' contaminated vaccines were responsible for infections in at least 220,000 people, of whom 70,000 developed some muscle weakness, 164 were severely paralyzed, and 10 died.

In the subsequent class-action lawsuit against the company, *Gottsdanker v. Cutter,* the jury ruled that Cutter Laboratories was not negligent in producing the vaccine but was still liable for the harm the vaccines had caused (the ruling was subsequently upheld when the Supreme Court declined to hear the appeal). A new legal standard for litigation was born: companies could be held responsible for the damages they caused even if the products they produced were not improperly made. This standard of "liability without negligence" had monumental importance for the business of vaccination. Because vaccination introduces foreign material into the human body, there can be no absolute guarantee for individuals' reactions. If they occur, vaccine reactions tend to be mild, usually limited to fevers or transitory soreness. But occasionally inoculations prompt more dire reactions, even resulting in death. The adverse reaction rate is part of the calculation that goes into deciding vaccine recommendations. The calculation is based on analyzing the risk of inoculating versus not inoculating and thus always rests on a tradeoff between potential harms. A good vaccine may cause harm or even death in a few cases, but not nearly to the extent seen in natural infection by disease agents. In addition, not everyone who receives a vaccine is protected, and others cannot take the vaccine for various medical reasons, but high levels of vaccination in a community serve to dampen or prevent continued disease transmission, thus protecting those who are not directly protected by vaccination. Public health researchers call this herd immunity. Hence, vaccination promotes the greater good of the public but occasionally does so at great cost to the individual.

Over the next few decades the duties of pharmaceutical companies in producing vaccines were further fleshed out in a series of court rulings. Recognizing that biological products occasionally prompt adverse reactions, courts declared vaccines to be "unavoidably unsafe products."[8] In a landmark 1968 case, *Davis v. Wyeth,* a federal appeals court ruled that although the vaccine in question (Sabin's live-virus polio vaccine) fell under the category of "unavoidably unsafe product," the manufacturer still had a duty to warn the consumer of the potential ill effects of taking it. The court rejected Wyeth's plea that a "one in a million" chance of adverse effects was so minor as to remove the company's duty to warn. The appellate court also ruled that the list of warnings packaged with the materials was insufficient notice, because the plaintiff had received his inoculation as part of a mass campaign against polio and not through a private physician. The case held the pharmaceutical company liable for the way its properly made product was used by a government agency in a mass vaccination campaign.

A similar case upheld by a federal appellate court in 1974, *Reyes v. Wyeth Laboratories,* further alarmed pharmaceutical manufacturers. As in the *Davis* case, the plaintiff in *Reyes* contracted polio following the administration of Sabin live-virus vaccine, and the eight-month-old child was subsequently paralyzed from the waist down. The child was inoculated as part of a mass immunization campaign, and the dose was delivered by a registered nurse. The vaccine was packaged with an insert listing the potential dangers of the vaccine, and the nurse had read the insert. Still, even though the child's mother had signed a waiver of liability for the state of Texas, and a wild strain of polio was circulating in the community and likely caused the child's infection, the jury found in favor of the plaintiff against Wyeth.[9]

Manufacturers and public health officials rightly feared the effect such court rulings would have on vaccine manufacturers and immunization campaigns. Vaccine manufacturing was already a low-profit enterprise, and manufacturers purchased liability insurance to guard against adverse judgments. The outcome of *Reyes* and similar cases suggested that pharmaceutical manufacturers would likely lose lawsuits charging damage caused by a vaccine; this prompted insurance firms to raise their liability rates, further eroding the profitability of the vaccine manufacturing sector. Public health officials identified several manufacturing firms that had already abandoned the field of vaccine production, and it was likely that others would soon follow. These officials dreaded the fact that vaccine production might soon be limited to a few companies or even only one, which would put production on a precarious footing: supplies could easily be disrupted by trouble in just one firm or facility.[10]

By January 1976, recognizing this potentially dangerous reduction of vaccine producers and the likelihood that cases such as *Reyes v. Wyeth* would accelerate, the CDC was drafting proposals to have the federal government indemnify manufacturers for any vaccine approved by the federal government and administered by either public health workers or private physicians. Since the federal government was "carrying out the responsibility to prevent and control communicable diseases," the CDC argued, it should bear the responsibility to "support persons seriously injured as a result of the inherent risks in vaccines recommended and taken for both personal and community protection."[11] But the speed of events outstripped the CDC's preparation for the contentious issue. Federal liability for vaccines would have to be authorized by Congress, but drafts of the CDC's liability proposal had not yet circulated outside public health circles by the onset of the swine flu whirlwind.

As vaccine manufacturers ramped up production, they began to seek insurance coverage for the vaccines they were producing.[12] They soon discovered that no insurance company would sell them a policy covering the vaccines they were making for the Swine Flu Program. Insurance companies calculate the risk of an event and offer insurance priced to that risk. But insurers looked at the scope of the program—more than 200 million doses in a judicial environment that had just ruled for the plaintiff in the *Reyes* case and a society they saw as increasingly litigious—and feared they could not adequately divine the potential expense involved. The insurers were afraid that given the sheer number of people receiving injections, many would sue even if the vaccine caused few or even no ill effects. Therefore, they refused to assume the risk of vaccine-related lawsuits under any price. Vaccine manufacturers declined to self-insure their vaccines because they feared that even frivolous lawsuits would result in enormous expenses in court costs. And without insurance, manufacturers refused to sell vaccine to the federal government.

The only resolution to this stalemate would have to come from Congress. Lawyers at the Department of Health, Education, and Welfare drafted an indemnity bill that the Office of Management and Budget approved, and it was submitted to Congress—where it stayed. The bill remained in committee for several reasons. First, some legislators suspected that pharmaceutical companies were seeking to shift responsibility for vaccine manufacturing onto the federal government. Second, some believed that insurance companies were hoping to shunt all the risks to the government, leaving them to make a profit on other, far safer policies they were willing to sell to vaccine makers. The overriding concern, however, seems to have been the fear that indemnifying vaccine manufacturers would set an unfortunate precedent, so that other industries doing business with the government would start asking it to shoulder their risks. Whatever the reasons, vaccine manufacturers, insurers, and Congress were at an impasse, and influenza vaccine manufacturing had stopped. It would take a dramatic event to restart it.

Canada's Problems

Canada too was having problems acquiring the doses required for its vaccination campaign, but unlike the United States, Canada's problems did not stem from manufacturers refusing to make vaccine. Rather, Canada had little if any influenza vaccine production capacity at all. Estimates place the production of Canadian-based pharmaceutical firms at only 100,000 doses a year, a mere 5 percent of the nation's annual use. Even with an extraordinary effort, Canadian firms could produce only 300,000 doses for a given flu season. To carry out the large-scale vaccination campaign they envisioned, Canadian health officials would need to find additional sources of A/New Jersey vaccines.[13]

In some ways the Canadian vaccination plan was simpler than the one proposed by the United States. Canadian health officials had explicitly tied their vaccination decision to A/New Jersey's presumed relationship to Spanish flu. Spanish flu's mortality blow had fallen hardest on young adults. Therefore, Canadian officials decided to inoculate young adults, with an emphasis on reaching those between the ages of twenty and fifty. Because children younger than sixteen had higher reaction rates to the shots, Canadian health officials decided they would not vaccinate those fifteen or younger. When the Canadian health official John Furesz announced his country's plan to not inoculate children at the joint influenza meeting in Washington, D.C., on 25 March 1976, the American pediatrician Samuel Katz was "horrified."[14] The Canadian program would not need to craft different recommendations and dose schedules for their population; instead, they needed a bivalent dose (A/New Jersey and A/Victoria) for their high-risk patients and a monovalent (A/New Jersey) for the rest of their adult population.

Canadian health officials hoped to acquire these vaccines from the same source that provided 95 percent of their yearly vaccine: the United States. Initially that hope seemed reasonable. In mid-April 1976 the U.S. State Department informed Canadian health officials that the United States would make up the difference between the amount of vaccine Canada needed and the amount it could obtain from other sources. But promises made to its northern neighbor raised questions about what the United States should do for its southern neighbor. Some U.S. officials wondered why vaccine would be made available to Canada but not to Mexico. Eventually President Ford was forced to intervene in the dispute. Canada and Mexico would receive doses only after U.S. demand was met. Canadian and Mexican health officials would have to find other sources of vaccine if they wanted to protect their citizens.

With U.S. pharmaceutical firms cut off as a source for vaccine, at least until the more than 200 million U.S. citizens had received their doses, Canadian health officials searched abroad. They contracted with Commonwealth Serum Laboratories, in Australia, for 8 million doses and purchased an additional 2–3 million doses from Evans Medical, in the United Kingdom. Even piecing together vaccine supplies in this way, Canada seems to have been a few million doses short of the amount its planned vaccination program required.[15]

Canada's travails in acquiring vaccine for its immunization program illustrate the larger problem of pandemic response in 1976. Vaccine manufacturers in the United States produced the lion's share of vaccine for the export market. When that production was commandeered for domestic consumption, other national health programs were left to scramble to find vaccine. Canada was able to purchase vaccine for its immunization program only because other nations had declined to mount large-scale vaccination campaigns. The 8 million doses purchased from an Australian firm and the 2–3 million from the British firm would not have been available if these nations had opted for crash immunization programs. Canada would have been forced to make hard ethical and practical choices in determining which of its citizens should receive its meager supply of vaccine, and these decisions would have been further complicated by the fact that its southern neighbor was vaccinating its entire population.

The NIIP Jump-started

In 1976 the United States celebrated the bicentennial of its national independence, and 4,400 members of Pennsylvania's American Legion, along with relatives and other guests, celebrated in Philadelphia's Center City, at the Bellevue-Stratford Hotel.[16] The raucous meeting ended on 24 July 1976, and members dispersed to their hometowns around the state. On Friday, 30 July 1976, a physician in Bloomsburg, Pennsylvania, discovered that three patients he was treating for high fevers and pneumonia had all attended the Legionnaires' convention the week before. He contacted the Pennsylvania State Department of Health to inquire whether other cases had been reported but was informed that the department was closed for the weekend. By the following Monday morning, when it reopened, several additional cases had been reported. The state health department immediately contacted the CDC to report the unusual cluster of pneumonia cases.

The symptomology of the illness—acute onset of fever, chills, headache, body aches, and eventual development of a cough—had the CDC considering influenza. They quickly solicited blood and other samples and dispatched epidemiologists to assist Pennsylvania's health department in its investigation. Laboratory workers from the CDC immediately put samples collected from the patients through a battery of diagnostic tests to determine whether influenza was the cause, and the answer was quickly clear: whatever had caused the illnesses among the Legionnaires was not influenza. By 5 August 1976 the CDC announced that the affliction was definitively not swine flu. Although not related to the Swine Flu Program, the CDC would be under intense pressure over the ensuing months to determine the cause of "Legionnaires' disease" (as the illness was dubbed).[17]

Public health officials were not the only ones to think of swine flu when the Legionnaires' cases were first reported. Federal legislators also thought a swine flu pandemic had arrived and were not mollified by the CDC's announcement that the illnesses were not caused by influenza.[18] They could easily envision that the media frenzy currently enveloping the Legionnaires' mystery would be the same if a swine flu pandemic appeared. And when the media came to public health officials to inquire why there was no vaccination program protecting the public, USPHS officials would point the finger right at Congress and the stalled liability bill. The subcommittee chairs, Rogers and Kennedy, immediately took action. The Federal Tort Claims Act, which had been mired in Senate and House subcommittees, was quickly passed out for consideration, first on the floor of the Senate. After passage there, the bill was brought to the floor of the House of Representatives. After a vigorous but short debate, the bill passed the House on a vote of 250 to 83 and was delivered to the president for his signature. President Ford signed the Tort Claims Act (Public Law 94–380) into law on 12 August 1976. The National Influenza Immunization Program was back in business, but a new timetable would have to be created.

The original plan had called for a two-stage vaccination process, with high-risk patients being vaccinated in late July and early August. The program would then inoculate the general population in early September. The nearly two-month hiatus had wrecked these plans, and so the program administrators telescoped the two-phase operation into a single massive effort. The logistics of managing two streams of vaccine (bivalent for high-risk and monovalent for the general population) were further complicated by the lack of any recommendation about the dose schedule for children, which had not yet been determined. But far and away the biggest problem for the program would be the availability of the vaccines.

The nearly two-month impasse over liability issues had slowed production by the four pharmaceutical firms. Although the firms had made vaccine prior to the liability impasse, and most had maintained at least some production during the halt, the new manufacturing schedules required the companies to ramp up production. Other factors further affected the anticipated delivery schedule. One pharmaceutical firm, Parke, Davis, had initially manufactured its vaccine using the wrong viral strain. Instead of using A/New Jersey/76, Parke, Davis had mistakenly used the A/Swine/1976/31 "Shope-like" virus. This forced the rejection of forty-three lots, more than four million doses of vaccine. Precious time was also lost, for Parke, Davis had to restart the production process from the initial step, growing seed stock.[19] Other firms also suggested that their production lagged because the number of vaccine doses generated per egg was unexpectedly low.

There was one final delay before the program could begin. Administrators for the NIIP had hoped to begin vaccinating by late September, but they were forced to wait until 1 October because the vaccine manufacturers' lawyers interpreted the new law as granting federal liability protection only after the start of the fiscal year, 1 October. Finally, with great fanfare, the inoculations began.

The injection programs started slowly (not all states had received their allotments of vaccine by the first of October) but steadily began to pick up speed. By the tenth day of the immunization schedule, one million Americans had received their shots, and the per-day rate of inoculations was accelerating. The star-crossed immunization program then suffered another setback, one that clearly could have been avoided.

On 11 October 1976, three elderly people in Pittsburgh, Pennsylvania (Allegheny County), died suddenly hours after receiving their swine flu shots. All three had received their injections at the same clinic, along with 1,239 other people. The Allegheny County coroner stated that he wanted to test whether the vaccinations had played a role in the victims' sudden demise. On 12 October the Allegheny Department of Health suspended its vaccination program until the vaccine was cleared. The media quickly picked up on this story, and it became national headline news. All the major news networks had prominent features, and some media outlets created hyperbolic stories of the course of events in Pittsburgh. The nadir was reached by the *New York Post,* which described (or invented) a lurid account of the scene at the clinic. Public health officials decried the "body count" mentality of the press even as they searched for additional sudden deaths associated with the swine flu injections.[20]

Following the widespread media coverage, nine states suspended their swine flu vaccination program. On 14 October 1976, Assistant Secretary of Health Theodore Cooper announced that an investigation of the vaccine used at the clinic showed no contaminants or problems and that the victims' deaths were due to previous heart conditions. In a visible vote of confidence for the vaccine and the program, President Ford and his family were inoculated with the vaccine at the White House. The CDC reported that temporally associated deaths (illness or deaths within forty-eight hours of inoculation) occurred at a rate of 5/100,000. Because the anticipated death rate per day for all causes among citizens in Pennsylvania was 17/100,000, it was to be expected that a number of deaths would occur shortly after the influenza injection, and though the temporal connection might seem to imply a causal connection between the injection and the deaths, they were unrelated.

But the damage to the Swine Flu Program had already been done. Time and momentum had been lost because of clinic closures in several states and the publicity that suggested the shots were deadly. Whereas earlier polls had shown the percentage of people who intended to receive the vaccine as steadily rising, in the weeks following the Pittsburgh deaths, polls showed a drop in the acceptance rate, from 57 percent to 42 percent of people interviewed. During the same period, those intending not to be vaccinated climbed from 18 percent to 36 percent of the individuals surveyed.[21]

The deaths of these three elderly residents of Pittsburgh may have been uncontrollable, but the media response was not. The epidemiologists at the CDC had anticipated coincidental deaths but had failed to warn the public or the media about the likelihood of these events. Worse, the Department of Health, Education, and Welfare had responded slowly to the first reports out of Pittsburgh and seemed surprised by the ensuing frenzy. Apparently the lessons of the intensity of the media response to Legionnaires' disease had not made a lasting impression on the department's public relations officers.

Despite the Pittsburgh setbacks, the program continued on, with the number of vaccinations given per week steadily increasing, reaching a peak of over 6 million injected during the week ending 20 November. The number dropped slightly below 5 million during the week of Thanksgiving, but by 27 November 1976 more than 30 million people had received swine flu immunization, and manufacturers had shipped nearly 110 million doses of the vaccine. The program was still running behind schedule in terms of production and injections but appeared to be picking up speed in both areas.[22]

Remarkably, the campaign was succeeding despite the fact that a swine flu pandemic had not appeared. In fact, the fall and early winter of 1976 was marked by little influenza activity anywhere in the world, a point not overlooked by the campaign's critics. The program was created to protect the American public from a pandemic of swine flu. The costs of a pandemic—both in human and economic terms—justified certain risks inevitable in introducing biological materials into such a large number of people. But absent the pandemic risk, the effects of vaccination outweigh the benefits. The trigger for this reassessment of risk was an unexpected and poorly understood affliction with an exotic name.

Guillain-Barré Syndrome

Guillain-Barré syndrome (GBS) is a notoriously difficult affliction to diagnose. The condition usually begins with a tingling sensation in the extremities and a gradual weakening in the muscles or reflexes moving up into the trunk of the afflicted person's body in a process known as "ascending paralysis." The condition may persist for weeks before abating, and most patients do make a complete recovery. There is no absolute laboratory test for the affliction; diagnosis is made by assessing symptoms. The condition was rarely identified prior to the 1970s because most cases were masked by its symptoms similarity to those of a polio infection. Currently, neurologists believe that either infections, especially respiratory or intestinal ones producing high fevers, or an immune response to certain vaccines may trigger the condition. In 1976 GBS was quite poorly understood, with only spotty estimates of the number of cases in a year. Its etiology was even more poorly understood. A search of the medical literature on GBS conducted at that time revealed only one case temporally associated with influenza A vaccination and four associated with being struck by lightning, hardly enough evidence to predict the rate of GBS cases.[23]

Collecting a list of possible side effects to influenza vaccines prior to the onset of the program, CDC epidemiologists had listed "neurological disorders" as a rare complication but had not specifically identified Guillain-Barré as a possible complaint. Therefore, when a Minnesota public health worker called the CDC's surveillance line for tracking reactions to swine flu inoculations to report a temporal association of the vaccine with a GBS case, CDC epidemiologists attached little importance to the information. However, they began to become interested in the question when a report from Minnesota issued on 19 November 1976 listed four more GBS cases among individuals who had received the vaccine. The Minnesota Department of Health subsequently forwarded the preliminary results of its investigation to the CDC and reported no association between the affliction and the vaccine. On 2 December 1976, however, a physician from Alabama called to report three cases of GBS in people from that state who had received the swine flu vaccine. The CDC initiated a formal investigation of Alabama and Minnesota, uncovering additional cases among the vaccinated and unvaccinated alike over the next seven days.[24]

Epidemiology is a numbers game—counting up the afflicted, comparing the number against baseline incidence, and projecting or detecting trends. The CDC epidemiologists were gathering numbers, but they had no baseline incidence of GBS cases against which to compare these numbers. The CDC did not list GBS as a reportable disease, so officials there had no clear idea of how many cases to expect, and the only systematic assessment on GBS incidence covered a single county in Minnesota (Olmstead). To remedy this lack, CDC investigators solicited information from several states and soon had a pool of cases. Although the GBS cases identified were equally split between the vaccinated and unvaccinated, the number of GBS sufferers who had been vaccinated were overrepresented as part of the total number of those diagnosed, because at the time of the identification of the afflicted, only 30 percent of the adult population had received the swine flu vaccine. Plotting vaccinated GBS cases revealed that the date of the condition's onset peaked two to three weeks after inoculation, a pattern that marked the presumed course of GBS onset. Based on this small amount of available data, it appeared that swine flu vaccination prompted elevated cases of GBS.[25]

If a pandemic had been occurring, the increased risk of GBS cases would be an acceptable risk. In the absence of a swine flu pandemic, the risks of increased GBS cases was completely unacceptable. On 16 December 1976, Assistant Secretary of Health Theodore Cooper announced the temporary suspension of the Swine Flu Program to investigate the association of inoculation and elevated GBS cases. The program never restarted.[26]

In the present day, it remains unclear whether the Swine Flu Program prompted increased numbers of GBS cases, and neurologists still debate the point. In 2004 the National Academy of Sciences concluded in its report *Immunization Safety Review* that "the evidence favored acceptance of a causal relationship between the 1976 swine influenza vaccine and GBS in adults," but this investigation does not appear to have settled the dispute. Those who believe the inoculations caused increased GBS cases point to the numbers of cases the CDC epidemiologists reported and the patterns they described. Those who deny the connection point out that there is no widely accepted standard for diagnosing GBS and question the reliability of the case identification rate underlying the CDC investigation. More specifically, they argue that actively soliciting reports of GBS complications and the influenza vaccine could create a bias in favor of identifying neurological complaints among the vaccinated, a concern that was pointed out by the Mayo Clinic neurologist Peter Dyck and shared by Michael Gregg, a deputy director of the CDC's Bureau of Epidemiology to whom Dyck mentioned the matter in a letter from 28 December 1976. Dyck suggested that questionnaires soliciting GBS symptoms would result in an inflated response rate from those receiving the vaccines and that the only sure way to assess the relationship between the vaccine and GBS would be by "some field epidemiological studies"; in an annotation, Gregg appended "agree." Nonetheless, the numbers generated by the CDC for its assessment of vaccine-caused GBS cases did not include field epidemiological studies.[27]

Settling this contentious issue falls beyond this book's scope, but it is suggestive to examine the discovery mechanisms in play for the earliest cases of GBS identified in relation to swine flu. The initial identification of the relationship was a mistake. One of the first clinicians to look for an association between influenza vaccination and GBS incidence did so because he misheard an audiotaped report. "The tape (Audio-Digest Foundation, Family Practice, Volume 24, Number 38) was recorded at a conference held at the University of California, Los Angeles, just as vaccinations were getting under way in October 1976. On the tape, Dr. Paul F. Wehrle tells how difficult it is to distinguish incidental illness from true side effects . . . the listening clinician *mistakenly* believed that he had been alerted to a *likely* complication [instead of a false association]. He looked for it and found it and was right for the wrong reasons."[28]

Regardless of whether the swine flu shots resulted in increased rates of GBS, the target of the campaign had not appeared; there was no swine flu pandemic to justify the expenditure of time, effort, and money—and the possible injuries and deaths. The resulting judgment of the campaign was harsh, led by the *New York Times,* whose editorial page had consistently criticized the campaign. Writing in the paper, Harry Schwartz famously labeled the program a "fiasco," an assessment shared by the incoming secretary of Health, Education, and Welfare, Joseph Califano Jr., appointed by the newly elected president,

Jimmy Carter, came in with the mandate of change, and he made his mark right off the bat by requesting the resignation of Assistant Secretary Theodore Cooper. On 4 February 1977 Califano also called CDC director David Sencer to Washington, where Califano's undersecretary requested his resignation. Sencer asked for, and was given, time to consider his options. Unfortunately, the information of his impending dismissal began to leak to the press. On 7 February 1977 the two men appeared at a meeting on the moratorium on the Swine Flu Program that received extensive media coverage; while there, Califano called Sencer aside, doing so in full view of the cameras. Shortly thereafter Califano announced Sencer's resignation, creating the impression he had just publicly fired Sencer. This was shabby treatment for a man who had given sixteen years of service to the CDC, eleven years as its director. Califano explained the firing by saying, "The Communicable Disease Center could do with some fresh air, with some fresh faces"; it was clear, however, that Sencer was taking the fall for the failed Swine Flu Program.[29]

Califano also commissioned a report on the Swine Flu Program to assess the process from inception to conclusion. Califano tapped Richard E. Neustadt, of the John F. Kennedy School of Government at Harvard University, and Harvey F. Fineberg, director of the graduate program in health policy and management at Harvard's School of Public Health, to do the study. Neustadt and Fineberg's exhaustive investigation utilized many interviews, both on and off the record, to construct a narrative and analysis of the project with an eye to producing recommendations for future programs from the lessons learned. The report, subsequently published as a book, provoked controversy among many of those involved in the Swine Flu Program. While appreciating the detailed chronology and acknowledging the need for periodic programmatic reassessment to determine the continued necessity of previous decisions— dubbed "Alexander's questions," after E. Russell Alexander, who had raised this suggestion at the 10 March 1976 ACIP meeting—many decried how the report characterized the motives of the officials involved in deciding for the vaccination campaign. Nevertheless, the book remains the signal touchstone for examining the Swine Flu Program.

The National Influenza Immunization Program was a public failure of the interventionist approach to controlling influenza. Scientists had failed by incorrectly predicting a pandemic, leading officials to create a program to protect against a threat that never appeared. Moreover, the science failed again in the following year, 1977, but this time the scientists involved prompted an epidemic instead of guarding against one. And though not as well publicized as swine flu, the incident would shape public health preparation for pandemic influenza for the next two decades.

Russian Flu, 1977

The 1976–1977 influenza season in the Northern Hemisphere was quiet. Swine flu did not reappear, and only the A/Victoria strain from the previous year circulated in any great volume. Ironically, administrators at the U.S. Department of Health, Education, and Welfare were forced to lift their moratorium on swine flu doses for high-risk patients because all vaccine for A/Victoria strain had been combined with A/New Jersey in bivalent doses. But aside from the flare-up of A/Victoria strains, the spring of 1977 ended with a low amount of overall influenza activity.[30]

The onset of the next flu season, in the fall of 1977, was much the same as the preceding year. Then, on 7 December 1977, the WHO notified the CDC of isolates of a strain of H1N1 forwarded by the Soviet Union. The virus was recovered on 21 November 1977 in the midst of a localized influenza epidemic. The Soviet report confirmed a previous report the CDC had received from Hong Kong on 25 November 1977 that also suggested an H1N1 strain was in circulation. The CDC requested that samples be sent to it for study, and these samples arrived on 14 December 1977.[31]

The new influenza strain, subsequently (and incorrectly, as it would turn out) dubbed "Russian flu 1977," was puzzling. Historically, when a new viral type appeared, it drove the prevailing strain out. But this virus showed no sign of doing that; instead, both the new strain and the prevailing one (the H1N1 Russian flu and H3N2 Texas, a drifted variant of A/Victoria) circulated through the population. Although the new strain fit the eleven-year-cycle theory, it did not fit the recycling theory. According to the latter, the next strain to appear should be related to Spanish flu, and Russian flu was not. The new virus also had an unusual infection pattern. Instead of striking all the population, it seemed to disproportionately infect those under the age of twenty. Finally, tests showed the virus to react strongly to reagents from the early 1950s, suggesting that it was closely related to strains that had circulated from 1947 through 1957.[32]

The reason for the virus's unusual infection and reaction pattern was soon discovered. The virus was not simply *like* a strain that had circulated in the 1950s; the virus *was* a strain that had circulated in the 1950s, specifically, the H1N1 "Scandinavian" strain that had been isolated in 1950–1951. The Russian flu of 1977 was caused by the same strain that had circulated twenty-seven years earlier. Because of the high mutation rate of the influenza virus—especially under the pressure of the human immune system—the only explanation was that the virus had accidentally escaped from a laboratory. In addition, because the first cases were seen in China between May and October 1977, the epidemic likely originated there. As was previously mentioned, Chinese researchers were working on live-virus strains as early as 1972, and they no doubt had been pursuing influenza research since that date. The H1N1 strain that was prompting elevated cases of influenza sickness and death around the world (the drifted descendants of which still circulate in the world today) likely resulted from a Chinese laboratory mistake.[33]

Legacies

The supporters of the National Influenza Immunization Program point to the successes of the crash-immunization effort. More than 42 million doses of vaccine were injected in the eleven weeks from 1 October to 16 December 1976. This total was more than twice the number of people receiving the vaccine in any previous year in the United States. Despite a number of setbacks and delays, manufacturers quickly produced over 157 million doses of a vaccine that met high quality standards for influenza vaccine, and they no doubt could have produced more if the demand for the vaccine had continued. Finally, some of the key experts involved in the program stated that faced with the same evidence, they would make the same recommendations.[34]

The public, however, viewed the Swine Flu Program as a failure. In addition, the pointed fingers and assignments of blame that trailed in the wake of the program must have given public health experts pause. They must have been similarly concerned by the inadvertently triggered Russian flu of 1977. A global epidemic had been sparked by a laboratory error, and influenza scientists all knew it. The WHO meeting in Geneva on 7–8 April 1976 illustrated that laboratories were engaging in potentially risky research, such as the deliberate infection of humans with novel strains and the use of unstable attenuated live-virus vaccines. Such risky research might be justified if the scientific community was certain that a pandemic was imminent, but nobody could make such a prediction.

The back-to-back failures of pandemic planning and research—one public and the other widely known in the research community—discredited the activist approach to preparing for a pandemic. The superheated atmosphere of international conferences and workshops to plan for the "forecast" pandemic of 1978 dissipated. The eleven-year-cycle theory of influenza pandemics was abandoned, and the logic of the recycling theory came into question. Influenza researchers were chastened; the wily influenza virus had tricked them again.

The events in 1976 and 1977 demonstrated the failure of a nation-centered approach and the danger of risky, unregulated vaccine research. The two years also demonstrated the inherent limitations of nation-centered approaches to international pandemic events. The international technical elites were evaluating the science surrounding new viral strains, but they recommended courses of actions that only a handful of states could even attempt. And the difficulties encountered by the United States, the largest producer of influenza vaccines at the time, left it unclear whether any state could pursue the recommended courses of action. Clearly the nation-centered model had failed, and new methods would have to be developed.

Over the next few years the WHO faced an institutional crisis. Proponents of "health for all" argued that the WHO should concentrate on improving basic health care for all its member states, which in effect meant a focus on the "developing" nations. This type of approach emphasized social and economic support for health. Advocates for technical solutions, mainly in the "developed" nations, pushed for a continued focus on specific disease eradication and control and promoted the use of vaccines and medicants to improve health. These split goals and methods created great turmoil in the WHO and prompted a bitter and far-reaching financial crisis as wealthy nations began to designate funds they sent the WHO as being earmarked for specific programs, not as general dues paid to the organization.[35]

The financial crisis affected the WHO throughout the 1980s and 1990s and still remains a thorny issue, but by far the biggest challenge to the organization was found in the issue of emerging diseases. The resurgence of tuberculosis and other such age-old health threats, the increasing trend of antibiotic-resistant bacterial infections, and the explosive appearance of AIDS has demolished the faith of imminent mastery over disease so prevalent among the previous generation of public health administrators. The failure of technical solutions and "magic bullet" approaches to public health has prompted a reevaluation of global public health. Nowhere were these ideas more strongly crystallized than in the response to the AIDS crisis, which created both the technical solution of multidrug therapy and vaccine research and the more social approach that emphasized generalized health care development, including education on avoidance techniques and support for clinics overwhelmed by the disaster. The expensive multidrug regimes, though relatively successful, were priced well outside what impoverished nations could afford, prompting intense negotiations to make the treatment available through generic drug and subsidy programs for poorer nations, where the pandemic hit with the most devastating force. The AIDS pandemic drew attention from both technical and social medicine proponents.

In the ensuing two decades, influenza pandemic planning was ignored or placed at a low priority. Manufacturing capacity declined as pharmaceutical firms abandoned the low-profit, high-risk business of vaccine production, and the number of firms in the industry contracted through buyouts and mergers.

The merger process resulted in a truly globalized vaccine production system with a corporation headquartered in one nation, producing vaccine in another, and selling the vaccine all over the world. At the same time, surveillance capacity and research on the influenza virus continued to expand. Speedier and more powerful tests allowed for rapid identification of new strains, and breakthroughs in genetics allowed influenza experts to discuss the code of the influenza virus in exquisite detail. New and revived infections commanded the attention of national and international health officials, and concern over a possible influenza pandemic retreated to the background. In 1997, however, public health experts would receive a sharp wakeup call that would prompt them to reevaluate influenza pandemic planning. The response to an influenza pandemic was moving into a new era, and with it came new ideas and approaches. But the history of influenza pandemics and previous public health responses still informed strategic preparations.

CHAPTER 11

The Continuing Lessons of Influenza's History

Pandemic influenza remains a threat to human health in the twenty-first century, just as it was in preceding centuries. Combating or mitigating the impact of influenza epidemics continues to rely on the procedures whose value lay behind the establishment of the World Influenza Centre in 1947: detecting a novel strain of influenza in order to manufacture and distribute a protective vaccine against it. But for decades following the events in 1976 and 1977, the effectiveness of these twin elements traveled in opposite directions. Nothing illustrates this divergence better than pointing out that manufacturers still use fertilized egg production methods developed in the 1930s to produce vaccines against viruses now identified by powerful twenty-first-century machines that sort genes through reverse transcription–polymerase chain reaction (RT-PCR). Globalization of vaccine manufacturers and contraction in the number of such firms reshaped the landscape of national and international vaccine production, a process that occurred largely unacknowledged by public health officials, who have faced mounting challenges posed by afflictions including AIDS and tuberculosis. Events in Hong Kong in 1997 and in the years that followed reasserted the threat posed by novel influenza strains and prompted a reassessment of national and international plans for pandemic influenza. Effective, new responses would have to operate on a new global model. Influenza infections simply move too quickly to be combated by a nation-centered vaccination approach.

Hong Kong, 1997

On 6 September 1997, the *Lancet* reported that a small boy in China had died of a new strain of influenza identified as H5N1. This human case of a strain previously found only in birds closely followed scattered reports concerning localized epidemic outbreaks of an illness that was killing chickens and geese in southeastern China throughout the winter and early spring of 1997. A small group of researchers from the CDC joined with Hong Kong's health department to survey the region and determine whether a new influenza virus was circulating. Suddenly, in November and December 1997, the number of cases of people stricken with the H5N1 virus began to pick up. Eighteen people were diagnosed with this strain in Hong Kong, and six of them died. To that point the virus was not well adapted to human transmission, and it seemed that all the infected had contracted the illness from direct contact with infected birds. A survey of the local "wet markets," which were stocked with live chickens, geese, and ducks, showed widespread, albeit low, levels of H5N1 infection in these birds. Close genetic examination of samples gathered from the markets suggested that the virus was developing mutations that had been associated with greater transmission in the human population. Faced with this evidence of a novel influenza strain that appeared to be adapting for human infection, Hong Kong officials ordered the closure of the wet markets and the slaughter of all the poultry and waterfowl there. In dramatic fashion, officials garbed in masks and robes killed all the birds in the market area. The action appeared to have worked; the emerging chain of infection in Hong Kong was broken.[1]

The events in Hong Kong had shaken WHO officials, who realized that the actions taken had served only as a stopgap measure. Many health officials believed that the new H5N1 strain continued to circulate in the rural areas of China and was likely to reemerge. The officials were correct; by 2004 the H5N1 avian strain—dubbed bird flu—was circulating widely throughout Southeast Asia and had been identified in Europe and Africa. The highly pathogenic but poorly transmitted virus continues to be an item of intense concern for influenza researchers and public health officials.

The events in Hong Kong showed that a new and potentially deadly type of influenza had appeared, but there was further reason for alarm, because WHO officials realized that they had no coherent mitigation strategy. Slaughtering poultry and waterfowl was an act of desperation, for few other solutions to the problem were available. The apparent success of this gamble in Hong Kong did not offer a model that could be readily copied in other events, leading public health officials to realize that their outdated pandemic influenza plans needed to be revised.

In examining pandemic planning following the Hong Kong incident, WHO officials concluded that the surveillance system was still insufficient to provide an early warning of an emerging pandemic influenza strain. The powerful new genetics technology had provided vital information, revealing that the new virus seemed to be acquiring potentially dangerous mutations, but surveillance had failed to detect the virus as it circulated through the rural areas of China for months or even years.

The surveillance system was only as strong as its weakest link, and influenza monitoring depended completely on national health programs to provide information about and access to new infections or viruses in a timely fashion. The WHO's concerns with tardy reporting of infections were amply validated just a few years later. In February 2003 Chinese health officials reported that an unidentified agent—subsequently called severe acute respiratory syndrome (SARS)—was causing infections in the country's southeastern provinces. This disease propagated, with clusters of infections popping up throughout Southeast Asia and as far away as Canada. The sudden appearance of a new infectious agent was concerning, but what really disturbed WHO officials was the fact that the Chinese had identified the outbreak as early as November 2002 but had not informed their organization until the affliction began to spill out to surrounding nations.[2] Delayed or suppressed public health information threatens all nations, not just the nation where an infection is circulating.

The WHO officials realized that inadequate or incomplete surveillance endangered global health with respect to a variety of infectious organisms, but based on nearly six decades of experience with the influenza virus, they recognized the special relationship between surveillance and protection against influenza pandemics. As concerned as they were with the surveillance limitations suggested by China's experience with SARS, health officials were even further alarmed by the trend in the manufacturing of influenza vaccines. Two decades of combination in this sector of the pharmaceutical industry had left only a few firms that produced the overwhelming majority of vaccines for the global market. The dangers of this type of arrangement are twofold: first, the fact that much of the manufacturing capacity is in the hands of a few producers makes the supply of vaccine vulnerable, since localized problems can have a widespread impact. Second, because the manufacturers seek to maximize efficiency, they have little room to ramp up production in an emergency. Events would soon illustrate both these dangers.

In 2004 British pharmaceutical inspectors condemned the entire production lot of inactivated influenza doses from the vaccine-maker Chiron for having failed tests of sterility and contamination. Chiron was one of two major manufacturers for the seasonal U.S. influenza vaccine market. The sudden loss of nearly 50 percent of the supply for the U.S. market triggered a hurried scramble for additional vaccines, but there was little to be had, for other vaccine manufacturers were already operating at or near full capacity. Contrary to the situation in 1976, the United States had to solicit access to vaccine production commanded by other nations. In an example of "turn about is fair play," Canadian health officials informed their southern neighbor that they would provide the United States with vaccine only "after Canadian needs [had been] met." Acknowledging the limitations the nation's lack of production capacity had imposed in 1976, Canadian health officials had sought to increase domestic sources by bolstering the use of seasonal vaccines among its citizens. As a result, influenza vaccine was rationed in the United States during the influenza season of 2004–2005.[3]

New Approaches

The combination of events in the late 1990s and early 2000s prompted the WHO to reexamine its tactics regarding pandemic influenza, and this led it to craft a new program. Surveillance and manufacturing, however, remained the key elements for public health action against the influenza virus. To be effective, any response to a pandemic strain must be quick enough to stay ahead of the rapidly transmissible influenza virus, a consideration even more important in today's increasingly interconnected world. Accordingly, the WHO has sought to reverse its traditional surveillance relationship with its member states. Instead of having its experts wait for samples to be sent to the organization's influenza centers, the WHO has sought to provide national health centers with the diagnostic tools to identify emerging strains as quickly as possible on site. Once a new strain is identified and confirmed, the new WHO system calls for sending experts to the area where the virus was first detected. When these experts arrive, they are empowered to take action to choke off the emerging strain by quarantine and widespread use of antivirals and protective vaccines, halting the chain of transmission before it can become established in the human population. The new policy reflects the fact that fast-moving influenza infections will always outstrip manufacturers' abilities to provide protective inactivated influenza vaccines. Also, in 2005 the WHO passed new international health regulations that require all member states to facilitate global cooperation and communication for events deemed "public health emergencies of international concern." As with all WHO edicts, however, this one relies on the voluntary cooperation of nation-states.[4]

This new pandemic response was implicitly geared to interrupting a pandemic of bird flu, or avian H5N1. The H5N1 influenza strain circulating throughout Eurasia and Africa has been marked by poor human-to-human transmission and high mortality in domesticated birds. The sudden die-off of flocks of chickens was seen as an early warning that bird flu was circulating in an area. When health officials detected the likely appearance of bird flu, they could intensively watch the citizens of that region to uncover any infection in the human population. If instances of bird-to-human or human-to-human transmission were detected, WHO officials could rapidly dose the community with antivirals and inoculate the people in the region with an experimental vaccine to prevent the virus from adapting to the human host through serial passage. The design underlying this approach is manifest in the WHO's new pandemic influenza alert system, which notes in its discussion of its first phase that "no animal influenza virus circulating among animals have been reported to cause infection in humans" and stipulates that its phase 4 will be triggered "when human-to-human transmission of an animal or human-animal influenza reassortant virus able to sustain community-level outbreaks has been verified." In response to bird flu, WHO officials were vigilant for infections that would trigger phase 4.[5]

In the spring of 2009 a pandemic strain did appear, but despite their preparations, health officials were still surprised. The pandemic strain was not the feared H5N1 bird flu but an unanticipated reassortant H1N1 swine flu. The virus had cycled through populations undetected at the levels specified in the first stages of the WHO pandemic alert system and was discovered only when it was circulating at the community or regional level. The efficient and widespread transmission of the virus rendered any interdiction campaign moot, and the WHO recognized this reality by quickly raising its pandemic alert level to six (the highest). The novel virus was a pandemic. In the absence of international containment efforts, national health organizations relied on advocating proper hygiene techniques and pushing manufacturers to produce and distribute a protective vaccine. These responses would have been familiar to previous health officials.[6]

Although at this writing a full assessment of the 2009 H1N1 pandemic is not clear, the available accounts suggest that the vaccination effort repeated the course of events from generations before. There was a desperate scramble for vaccine at the outset of the influenza season, but little was available, leading to rationing and shortages. As the pandemic wave crested, manufacturing began to catch up with demand and increasing stocks of vaccine were released. But as the number of new infections declined, so too did the public clamor for the shots. With the end of the influenza season, a large percentage of the year's vaccine sat in inventory, unused and unsellable, and had to be destroyed. The events surrounding the pandemic, which turned out to be mild, engendered charges of conspiracy on the part of health organizations, which were accused of creating hysteria to inflate vaccine manufacturers' profits. It seems that all that is old is new again.[7]

Influenza Pandemics in Perspective

In examining the 120-year history of influenza pandemics and public health response, one can marvel at how much has been learned about the virus and be humbled by how much more there is still to know. Influenza pandemics are relatively rare events. This infrequency is a boon to the human population, which does not often have to face the steep rise of illness and death associated with an epidemic, but means that influenza researchers have few opportunities to study the virus in its pandemic manifestation. Accordingly, researchers must rely on the experience of preceding influenza pandemics to shape public health policies concerning new or anticipated influenza pandemics. History is often a useful guide for scientific researchers, but rarely is history as pertinent as it is in studying influenza epidemics. The information gathered from the 1889 Russian flu shaped the expectations of medical researchers in 1918. The disastrous Spanish flu informed the creation of surveillance systems and spurred the development of protective vaccines. The failure of vaccination campaigns in 1957 and 1968 led to a hyperalert public health system in 1976. The "fiasco" of 1976 and the human culpability in the release of the 1977 Russian flu prompted an abandonment of pandemic intervention planning for a generation. Preparation for a potential bird flu pandemic created a structure that, while innovative, drew on a century's worth of experience with the influenza virus. The 2009 H1N1 swine flu will undoubtedly both reinforce previous lessons on influenza pandemics and educate health officials on some new ones. Public health responses in 2009 will serve as a model for future public health programs.

The Swine Flu Program of 1976 merits a special position in the history of public health responses to pandemic influenza because it was a large-scale effort to protect all the nation's citizens against an influenza pandemic, and to do this on an emergency basis. In many ways, the program was and probably will remain unique, the product of a particular historical context. Only the United States had the productive capacity, administrative experience, and hubris to attempt such a large-scale vaccination campaign. United States Public Health Service officials thought they could rapidly implement a universal vaccination program to inoculate every citizen, and despite a host of delays and setbacks, they nearly did. Although events pushed the program beyond its initial vaccination target dates, it clearly could have achieved its goal. More than 150 million doses were prepared and submitted to the Bureau of Biologics for certification and release by 16 December 1976.[8]

The Swine Flu Program represented the pinnacle of the national vaccination response. But the fallout from the program combined with the accidental laboratory release of virus in 1977 prompted a reassessment of such feverish preparations for a pandemic. Soon the changing landscape of pharmaceutical manufacturing rendered massive, nation-based vaccination campaigns an impossibility.

In the present day no nation could attempt the same type of program as the United States did. Vaccine manufacturing firms are truly globalized, with companies headquartered in one nation, producing the vaccine in a second, and selling it around the world. Who would be able to command such production—the nation where the firm is headquartered, the nation where it is produced, or the nations that have ordered the vaccine? This question has no clear answer at the moment.

The spectacular nature and perceived failure of the 1976 effort prompted retrospective evaluations of the United States' decision and program. Some of this assessment has harshly criticized the intentions and capabilities of scientists and health officials involved in the inoculation campaign. Both critics and supporters of the vaccination effort have sifted through the ashes of the program with an eye toward drawing useful lessons from the events for use in the next public health alert. Analysts who have reexamined the Swine Flu Program of 1976 have rightly pointed out its lack of a built-in reassessment of the program's continuing necessity. After considering and discarding the concept of stockpiling the vaccine early in the program, USPHS officials never revisited the decision to undertake the vaccination effort, even when the pandemic had not appeared.[9] But these retrospective critics have failed to appreciate the very factor that drove the decision in the first place. The experts who made their recommendation for a vaccination program did so because of the experiences of 1957 and 1968 and not because of presidential politics, or vainglory, or panic. The pandemic years of 1957 and 1968 demonstrated that public health officials must make vaccination decisions rapidly if they are to stay ahead of an emerging virus. The period after the failed 1968 vaccination campaign was marked by conferences and workshops dedicated to improving surveillance, speeding up and increasing the volume of vaccine manufacturing, and shoring up interstate planning to coordinate massive vaccination campaigns. When the A/New Jersey virus appeared, researchers and health officials felt compelled by the previous history of the influenza virus to make a quick decision, seeking to apply the lessons they had learned from previous pandemics.

Strangely, the WHO's recommendation to its member states in 1976 has not received the same intense scrutiny as the U.S. decision. Officials at the WHO drew on the same evidence and experience of past influenza pandemics as had the USPHS officials, but their organization's member states operated under manufacturing constraints that the United States did not face. The ambiguous nature of the evidence for a pandemic, most nations' inability to manufacture inactivated influenza vaccines in large quantities, and fears about the use of unstable live-virus vaccines prompted the WHO to recommend "watchful waiting." Analysts examining these events, however, have overlooked the fact that the feasibility of the WHO's recommendation rested on a surveillance system that did not justify such faith. It is highly unlikely that an influenza pandemic would have been detected prior to community-wide spread. If A/New Jersey had indeed prompted a pandemic, the nations that had followed the WHO recommendation would have been ill prepared to mount a vaccination campaign. The WHO recommendation re-created the situation that existed in 1957 and 1968 because that was all these nations could do.

The events of 1976 are more than a historical curiosity; they illustrate a difficulty that faces all public health recommendations and speak to a broader issue that confounds governmental planning: analyzing risk. Predicting the likely outcome of complex systems is an imprecise venture, and the randomness inherent in biological systems further complicates the effort. Scientists are forced to speak of probabilities, possibilities, and contingency because predictions about biological phenomena can never be absolutely certain. Policy makers, however, must speak in absolutes. Worthy programs always outnumber resources, and short-term programs to address immediate concerns often trump efforts to prepare for an event that might or might not happen in the future. The recent experience of New Orleans and Hurricane Katrina is a case in point. In retrospect, spending the money to bolster the levees would have been a sound investment. But justifying such an expenditure to prepare for an event that had a low probability of occurring in any one year was difficult. The poor citizens of New Orleans and the taxpayers of the nation continue to pay for this shortsighted decision.

In 1976, the reality of this fight for funding was recognized by the CDC's director, David Sencer. To increase the likelihood that the vaccination program would be funded, he escalated the rhetoric used to describe the probability that a dangerous pandemic would appear by speaking of it as a "strong possibility." The senior advisers at the Department of Health, Education, and Welfare recognized this funding reality, too. To ensure that the program was authorized by the Ford administration and by Congress, they changed "strong possibility" to certainty, saying, for example, "There will be a major flu epidemic." Both sets of administrators thought that the need for the program justified this escalation. As Sencer later related it, the vaccine decision was a "technical decision," but the "funding of course [was] political."[10] But the inflated assessment of the risk of the new virus left the public health sector vulnerable to charges of incompetence or malfeasance if the pandemic did not emerge. In retrospect, the short-term benefits of achieving funding for the vaccination program were outweighed by the long-term costs to the authority of public health officials in predicting health emergencies.

The final element to consider in assessing influenza pandemics is the virus itself. Biological organisms are unpredictable and encompass so many variables that even the most powerful models of an organism's behavior must incorporate an element of chance. Influenza viruses have significantly unpredictable outcomes simply because of their high mutation rate, but their tendency for recombination exacerbates this unpredictability. The fact that one influenza virus strain can swap genetic segments with any other strain makes predicting the future pathway of an influenza virus highly uncertain. Although no samples of the 1889 Russian flu virus still exist, it was presumably created by a recombination event. Influenza scientists can state conclusively that the 1957 Asian and the 1968 Hong Kong flu pandemics were sparked by recombinant strains. The calamitous 1918 Spanish flu virus appears to have been an avian influenza strain that mutated into one readily transmissible by human hosts, which explains why public health officials are concerned about bird flu. These combination events and high mutability rate make predicting influenza pandemics enormously difficult and ensure that the virus has a say in any future discussions about control outbreaks.

National and international health organizations have been alert to the possibility of a novel influenza strain sparking an epidemic and were especially vigilant for the appearance of H5N1. Accordingly, their surveillance emphasis for the appearance of a new human-transmissible strain was focused on those regions where bird flu was known to be circulating and where many influenza researchers had increasingly suggested a new virus was likely to emerge: Southeastern Asia. But the wild-card feature of the influenza virus was played again. In early June 2009, the WHO did raise its pandemic alert level to 6, which designates that a global pandemic of influenza is under way. The alert, however, was raised not for the anticipated bird flu but for a new H1N1 virus dubbed "swine flu." The novel H1N1 swine flu comprises genetic segments from human, avian, and two types of swine strains (Eurasian and North American). The locus of appearance (North America) and parentage (a mixture of swine, avian, and human donor strains) were completely unexpected. A new influenza strain had emerged and spread into community-wide outbreaks prior to detection. At this writing, the explanation for the virus's emergence and its genetic makeup remain a mystery.[11]

The 2009–2010 swine flu's ability (shared by its predecessors) to outstrip manufacturing and distribution methods of protective vaccines underscores the global population's vulnerability to influenza pandemics. The planet's growing population and the acceleration of interconnectedness that marks the current era continue to increase the gap between the rapid spread of infectious agents and the abilities of health systems to protect their charges. In the case of the influenza virus, researchers herald new breakthroughs in vaccine production, reverse genetics, and potentially universal vaccines that would preclude the necessity of yearly updated vaccines.[12] Perhaps these technological advances will render influenza pandemics quaint relics of the past. But these new methods are for the future, and although they hold great promise, they remain in the laboratory or on the drawing board. In the present we are faced with the same concerns that have faced generations before. How do we control pandemic influenza? As events in 2009 demonstrate, we have not yet found a satisfactory answer to this question.

The story of influenza pandemics in the long twentieth century has been the story of science as well, both reflecting and illuminating scientific breakthroughs and missteps. The 1889 Russian flu provided an opportunity to test the germ theory of disease. Although researchers at that time were trying to track the wrong causative agent, the careful elucidation of the pandemic's appearance and spread sketched out the broad pattern of an influenza pandemic and its unmistakable relationship to transportation, its connections, and the virus's ability to rapidly cycle through a population. The disastrous Spanish flu shattered the medical complacency that had surrounded influenza epidemics and shook the faith early-twentieth-century scientists held in their abilities to control infections. Although the pandemic may have been "forgotten" by the larger public and deliberately omitted by physicians in their retrospective histories, those involved in the pandemic carried vivid personal memories of the tragic event.[13] As if it were a crazy aunt in the attic, public health experts recalled the catastrophe even if they rarely talked about it. The postwar, technologically driven capacity to detect, understand, and control the natural world was reflected in astonishing breakthroughs in studying the influenza virus and in the development of methods to protect the public from infection. Combined with an increasing appetite for large-scale, government-led approaches to national problems, the partnership between science and government underlay responses to the Asian, Hong Kong, and swine flu events of 1957, 1968, and 1976, respectively. The public recriminations that followed the Swine Flu Program and the private recriminations that trailed the artificially produced

Russian flu epidemic in 1977 undercut the optimistic belief of those in public health who predicted an imminent mastery of infectious diseases. The emergence of new infections and the reemergence of old scourges occurred against a backdrop of the perceived failure of other technologically driven approaches to human problems. Whether the intransigent factor took the form of environmental degradation and pollution or stubborn inequalities in health and economic well-being, mastery of the world we inhabit seemed nowhere near imminent and perhaps not even a desirable goal.

In similar fashion, influenza pandemics have shed light on the evolving trajectory of international public health and the World Health Organization. Mirroring national concerns with border-defying infections in the late nineteenth and early twentieth centuries, which rested on narrow self-interest, the WHO influenza surveillance system originally benefited only a handful of nations. Building on a technical, state-centered approach patterned after programs in the League of Nations Health Organization, the WHO developed programs that relied on extensive equipment and training that suited a small, elite group of experts. The uneven mix of success (smallpox eradication) and failures (malaria eradication) and the expense of specialized solutions prompted a revolt from the nations that lacked the infrastructure and other resources to benefit from these high-tech approaches. The desire for generalized improvement for health needs clashes with a focused attack on selected diseases and conditions. Complicating matters is the rise of private philanthropic entities (e.g., the Gates Foundation) with deep pockets and generally narrow, disease-specific targets.

In many ways this, argument over the appropriate focus for international health programs, whether targeted disease mitigation or a generalized improvement of conditions, evokes the "seed versus soil" debate that animated contagionist and anticontagionist conflict in the nineteenth century. For the bulk of the twentieth century, the seed, or germ, of a disease would hold pride of place in scientific and medical research on health. And this approach produced astounding health improvements. But in the later twentieth century, it increasingly became apparent that the health circumstances of living arrangements can provide fertile soil for diseases to sprout and that successful efforts to protect health have included targeting the situations (poverty, lack of clean water, squalor) that allow diseases to thrive.[14] Addressing both facets of illness, causative agents and the circumstances in which they flourish, is the legacy of the twentieth-century contest against disease. In the twenty-first century, however, a new global model of public health has begun to emerge. Again, influenza pandemics help to illustrate these changes.

The failure of the 1957 and 1968 vaccination programs, combined with the steady increase in population and the concentration of manufacturing into global corporations, has rendered national vaccination efforts impracticable. Vaccine production is currently unable to keep up with the rapid spread of the influenza virus, and it will remain so for the foreseeable future. In recognition of this reality, the WHO reorganized pandemic planning. First, it pushed through a new version of its International Health Regulations that underscores the global nature of health threats. Second, it reworked pandemic mitigation plans to catch the virus in its first halting steps of human transmission, at which point antivirals and experimental vaccines globally stockpiled would be rushed to the site of a potentially emerging pandemic. The plan recognizes that the health and well-being of a nation's citizens relies on a global commitment to the health of all.

The new influenza pandemic response plan, in addition to being our current best hope to interdict an emerging influenza pandemic, can also serve as a template for international partnerships for health protection more broadly. Nation-centered, or nation-only, responses to influenza pandemics do not work, as history and current-day capacities make abundantly clear. A global approach to protecting the public against a pandemic of influenza, one that draws on the abilities of all nations and benefits all nations, offers the design most likely to succeed in combating this dangerous virus. Whereas powerful states in the early twentieth century pursued health goals that sought to keep the diseases of "Others" away from their home populations, it has now become apparent that there is no "Other." We are all swimming in the same disease pool. It is not only compassion that should have us concerned about the health of our fellow planet inhabitants—and compassion has done mighty work in alleviating misery around the globe—but also enlightened self-regard: global health is a matter of dire national interest.

The reality of the interconnected twenty-first-century world and its relation to health has motivated a number of national health organizations and a bewildering mixture of nongovernmental organization to address matters of global health. Some of these global organizations and private approaches have deep pockets indeed, but at present, the autonomous programs lack any coordination, resulting in a wasteful duplication of plans and a confusing mix of programs. The organization most suited to taking the lead in these new approaches to international health appears to be the World Health Organization. To its credit, the WHO seems to have recognized this responsibility and opportunity. Although it seems unlikely that any of these organizations will give up their autonomy completely, some sort of coordination of effort is required. If the WHO fails in this harmonizing endeavor, some other agency or organization must emerge or be propelled to take on this coordinating role. The stakes are too high to allow the current push for international health to fail.

The evolving WHO policies are not a perfect solution, as the 2009 H1N1 swine flu pandemic reminds us, and some organizations are justifiably suspicious of the WHO's ability to deliver on the promises of international health. But the new WHO policies do represent a promising model for public health. The problems that we now face—infectious diseases, environmental degradation, and climate change—are global ones. So too need to be our solutions.

NOTES

Introduction: Wagers and Unexpected Outcomes

1. The following account of the Fort Dix outbreak was drawn from Richard E. Neustadt and Harvey V. Fineberg, *The Swine Flu Affair: Decision-Making on a Slippery Disease* (Washington D.C.: U.S. Department of Health, Education, and Welfare, 1978), 5–9; Arthur M. Silverstein, *Pure Politics and Impure Science: The Swine Flu Affair* (Baltimore, Md.: Johns Hopkins University Press, 1981), 1–5; Phillip Boffey, "Anatomy of a Decision: How the Nation Declared War on Swine Flu," *Science* 192 (14 May 1976): 636–41; Lawrence Wright, "Sweating Out the Swine Flu Scare," *New Times,* 11 June 1976, 28–38; and Martin Goldfield et al., "Influenza in 1976: Isolations of Influenza A/ New Jersey/76 Virus at Fort Dix," *Journal of Infectious Disease* 136, suppl. (Dec. 1977): S347–55.

2. The level of stress among military basic trainees is nicely illustrated by a nearly contemporaneous study. The U.S. Army discovered that stress markers were higher in basic trainees than in Green Beret troops and Army helicopter medics during the Vietnam War. The levels of stress in these recruits were comparable to those in schizophrenics at the moment of "total psychic disorientation." See Wright, "Sweating," 31.

3. "Testing" a sample to determine whether it contained influenza took several days. Chapter 1 will provide a description of influenza strains and their nomenclature.

4. President Gerald Ford, "The President's Remarks Announcing Actions to Combat the Influenza," *Weekly Compilation of Presidential Documents* 12, no. 13 (24 Mar. 1976): 484.

5. "Number of Persons Receiving Influenza Vaccine, United States 1972–1977," box 21, folder titled "1975–76 Flu Handbooks (2)," Record Group 442, National Archives and Records Administration, Southeast Region, FRC Accession Number 442–91– 0075 (further references to this collection are shown as RG 442, NARA SE Region).

6. This is a simplistic summation of the challenges in developing a scientific worldview of course, for Newton could not literally "see" the gravitational forces so central to his theory of the universe.

7. Thomas Kuhn originated the notion of paradigm shifts in science; see his semi-

nal work *The Structure of Scientific Revolutions,* 2d ed., enlarged (Chicago: University of Chicago Press, 1970 [1962]). See also Erich Von Dietze, *Paradigms Explained: Rethinking Thomas Kuhn's Philosophy of Science* (Westport, Conn.: Praeger, 2001).

8. Even Sir Isaac Newton maintained a fervent belief in alchemy throughout his magnificent life, an inconvenient fact often omitted by his early chroniclers. See Patricia Fara, *Newton: The Making of Genius* (New York: Columbia University Press, 2002), 29. As Bruce T. Moran points out, the line between chemistry and alchemy was not so clear in the past. See Bruce T. Moran, *Distilling Knowledge: Alchemy, Chemistry and the Scientific Revolution* (Cambridge, Mass.: Harvard University Press, 2005).

9. "Variolation" differs from "vaccination"; in the former, the recipient is infected with a (one hopes) mild strain of the virus, whereas in the latter the recipient is infected with a closely related but generally benign strain of the virus in question, such as cowpox for smallpox, in the hope of providing cross-immunity. See F. Fenner et al., *Smallpox and Its Eradication* (Geneva: World Health Organization, 1988), 245–76.

10. K. David Patterson, *Pandemic Influenza 1700–1900: A Study in Historical Epidemiology* (Totowa, N.J.: Rowman and Littlefield, 1986); Gerald F. Pyle, *The Diffusion of Influenza: Patterns and Paradigms* (Totowa, N.J.: Rowman and Littlefield, 1986).

11. W. I. B. Beveridge, *Influenza: The Last Great Plague: An Unfinished Story of Discovery* (New York: Prodist, 1977); June E. Osborn, ed., *History, Science, and Politics: Influenza in America, 1918–1976* (New York: Prodist, 1977).

12. See Neustadt and Fineberg, *Swine Flu Affair*; Arthur Silverstein, *Pure Politics.* Silverstein was a congressional science fellow with the Senate's health subcommittee during the swine flu crisis.

13. Purportedly, even President Gerald Ford read the book during this time. Crosby's book remains the best work on the subject. See Alfred Crosby, *Epidemic and Peace, 1918* (Westport, Conn.: Greenwood, 1976). The claim that Ford read the book comes from Neustadt and Fineberg, *Swine Flu Affair,* 19.

14. John M. Barry, *The Great Influenza: The Epic Story of the Deadliest Plague in History* (New York: Viking, 2004); Howard Phillips and David Killingray, eds., *The Spanish Influenza Pandemic of 1918–19: New Perspectives* (London: Routledge, 2003); Carol R. Byerly, *Fever of War: The Influenza Epidemic in the U.S. Army during World War I* (New York: New York University Press, 2005); Kirsty E. Duncan, *Hunting the 1918 Flu: One Scientist's Search for a Killer Virus* (Toronto: University of Toronto Press, 2003).

15. The publication record of the calamity perhaps tells us something about the public's confidence in medical triumphs in the middle twentieth century and our own anxieties about emerging diseases in the twenty-first century.

16. See Stephen S. Morse, ed., *Emerging Viruses* (New York: Oxford University Press, 1993); Stephen S. Morse, *The Evolutionary Biology of Viruses* (New York: Raven, 1994); and Institute of Medicine, *Emerging Infections: Microbial Threats to Health in the United States* (Washington, D.C.: National Academies, 1992). This rapid adoption of disease threats as destabilizing nation-states is not without its critics. In somewhat parallel arguments, Sara Davies and Nicholas King identify the "emerging infectious disease" model as a repackaging of colonial medical practices that sought to keep the diseases of the lesser-developed states (colonies) from infecting the developed (colonizing) states. See Sara E. Davies, "Securitizing Infectious Disease," *International Affairs* 84,

no. 2 (2008): 295–313; and Nicholas B. King, "Security, Disease, Commerce: Ideologies of Postcolonial Global Health," *Social Studies of Science* 32, no. 5–6 (Oct.–Dec. 2002): 763–89.

17. See Akira Iriye, *Global Community: The Role of International Organizations in the Making of the Contemporary World* (Berkeley: University of California Press, 2002); Akira Iriye, *Cultural Internationalism and World Order* (Baltimore, Md.: Johns Hopkins University Press, 1997); and F. P. Walters, *A History of the League of Nations* (London: Oxford University Press, 1952).

18. See Norman Howard Jones's extended essay on international public health serialized in *WHO Chronicle* 31–32 (1977–1978).

19. Elizabeth W. Etheridge, *Sentinel for Health: A History of the Centers for Disease Control* (Berkeley: University of California Press, 1992).

20. Kent Buse, Wolfgang Hein, and Nick Drager, eds., *Making Sense of Global Health Governance: A Policy Perspective* (Basingstoke, U.K.: Palgrave Macmillan, 2009); Michael H. Merson, Robert E. Black, and Anne J. Mills, eds., *International Public Health: Diseases, Programs, Systems and Policies*, 2d ed. (Sudbury, Mass.: Jones and Bartlett, 2006).

21. Harry Schwartz, "Swine Flu Fiasco," *New York Times,* 21 December 1976, p. 33, col. 2.

22. Jeffrey K. Taubenberger et al., "Initial Genetic Characterization of the 1918 'Spanish' Influenza Virus," *Science* 275 (21 Mar. 1997): 1793–96.

23. Rene Snacken, Alan P. Kendal, Lars R. Haaheim, and John M. Wood, "The Next Influenza Pandemic: Lessons from Hong Kong, 1997," *Emerging Infectious Disease* 5, no. 2 (Mar.–Apr. 1999): 195–203; Kennedy Shortridge, interview by author, 19 June 2011.

24. David L. Heymann and Guenael Rodier, "Global Surveillance, National Surveillance, and SARS," *Emerging Infectious Diseases* 10, no. 2 (Feb. 2004), available at http://www.cdc.gov/ncidod/EID/vol10no2/013–1038.htm (accessed 31 Oct. 2004).

25. "Summary of Probable SARS Cases with Onset of Illness from 1 November 2002 to 31 July 2003," Internet file, http://www.who.int/csr/sars/country/table2004_04_21/en/print.html (accessed 8 Aug. 2006).

26. Denise Grady, "Before Shortage of Flu Vaccine, Many Warnings," *New York Times,* 17 October 2004, p. 1, col. 1.

27. "Cumulative Number of Confirmed Human Cases of Avian Influenza A/(H5N1) Reported to WHO," Internet file, http://www.who.int/human_animal_interface/EN_GIP_LatestCumulativeNumberH5N1cases.pdf (accessed 3 Oct. 2011).

28. Dennis Normile, "Wild Birds Only Partly to Blame in Spreading H5N1," *Science* 312 (9 June 2006): 1451.

29. World Health Organization, Executive Board, "Influenza Pandemic Preparedness and Response: Report by the Secretariat," 115th Session, Agenda item 4.17, EB 115/44 (20 Jan. 2005), available at http://apps.who.int/gb/ebwha/pdf_files/EB115/B115_44-en.pdf (accessed 21 Aug. 2006).

30. See Lorna Weir and Eric Mykhalovskiy, *Global Public Health Vigilance: Creating a World on Alert* (New York: Routledge, 2010), 1–6 (global emergency vigilance system), 125–38 (2005 IHR). For Fidler, see Michael G. Baker and David Fidler, "Global Public Health Surveillance under New International Health Regulations," *Emerging*

Infectious Disease 12, no. 7 (July 2006): 1058–65; David Fidler, "Public Health and International Law: The Impact of Infectious Diseases on the Formation of International Legal Regimes, 1800–2000," in *Plagues and Politics: Infectious Disease and International Policy,* ed. Andrew T. Price-Smith (Houndmills, U.K.: Palgrave, 2001), 263–67; and David Fidler, *International Law and Infectious Diseases* (Oxford: Clarendon Press, 1999).

31. See the CDC reports in the *Morbidity and Mortality Weekly Report* for the chronology of events in 2009: "Swine Influenza (H1N1) Infection in Two Children—Southern California, March–April 2009," *MMWR* 58, no. 15 (24 Apr. 2009): 400–402; "Update: Swine Influenza A (H1N1) Infections—California and Texas, April 2009," *MMWR* 58, no. 16 (1 May 2009): 435–37; and "Outbreak of Swine-Origin Influenza A (H1N1) Virus Infection—Mexico, March–April 2009," *MMWR* 58, no. 17 (8 May 2009): 467–70. See also Fatima S. Dawood et al., "Emergence of a Novel Swine-Origin Influenza A (H1N1) Virus in Humans," *New England Journal of Medicine* 360, no. 25 (18 June 2009): 2605–15. For a description of pandemic phases, see "WHO Pandemic Phase Descriptors and Main Actions by Phase," Internet file, http://www.who.int/csr/disease/influenza/GIPA3AideMemoire.pdf (accessed 19 Aug. 2009).

32. Dawood et al., "Emergence"; Rebecca J. Garten et al., "Antigenic and Genetic Characteristics of Swine-Origin 2009 A (H1N1) Influenza Viruses Circulating in Humans," *Science* 325 (10 July 2009): 197–201.

33. For barricade vaccines, see Edwin Kilbourne, "Influenza Pandemics: Can We Prepare for the Unpredictable?" *Viral Immunology* 17, no. 3 (2004): 350–57.

Chapter 1. Influenza: Virus and History

1. The following information about the virus and illness it causes is drawn from Edwin Kilbourne, *Influenza* (New York: Plenum Medical, 1987); Karl G. Nicholson, Robert G. Webster, Alan J. Hay, eds., *Textbook of Influenza* (London: Blackwell Science, 1998); John M. Barry, *The Great Influenza: The Epic Story of the Deadliest Plague in History* (New York: Viking, 2004); and Washington C. Winn Jr., "Influenza and Parainfluenza Viruses," in *Pathology of Infectious Diseases,* vol. 1, ed. Daniel H. Connor (Stamford, Conn.: Appleton and Lange, 1997), 221–27.

2. The following information regarding the functioning of the immune system is drawn from Darla J. Wise and Gordon R. Carter, *Immunology: A Comprehensive Review* (Ames: Iowa State University Press, 2002); Mary S. Leffell, Albert D. Donnenberg, and Noel R. Rose, eds., *Handbook of Human Immunology* (Boca Raton, Fla.: CRC, 1997); and James A. Marsh and Marion D. Kendall, eds., *The Physiology of Immunity* (Boca Raton, Fla.: CRC, 1996).

3. This is a Darwinian process. For an overview, see Niall Shanks and Rebecca A. Pyles, "Evolution and Medicine: The Long Reach of 'Dr. Darwin,'" *Philosophy, Ethics, and Humanities in Medicine* 2, no. 4 (3 Apr. 2007), available at http://www.peh-med.com/content/2/1/4.

4. Mikhail Matrosovich et al., "Early Alteration of the Receptor-Binding Properties of H1, H2, and H3 Avian Influenza Virus Hemagglutinins after Their Introduction into Mammals," *Journal of Virology* 74, no. 18 (Sept. 2000): 8502–12.

5. Estimates of mortality due to "Asian" and "Hong Kong" flu are from Derek J. Smith, "Predictability and Preparedness in Influenza Control," *Science* 312 (21 Apr.

2006): 392. Some scientists speculate that the "Hong Kong" flu was less deadly because the similarity of the neuraminidase afforded some protection from the virus.

6. See Terence M. Tumpey et al., "A Two-Amino Acid change in the Hemagglutinin of the 1918 Influenza Virus Abolishes Transmission," *Science* 315 (2 Feb. 2007): 655–59.

7. Unless otherwise noted, the following information about influenza in the animal world is drawn from Robert G. Webster and William J. Bean Jr., "Evolution and Ecology of Influenza Viruses: Interspecies Transmission," in *Textbook of Influenza*, ed. Karl G. Nicholson, Robert G. Webster, and Alan J. Hay (London: Blackwell Science, 1998), 109–19.

8. Bjorn Olsen et al., "Global Patterns of Influenza A Virus in Wild Birds," *Science* 312 (21 Apr. 2006): 384.

9. That is why it would be so unusual if the Spanish flu was a largely unchanged avian flu strain. Several evolutionary changes would have to occur before the virus could infect, and be readily transmitted, to a new human host. See Terrence M. Tumpey et al., "Characterization of the Reconstructed 1918 Spanish Influenza Pandemic Virus," *Science* 310 (7 Oct. 2005): 77–80.

10. As I will discuss, the assorting tendency of combined viral replication underlies the technology of recombinant vaccine production. See Edwin D. Kilbourne, "Future Influenza Vaccines and the Use of Genetic Recombinants," *Bulletin of the World Health Organization* 41 (1969): 643–45.

11. Unless otherwise noted, the following discussion of the historical appearance of influenza is drawn from W. I. B. Beveridge, *Influenza: The Last Great Plague, an Unfinished Story of Discovery* (New York: Prodist, 1977); Christopher W. Patten, "Chronicle of Influenza Pandemics," in *Textbook of Influenza*, ed. Karl G. Nicholson, Robert G. Webster, and Alan J. Hay (London: Blackwell Science, 1998), 3–18; and K. David Patterson, *Pandemic Influenza 1700–1900: A Study in Historical Epidemiology* (Totowa, N.J.: Rowan and Littlefield, 1986).

12. See William H. McNeill, *Plagues and Peoples* (New York: Anchor/ Doubleday, 1976), especially chapter 3, "Confluence of the Civilized Disease Pools of Eurasia: 500 B.C. to A.D. 1200," 94–160.

13. An alternative origin for the name relies upon the seasonality of influenza infections, which seem to appear as soon as the weather turns cold. Hence the sickness was thought to result from the *influenza di freddo* (influence of the cold). See Beveridge, *Influenza*, 24.

14. Drawn from Beveridge, *Influenza*, 25.

15. Beveridge identified sixteen epidemic and pandemic years in 1700–1900; Patten identified ten and Patterson nine for the same period.

16. Patterson cautions however that ascribing influenza outbreaks as coming from the "East" may be more of a practice of identifying disease as the fault of an "Other," with the decadent and exotic East often blamed for diseases. He also believes that no pandemics can be definitively traced prior to the 1800s, making any association with Russia or China speculative; see Patterson, *Pandemic Influenza*, 84–85. Ann Jannetta argues that there were two regional disease systems—one centered in Europe and one in East Asia—that operated independently but with periodic transfer of diseases, includ-

ing pandemic strains of influenza. On this account, pandemics were as likely to move eastward as westward. She argues that this bifurcated influenza pattern extended from 1550 to at least 1800; see Jannetta, "Disease Dissemination in the Early Modern World: Connecting East and West," in *Higashi to Hishi No Iryo Bunka* (Medical culture East and West), ed. Yoshida Iadashis and Fukase Yasuaki (Tokyo: Shibunkaku, 2001), 390–410. My thanks to Patrick Manning for alerting me to this article.

17. It is not clear whether influenza appeared in the Americas prior to the arrival of Europeans, but it is certainly possible. The Americas are connected via the flyways of migratory birds that intermix populations of birds from Eurasia and the Americas. If there were influenza pandemics prior to the seaborne connection to Eurasia, they went unrecorded and are lost to history or as yet undiscovered.

18. For an overview of William Farr and the development of "life tables" in health statistics, see John M. Eyler, *Victorian Social Medicine: The Ideas and Methods of William Farr* (Baltimore, Md.: Johns Hopkins University Press, 1979).

19. See Alexander Langmuir, "William Farr: Founder of Modern Concepts of Surveillance," *International Journal of Epidemiology* 5, no. 1 (1976): 13–18.

20. But since no specific affliction could be tied to the "animalcules" van Leeuwenhoek observed, their potential significance was ignored. See J. N. Hays, *The Burdens of Disease: Epidemics and Human Response in Western History* (New Brunswick, N.J.: Rutgers University Press, 2000), 137–38.

21. For Philadelphia, see Hays, *The Burdens of Disease,* 130–34; for the development of miasmic theories of yellow fever, see Margaret Humphreys, *Yellow Fever and the South* (Baltimore, Md.: Johns Hopkins University Press, 1992), 17–44.

22. See generally John Duffy, *The Sanitarians: A History of American Public Health* (Urbana: University of Illinois Press, 1990). For Villermé, see William Coleman, *Death Is a Social Disease: Public Health and Political Economy in Early Industrial France* (Madison: University of Wisconsin Press, 1982); and Nancy Krieger, "The Making of Public Health Data: Paradigms, Politics, and Policy," *Journal of Public Health Policy* 13, no. 4 (Winter 1992): 412–16. For Shattuck, see Lemuel Shattuck and others, *Report of the Sanitary Commission of Massachusetts* (Boston: Dutton and Wentworth, 1850); and Barbara Gutmann Rosenkratz, *Public Health and the State: Changing Views in Massachusetts, 1842–1936* (Cambridge, Mass.: Harvard University Press, 1972), 8–36. For Chadwick, see Edwin Chadwick, *Report on the Sanitary Condition of the Labouring Population of Gt. Britain* (Edinburgh: Edinburgh University Press, 1965 [1842]); George Rosen, *A History of Public Health* (New York: MD Publications, 1958), 199–232; and Christopher Hamlin, "State Medicine in Great Britain," in *The History of Public Health and the Modern State,* ed. Dorothy Porter (Amsterdam: Rodopi, 1994), 132–64.

23. It should be noted that for Villermé, cleanup offered only a partial solution to the higher death rates. As he saw it, the true key to improve the health of the citizenry lay in eradicating poverty, which he took to be the underlying reason for the filth and sickness. Interestingly, this is a theme to which global health would return in the later twentieth century.

24. *Encyclopedia Britannica* (online), s.vv. "Albert, Prince Consort of Great Britain and Ireland."

25. Unless otherwise noted, the following information about cholera is drawn from

Hays, *Burdens of Disease,* 135–53; R. Pollitzer, *Cholera* (Geneva: World Health Organization, 1959); R. S. Bray, *Armies of Pestilence: The Impact of Disease on History* (New York: Barnes and Noble Books, 1996), 154–92; and Charles Rosenberg, *The Cholera Years: The United States in 1832, 1849, and 1866* (Chicago: University of Chicago Press, 1987 [1962]).

26. For discussion of the British Empire's interaction with the sultan of Oman, see Philip D. Curtin, *Disease and Empire: The Health of European Troops in the Conquest of Africa* (Cambridge: Cambridge University Press, 1998), 32–35.

27. The United States National Library of Medicine has a wonderful web site of period images and pamphlets accessible through its home page. See http://www.nlm.nih.gov/exhibition/cholera/index.html.

28. As Charles Rosenberg reports in *The Cholera Years* (46–53, 121), Andrew Jackson resisted cries for a national day of prayer and fasting in 1832, but President Zachary Taylor had no such qualms in 1849.

29. See Rosenberg, *The Cholera Years,* 193–94; Hays, *Burdens of Disease,* 146–47; and Steven Johnson, *The Ghost Map: The Story of London's Most Terrifying Epidemic and How It Changed Science, Cities, and the Modern World* (New York: Riverhead, 2006).

30. See Norman Howard Jones, "The World Health Organization in Historical Perspective," *Perspectives in Biology and Medicine* (Spring 1981): 467–68; David Fidler, "Public Health and International Law: The Impact of Infectious Diseases on the Formation of International Legal Regimes, 1800–2000," in *Plagues and Politics: Infectious Disease and International Policy,* ed. Andrew T. Price-Smith (Houndmills, U.K.: Palgrave, 2001), 263–67; and Virginia Berridge, Kelly Loughlin, and Rachel Herring, "Historical Dimensions of Global Health Governance," in *Making Sense of Global Health Governance: A Policy Perspective,* ed. Kent Buse, Wolfgang Hein, and Nick Drager (Basingstoke, U.K.: Palgrave Macmillan, 2009), 30–34.

31. Quarantining suspect individuals was not a problem, however, especially the "wrong" sorts of individuals from lower classes or "lesser" ethnic groups. See Howard Markel, *Quarantine! East European Jewish Immigrants and the New York City Epidemics of 1892* (Baltimore, Md.: Johns Hopkins University Press, 1999). Exclusion was another option; see Howard Markel, *When Germs Travel: Six Major Epidemics That Have Invaded America since 1900 and the Fears They Have Unleashed* (New York: Pantheon, 2004); and Alan M. Kraut, *Silent Travelers: Germs, Genes, and the "Immigrant Menace"* (New York: Basic Books, 1994).

32. Philip Curtin has devoted decades of work to examining this belief, which he addresses in "'The White Man's Grave': Image and Reality, 1780–1850," *Journal of British Studies* 1, no. 1 (Nov. 1961): 94–110; "Epidemiology and the Slave Trade," *Political Science Quarterly* 82 (2 June 1968): 191–216; *Death by Migration: Europe's Encounter with the Tropical World in the Nineteenth Century* (Cambridge: Cambridge University Press, 1989); and "The End of the 'White Man's Grave'? Nineteenth-Century Mortality in West Africa," *Journal of Interdisciplinary History* 21, no. 1 (Summer 1990): 63–88.

33. As Max Planck pointed out, scientists do not easily give up their old beliefs; "it rarely happens that Saul becomes Paul." Instead, he suggests, opponents of a scientific innovation "gradually die out and . . . the growing generation is familiarized with the idea from the beginning" (Planck, *The Philosophy of Physics* [New York: Norton, 1936], 97). For Kuhnian revolution, see Thomas Kuhn, *The Structure of Scientific Revolutions,*

2d ed., enlarged (Chicago: University of Chicago Press, 1970 [1962]); and Erich Von Dietze, *Paradigms Explained: Rethinking Thomas Kuhn's Philosophy of Science* (Westport, Conn.: Praeger, 2001).

34. Von Pettenkofer's assistant did not fare quite as well when he duplicated the experiment, suffering debilitative diarrhea. In order to infect an individual, the cholera vibrio must survive the harsh environment of the stomach to colonize the intestinal tract. It seems that von Pettenkofer and his assistant were fortunate in having highly acidic stomach environments on the day of their exhibition. See Hays, *Burden of Disease,* 151–52.

35. See table 3 in Rosen, *History of Public Health,* 314.

36. The following discussion is drawn from Douglas M. Haynes, *Imperial Medicine: Patrick Manson and the Conquest of Tropical Disease* (Philadelphia: University of Pennsylvania Press, 2001); Curtin, *Disease and Empire*; Anne-Emanuelle Birn, Yogan Pillay, and Timoth H. Holtz, *Textbook of International Health: Global Health in a Dynamic World,* 3d ed. (New York: Oxford University Press, 2009), 26–46; David Arnold, "Introduction," in *Imperial Medicine and Indigenous Societies,* ed. Arnold (Manchester, U.K.: Manchester University Press, 1988), 1–26; David Arnold, *Warm Climates and Western Medicine: The Emergence of Tropical Medicine, 1500–1900* (Amsterdam: Rodopi, 1996); Roy Macleod, "Introduction," in *Disease, Medicine, and Empire: Perspectives on Western Medicine and the Experience of European Expansion,* ed. Roy Macleod and Milton Lewis (London: Routledge, 1988), 1–11; and David Fidler, "Public Health," 263–69.

37. Daniel Headrick, *The Tools of Empire: Technology and European Imperialism in the Nineteenth Century* (New York: Oxford University Press, 1981).

38. See Birn et al., *Textbook of International Health,* 46–50; Fidler, "Public Health," 265–69; David Fidler, *International Law and Infectious Diseases* (Oxford: Clarendon, 1999), 13–23; and Berridge et al., "Historical Dimensions," 28–34.

39. "The late epidemic of Influenza, like others that have preceded it, reached Western Europe by way of the Russian dominions in Europe and Asia. The first accounts of it reached this country [Great Britain] from St. Petersburg in the end of November, but it would seem to have existed there since September, and to have become prevalent in October" (H. Franklin Parsons, *Report on the Influenza Epidemic of 1889–90: Presented to Both Houses of Parliament by Command of Her Majesty* [London: Eyre and Spottiswoode, 1891], 9).

40. In the Northern Hemisphere, flu season runs from October to March; in the Southern Hemisphere, it is the reverse. Flu researchers now recognize that influenza circulates all year, but the overwhelming majority of infections occur during flu season. Experts generally agree that this seasonality most likely occurs because people are inside more in cooler weather, influenza virus remains suspended in air for longer periods in cool dry environments, the virus remains viable outside the host for a longer period in such an environment, and students return to schools. See, for example, Kilbourne, *Influenza*; and Jonathan S. Nguyen-Van-Tam, "Epidemiology of Influenza," in *Textbook of Influenza,* ed. Karl G. Nicholson, Robert G. Webster, and Alan J. Hay (London: Blackwell Science, 1998), 181–206. A recent series of experiments conducted at the Mount Sinai School of Medicine in New York provides experimental evidence for one explanation regarding the seasonality of the influenza infection. Peter Palese spotted

an article on Spanish flu that appeared in the *Journal of the American Medical Association*; the report's author noted that all his guinea pigs died when Spanish flu was raging in his town, and necropsy showed they had died of pneumonia. Palese posited that guinea pigs are susceptible to flu and so arranged to test transmission rates under various conditions of heat and humidity. Palese demonstrated that the virus spread most effectively in conditions of cold and low humidity, those generally prevalent during the winter months. See A. C. Lowen, S. Mubareka, J. Steel, and P. Palese, "Influenza Virus Transmission Is Dependent on Relative Humidity and Temperature," *PLoS Pathology* 3 (10), online journal, http://www.plospathogens.org/article/info:doi/10.1371/journal.ppat.0030151 (accessed 20 Oct. 2011); and Gina Kolata, "Study Shows Why the Flu Likes Winter," *New York Times,* 5 December 2007, 1.

41. Patterson, *Pandemic Influenza,* 50.

42. "In the Russian Empire epidemic Influenza appears to have been first recognized in Central Asia at Bokhara in the second half of May (Old Style) 1889, and before the middle of July half the Europeans dwelling at New Bokhara had been attacked. . . . The epidemic traveled westwards along the Central Asia railway, to break out at St. Petersburg in October" (Parsons, *Report on the Influenza Epidemic,* 14).

43. "In 1889–90 the epidemic, assuming it to have started from Russia in October, took about six weeks or two months to spread over Europe, and to reach North America; rather more than two months to reach the Cape; about three months to reach South America; about four months to reach India; five months to reach New Zealand and Australia and Arabia; nine months to reach Iceland, and ten months to reach St. Helena and Mauritius" (ibid., 71).

44. "In the press, the arguments of Drs. Proust and Brovandel hinged on the assertion 'It's only flu.' Readers of *Le Matin* and *Le Temps* were told daily that the epidemic was no cause for alarm"; "throughout the epidemic, medical authorities were reluctant to waver from their position that the disease was benign. Even as the number of persons dying from respiratory complications began to soar, medical and public health representatives held to their initial promises that the disease was neither deadly nor dangerous. This tendency was not just a French construction, [for] examples appeared across Europe" (Mari Loreena Nicholson-Preuss, "Managing Morbidity and Mortality: Pandemic Influenza in France, 1889–90," [master's thesis, Texas Tech University, 2001], 99, 62).

45. Advertisement for "Minard's Liniment," *New Hampshire Sentinel,* 2 December 1889, 1; for "Hood's Sarsaparilla," *Philadelphia Inquirer,* 2 January 1890, 3; for "Pond's Extract," *Chicago Daily Inter Ocean,* 1 January 1890, 8; for "Brad's Throat and Catarah Powder," *Baltimore Sun,* 31 December 1889, 2; for "West's Electric Cure," *Chicago Daily Inter Ocean,* 29 December 1889, 11. All available at *America's Historical Newspapers,* a digital collection at www.newsbank.com (accessed on 25 Aug. 2008).

46. "Examination of the bronchial sputum in Influenza led to very different results. Minute non-mobile bacilli having a characteristic appearance occur in greater or less amount in the sputum of all cases of Influenza; during the acute stage of the disease they are generally present in abundance, occasionally almost in pure culture; and they tend to disappear as the disease passes off. These bacilli, which are the same as those described by Pfeiffer and Kitasato, do not occur in the bronchial secretions

of any other disease; they must be regarded as pathognomonic of Influenza; and their life-history confirms, as Dr. Klein posits, with what we believe to be the facts about the contagion of the disease" (R. Thorne Thorne, "Introduction By the Medical Office, to Local Government Board," in *Further Report and Papers on Pandemic Influenza, 1889–92: Presented to Both Houses of Parliament by Command of Her Majesty,* by H. Franklin Parsons [London: Eyre and Spottiswoode, 1893], x).

47. Patterson, *Pandemic Influenza,* 72.

48. "Influenza is a disease comparatively harmless to young people after the first year and especially dangerous at the later periods of life, and therefore, like heart disease and cancer, most fatal in populations containing a larger proportion of elderly persons, and least so in those which contains the largest proportion of children and young persons" (H. Franklin Parsons, *Further Report,* 4).

Chapter 2. The Forgotten Pandemic Remembered

1. Spanish flu has generated a staggering amount of literature in the fields of medicine, science, and history in the last few years. The most accessible include John M. Barry, *The Great Influenza: The Epic Story of the Deadliest Plague in History* (New York: Viking, 2004); Howard Phillips and David Killingray, eds., *The Spanish Influenza Pandemic of 1918–19: New Perspectives* (London: Routledge, 2003); and a series of works from Jeffrey Taubenberger's laboratory at the U.S. Armed Forces Institute of Pathology, including Jeffrey K. Taubenberger, Ann H. Reid, Thomas A. Janczewski, and Thomas G. Fanning, "Integrating Historical, Clinical, and Molecular Genetic Data in Order to Explain the Origin and Virulence of the 1918 Spanish Influenza Virus," *Philosophical Transactions of the Royal Society of London,* ser. B, Biological Sciences, 356, no. 1416 (Dec. 29, 2001): 1829–39; and Jeffrey K. Taubenberger and David M. Morens, "1918 Influenza: The Mother of All Pandemics," *Emerging Infectious Diseases* 12, no. 1 (Jan. 2006): 15–22. Two earlier works may also greatly profit the reader. The first is Edwin O. Jordan's *Epidemic Influenza: A Survey* (Chicago: American Medical Association, 1927), in which Jordan organizes the voluminous contemporary medical literature on the Spanish flu pandemic and generates conclusions from the evidence that presage many of the scientific conclusions about influenza in the twenty-first century. The second book is Alfred Crosby's *Epidemic and Peace, 1918* (Westport, Conn.: Greenwood, 1976), which the Cambridge University Press reissued as *America's Forgotten Pandemic* in 1989. Crosby's book is a lively read and focuses attention on the overlooked pandemic. As I will show, Crosby's account had an impact on the United States' response to the 1976 swine flu.

2. Crosby, *Epidemic and Peace,* 26.

3. Specifically, according to John Barry, the point of origin was Haskell County, Kansas; see Barry, *The Great Influenza,* 92. An alternative account comes from the virologist John Oxford, who argues for an origin in the French and English military camps, where outbreaks of "purulent bronchitis" was identified in soldiers in infirmaries in 1916 and 1917. The symptoms described echoed later symptomology identified with Spanish flu; see J. S. Oxford et al., "Who's That Lady?" *Nature Medicine* 5, no. 12 (Dec. 1999): 1351–52; and J. S. Oxford, "The So-Called Great Spanish Influenza Pan-

demic of 1918 May Have Originated in France in 1916," *Philosophical Transactions of the Royal Society of London,* ser. B, Biological Sciences, 356 (2001): 1857–59.

4. This discussion of Camp Funston and the initial outbreak is drawn from Barry, *The Great Influenza,* and Jordan, *Epidemic Influenza,* unless otherwise noted.

5. What role, if any, the unusual circumstances of the trenches played in the emergence of the second, killer wave is unclear. The evolutionary biologist Paul Ewald argues forcefully, if not conclusively, that there would have been no deadly second wave without the trenches; see Ewald, *Evolution of Infectious Disease* (New York: Oxford University Press, 1994), 110–16.

6. Later in his memoirs, however, Field Marshall von Ludendorff blamed the failed July German offensive on the flu-weakened state of his army (Crosby, *Epidemic and Peace,* 25–27).

7. The outbreaks occurred at Brest on 22 August 1918, at Freetown on 24 August, and at Boston on 27 August. The following account of the second wave is drawn from Crosby, *Epidemic and Peace,* and Jordan, *Epidemic Influenza,* unless otherwise noted.

8. Taubenberger et al. estimate 28 percent were infected worldwide ("Integrating Historical," 1830). Other estimates of infections with Spanish flu range even higher.

9. For Gambia, see Donald R. Wright, *The World and a Very Small Place in Africa* (Armonk, N.Y.: M.E. Sharpe, 1997), 203. Wright erroneously has the date as 1919; it should read 1918. For the Yukon, see Crosby, *Epidemic and Peace,* 241–57.

10. Mortality among those who contracted Spanish flu has been estimated 2.5 percent, substantially greater than the 0.1 percent for other influenza epidemics. See Jeffrey K. Taubenberger, "Genetic Characterisation of the 1918 'Spanish' Influenza Virus," in *Spanish Influenza Pandemic,* ed. Phillips and Killingray, 39–46 (estimate on 40).

11. Figures drawn from table 32 in Jordan, *Epidemic Influenza,* 101.

12. Dr. Roy Grist qtd. in Barry, *The Great Influenza,* 187–88.

13. See Paul Starr, *The Social Transformation of American Medicine: The Rise of a Sovereign Profession and the Making of a Vast Industry* (New York: Basic Books, 1982), 112–27; Victoria A. Harden, *Inventing the NIH: Federal Biomedical Research Policy, 1887–1937* (Baltimore, Md.: Johns Hopkins University Press, 1986); and Elizabeth Fee, *Disease and Discovery: A History of the Johns Hopkins School of Hygiene and Public Health, 1916–1939* (Baltimore, Md.: Johns Hopkins University Press, 1987).

14. Abraham Flexner, *Medical Education in the United States and Canada: A Report to the Carnegie Foundation for the Advancement of Teaching* (New York, 1910).

15. The account of the medical team visit to Devens is drawn from Crosby, *Epidemic and Peace,* 3–11.

16. This example is from Malden, a small community outside Boston: "238 cases were admitted and 91 of them died—a mortality of 38%. Such a large mortality needs an explanation and it is found in a study of the cases admitted during the month of September and October, during which months, by a vote of the Board of Health, no case was admitted unless it was influenza complicated with pneumonia" (*Board of Health Minutes of Meetings* [logbook], 14, located at the Malden Public Health Department).

17. The figure 4,597 is drawn from Jordan, *Epidemic Influenza,* 101; on trolling for dead, see Barry, *The Great Influenza,* 327–28.

18. Comparative cities data has been drawn from table 23 in Jordan, *Epidemic Influenza,* 103; the data for Australia and American Samoa, from Crosby, *Epidemic and Peace,* 234–36.

19. Qtd. in Barry, *The Great Influenza,* 265. Pfeiffer's bacillus is now known as *Haemophilus influenzae.*

20. See chapter 23 of Barry, *The Great Influenza,* 266–80, for an account of these prodigious but futile efforts.

21. See Carol R. Byerly, *Fever of War: The Influenza Epidemic in the U.S. Army during World War I* (New York: New York University Press, 2005); Byerly discusses military physicians' confidence in their abilities and their later silence on the impact of the Spanish flu on 14–38 and 125–52.

22. George A. Soper, "The Lessons of the Pandemic," *Science,* n.s., 49, no. 1274 (30 May 1919): 501–6.

23. Commissioner of Public Health for Massachusetts, Eugene R. Kelly, from executive summary, *The Commonwealth of Massachusetts, Annual Report of the Department of Public Health for the Year Ending November 30, 1920* (Boston: Wright and Patten, 1921), 13.

24. Jordan's initial estimate is a heroic effort, but subsequent research has indicated higher numbers both for the United States and globally. These subsequent efforts will be discussed later. See table 64 of Jordan, *Epidemic Influenza,* 228.

25. A classic discussion of the graphed mortality patterns appears in Jordan, *Epidemic Influenza,* 47–48; and Crosby, *Epidemic and Peace,* 21. For South Africa and Chicago, see Barry, *The Great Influenza,* 239. See also Phillips and Killingray, eds., *Spanish Influenza Pandemic.*

26. James G. Ellison, "A Fierce Hunger: Tracing Impacts of the 1918–19 Influenza in Southwest Tanzania," in *Spanish Influenza Pandemic,* ed. from Phillips and Killingray, 221–29. More accurately, the area in question was the region of Africa now known as Tanzania, which was not founded until 1964.

27. In considering a puzzlingly low population reported in census figures for India and Pakistan, the demographer Kingsley Davis attributes the deficit to Spanish flu: "We find that the average growth of the population during the 1901–10 and 1921–30 decades was 8.35 per cent per decade. Applying this to the 1911 population, we get an expected growth of 25.3 million during the 1911–20 decade. Actually the population grew by only 2.7 million. The difference is 22.6, which, if attributed to influenza gives us an estimate that is higher than the figure of 19 million death arrived at above" (Davis, *The Population of India and Pakistan* [Princeton, N.J.: Princeton University Press, 1951], app. B, 237). It should be noted that Davis's 1951 estimate of 19 million dead in India and Pakistan is almost identical to the 18.5 million figure that is the current mortality estimate for the two nations. Both these estimates suggest a much higher global toll than Edwin Oakes Jordan's estimate of 21.5 million total fatalities, which was the accepted estimate at the time. See Niall P. A. S. Johnson and Juergen Mueller, "Updating the Accounts: Global Mortality of the 1918–1920 'Spanish' Influenza Pandemic," *Bulletin of the History of Medicine* 76, no. 1 (2002): 108.

28. It should be noted that some communities did protect themselves through heroic isolation—Gunnison, Colorado, for example, set up a perimeter to prevent outsid-

ers from entering the town—and that those communities that quickly and effectively instituted "social-distancing measures" (e.g., closing schools or banning public meetings) mitigated the second wave's impact. But the successfully isolated communities were small, and communities that avoided the second wave were hit harder by the third wave. See Stephen S. Morse, "Pandemic Influenza: Studying the Lessons of History," *Proceedings of the National Academy of Sciences* 104, no. 18 (1 May 2007): 7313–14; and Richard J. Hatchett, Carter E. Mecher, and Marc Lipsitch, "Public Health Interventions and Epidemic Intensity during the 1918 Influenza Pandemic," *Proceedings of the National Academy of Sciences* 104, no. 18 (1 May 2007): 7582–87.

29. Jordan, *Epidemic Influenza,* 3.

30. The following account of the reconstruction of the Spanish flu virus is drawn from Patricia Gadsby, "Fear of Flu: Pandemic Influenza Outbreaks," *Discover* 20, no. 1 (Jan. 1999): 82; Taubenberger et al., "Integrating Historical," 1829–39; Elizabeth Pennisi, "First Genes Isolated from the Deadly 1918 Flu Virus," *Science* 275 (21 Mar. 1997): 1739; Taubenberger and Morens, "1918 Influenza," 15–22; and Diane Martindale, "No Mercy," *New Scientist* (14 Oct. 2000): 2929.

31. Jeffrey K. Taubenberger et al., "Initial Genetic Characterization of the 1918 'Spanish' Influenza Virus," *Science* 275 (21 Mar. 1997): 1793.

32. The following account of Hultin's recovery of the Spanish flu virus is drawn from the following sources unless otherwise noted: Gina Kolata, *Flu: The Story of the Great Influenza Pandemic of 1918 and the Search for the Virus That Caused It* (New York: Farrar, Straus and Giroux, 1999); Elizabeth Fernandez, "The Virus Detective: Dr. John Hultin Has Found Evidence of the 1918 Flu Epidemic That Had Eluded Experts for Decades," *San Francisco Chronicle,* 17 February 2002, CM-8, available at http://articles.sfgate.com/2002-02-17/living/17532857_1_virus-deadly-organisms-alaskan (accessed 27 Nov. 2007); Ned Rozell, "Permafrost Preserves Clues to Deadly 1918 Flu," article 1386, *Alaska Science Forum* (29 Apr. 1998), www.gi.alaska.edu/ScienceForum/ASF13/1386.html (accessed 27 Nov. 2007); Ned Rozell, "Villager's Remains Lead to 1918 Flu Breakthrough," article 1772, *Alaska Science Forum* (1999), www.gi.alaska.edu/ScienceForum/ASF17/1772.html (accessed 27 Nov. 2007); and Ian Watson (producer), "The Next Pandemic," transcript of television program, Australian Broadcasting Corporation, 7 May 1998, available at www.abc.net.au/quantrum/scripts98/9808/script.htm (accessed 27 Nov. 2007).

33. For a sometimes bitter account of this star-crossed expedition from the organizer's point of view, see Kirsty E. Duncan, *Hunting the 1918 Flu: One Scientist's Search for a Killer Virus* (Toronto: University of Toronto Press, 2003).

34. Kolata, *Flu,* 100–120.

35. Crosby, *Epidemic and Peace,* 305–6.

36. Terrence M. Tumpey et al. "Characterization of the Reconstructed 1918 Spanish Influenza Pandemic Virus," *Science* 310 (7 Oct. 2005): 80.

37. The account of the experimental introduction of the re-created Spanish flu into cynomolgus macaque monkeys and the tentative conclusions drawn from the experiment are taken from Darwyn Kobasa et al., "Aberrant Innate Immune Response in Lethal Infection of Macaques with the 1918 Influenza Virus," *Nature* 445 (18 Jan. 2007):

319–23; Kerri Smith, "Concern as Revived 1918 Flu Virus Kills Monkeys," *Nature* 445 (18 Jan. 2007): 237; and Yueh-Ming Loo and Michael Gale Jr., "Fatal Immunity and the 1918 Virus," *Nature* 445 (18 Jan. 2007): 267–68.

38. For an excellent and accessible description of the process, see Barry, *The Great Influenza,* 242–53.

39. See Taubenberger et al., "Integrating Historical"; Taubenberger and Morens, "1918 Influenza"; Martin Enserink, "From Two Mutations, an Important Clue about the Spanish Flu," *Science* 315 (2 Feb. 2007): 582; and Terrence M. Tumpey et al., "A Two-Amino Acid Change in the Hemagglutinin of the 1918 Influenza Virus Abolishes Transmission," *Science* 315 (2 Feb. 2007): 655–59.

40. Data as of 19 August 2011. The WHO had recorded 565 confirmed cases with 331 deaths. See "Cumulative Number of Confirmed Human Cases of Avian Influenza A/ (H5N1) Reported to WHO," Internet file, http://www.who.int/human_animal_interface/EN_GIP_LatestCumulativeNumberH5N1cases.pdf (accessed 3 Oct. 2011).

41. Jordan, *Epidemic Influenza,* 228–29. Actually, Jordan offered the precise figure of 21,642,283, although he knew that no estimate could be that precise.

42. See K. David Patterson and Gerald F. Pyle, "The Geography and Mortality of the 1918 Influenza Pandemic," *Bulletin of the History of Medicine* 65 (1991): 4–21.

43. See Johnson and Mueller, "Updating the Accounts," 105–15.

44. The following discussion is drawn from Crosby, *Epidemic and Peace,* 311–25.

45. Gary Gernhart, "A Forgotten Enemy: PHS's Fight against the 1918 Influenza Pandemic," *Public Health Reports* 114, no. 6 (Dec. 1999): 559–61.

Chapter 3. Breakthroughs

1. Howard Phillips and David Killingray, "Introduction," in *The Spanish Influenza Pandemic of 1918–19: New Perspectives,* ed. Phillips and Killingray (London: Routledge, 2003), 13–14.

2. In a personal interview with the author (23 Aug. 2007), Claude Hannoun, former director of the WHO collaborating center for respiratory viruses at the Pasteur Institute, reported that René Dujarric de la Rivière, with whom Hannoun had worked in 1947, had claimed in a 1918 publication that influenza was caused by a virus. His work was overlooked. See René Dujarric de la Rivière, "La grippe, est-elle une maladie à virus filtrant?" (Is influenza a filtering virus disease?) *Comptes Rendus de l'Académie des Sciences* 167 (1918): 606–7.

3. Dorothy Crawford, *The Invisible Enemy: A Natural History of Viruses* (Oxford: Oxford University Press, 2000), 12–19.

4. And they were right. At that time scientists had no knowledge of the phenomena of genetic drift and genetic shift.

5. Edwin O. Jordan, *Epidemic Influenza: A Survey* (Chicago: American Medical Association, 1927), 512.

6. Donaldson and Scott qtd. in W. I. B. Beveridge, *Influenza: The Last Great Plague, an Unfinished Story of Discovery* (New York: Prodist, 1977), 3.

7. The following discussion of the Rockefeller Foundation's support for medical research is drawn from John Farley, *To Cast Out Disease: A History of the International Health Division of the Rockefeller Foundation (1913–1951)* (Oxford: Oxford University Press, 2004).

8. See Elizabeth Fee, *Disease and Discovery: A History of the Johns Hopkins School of Hygiene and Public Health, 1916–1939* (Baltimore, Md.: Johns Hopkins University Press, 1987).

9. For the Hygiene Laboratory, see Victoria A. Harden, *Inventing the NIH: Federal Biomedical Research Policy, 1887–1937* (Baltimore, Md.: Johns Hopkins University Press, 1986), 9–26; for Lawrence, see John Duffy, *The Sanitarians: A History of American Public Health* (Urbana: University of Illinois Press, 1990), 193–204.

10. See Philip J. Hilts, *Protecting America's Health: The FDA, Business, and One Hundred Years of Regulation* (New York: Knopf, 2003), 35–71.

11. Harden, *Inventing the NIH,* 71–91.

12. The following account of Shope's discovery comes from Beveridge, *Influenza,* 1–7; Richard Shope, "Swine Influenza I: Experimental Transmission and Pathology," *Journal of Experimental Medicine* 54 (1931): 349–60; Richard Shope, "Swine Influenza II: A Hemophilic Bacillus from the Respiratory Tract of Infected Swine," *Journal of Experimental Medicine* 54 (1931): 361–72; and Richard Shope, "Swine Influenza III: Filtration Experiments and Etiology," *Journal of Experimental Medicine* 54 (1931): 373–85.

13. Interestingly, Koen's observations were roundly denounced by pig farmers who feared that this association of Spanish flu and pigs would prompt people to reject eating pork products. The events of 1976 and 2009 elicited a similar response; pork producers objected to the inclusion of the word *swine* in the naming of viruses in these years. Apparently pork producers do not believe in the old maxim that there is no bad advertising.

14. The following account of the discovery of the transmission element in human influenza comes from Beveridge, *Influenza,* 7–10; and David Tyrrell, "Discovery of Influenza Virus," in *Textbook of Influenza,* ed. Karl G. Nicholson, Robert G. Webster, and Alan J. Hay (London: Blackwell Sciences, 1998), 19–26.

15. The head of the British Medical Research Council, Walter Fletcher, suggested that dog distemper offered an indirect way to address the "influenza problem" by studying filterable viruses. Funding for the distemper research came from subscribers to *The Field,* a magazine for the "country gentleman." See Michael Bresalier, "Neutralizing Flu: Immunological Devices and the Making of a Virus Disease," in *Crafting Immunity: Working Histories of Clinical Immunology,* ed. Keton Kroker, Pauline M. H. Mazumdar, and Jennifer Keelan (Aldershot, England: Ashgate, 2008), 107–44.

16. Ironically, it was later determined that the ferrets at the Wellcome Institute did not have influenza but had contracted distemper.

17. According to the eminent influenza vaccine pioneer Dr. Kilbourne, "There hasn't been any more efficient method. It just happens to be a tremendous production machine. I don't know whether it reflects the fact that these things all went way, way back and began in fowl or something like that. They seem to be very happy in the egg. . . . The yield per cells, embryonic tissue yield per cell has been relatively enormous, like a thousand particles or so compared to tissue culture systems. And one of the problems with cell culture systems is that if you use a primary material, you have the danger of picking up extraneous viruses and so forth, retroviruses and God knows what" (Kilbourne, interview by author, 20 Jan. 2004).

18. See John R. Paul, *A History of Poliomyelitis* (New Haven, Conn.: Yale University

Press, 1971), 107–25, 373–81; David M. Oshinsky, *Polio: An American Story* (Oxford: Oxford University Press, 2005), 121–27; Bernard Seytre and Mary Shaffer, *The Death of a Disease: A History of the Eradication of Poliomyelitis* (New Brunswick, N.J.: Rutgers University Press, 2005), 47–50.

19. Present-day thinking suggests that influenza B and C represent two separate avian influenza A viruses that were introduced into the human population centuries ago. The strong selective pressure of the human immune system over a prolonged period of time created new types of influenza (B and C) much different from their avian A ancestor, and both B and C remain human diseases. See Christopher Scholtissek, "Genetic Reassortments of Human Influenza Viruses in Nature," in *Textbook of Influenza,* ed. Karl G. Nicholson, Robert G. Webster, and Alan J. Hay (London: Blackwell Sciences, 1998), 120–25.

20. Alfred Crosby, *Epidemic and Peace, 1918* (Westport, Conn.: Greenwood, 1976), 62.

21. See Hans Zinsser, *Rats, Lice, and History* (Boston: Little, Brown, 1934); and William H. McNeill, *Plagues and Peoples* (New York: Doubleday, 1976).

22. See Allan M. Brandt, *No Magic Bullet: A Social History of Venereal Disease in the United States since 1880* (New York: Oxford University Press, 1987 [1985]), 52–121. Of course, soldiers always found a way around these restrictions. It should also be noted that tropical medicine did not have as large an impact on the health of colonial forces in the tropics as is commonly suggested. A significant decrease in the death rate of colonial troops stationed in tropical regions occurred in the middle to later nineteenth century, before the germ theory of disease was accepted. This decline in mortality is likely due to the cleanup of barracks and encampments suggested by sanitarian inclinations. See Philip D. Curtin, *Disease and Empire: The Health of European Troops in the Conquest of Africa* (Cambridge: Cambridge University Press, 1998).

23. Carol R. Byerly, *Fever of War: The Influenza Epidemic in the U.S. Army during World War I* (New York: New York University Press, 2005), 39–68; and Crosby, *Epidemic and Peace, 1918,* 121–200.

24. See Zinsser, *Rats, Lice, and History*; and R. S. Bray, *Armies of Pestilence: The Impact of Disease on History* (New York: Barnes and Noble Books, 1996), 144–47.

25. Unless otherwise noted, the following discussion of the LNHO is drawn from the essays collected in Paul Weindling, ed., *International Health Organisations and Movements, 1918–1939* (Cambridge: Cambridge University Press, 1995); and from Norman Howard Jones's series on international public health, "The Organizational Problems between the Two World Wars," parts 1–5 plus an epilogue, published in the *WHO Chronicle: WHO Chronicle* 31 (1977): 391–403; 31 (1977): 449–60; 32 (1978): 26–38; 32 (1978): 63–75; 32 (1978): 114–25; and 32 (1978): 156–66.

26. Unless otherwise noted, the following discussion of the League of Nations' epidemic commission is drawn from Marta Aleksandra Balinska, "Assistance and Not Mere Relief: The Epidemic Commission of the League of Nations, 1920–1923," in *International Health Organisations,* ed. Weindling, 81–108.

27. Bray, *Armies of Pestilence,* 149.

28. Rajchman qtd. in Balinska, "Assistance," 94.

29. See F. P. Walters, *A History of the League of Nations* (London: Oxford University Press, 1952).

30. The following information about the military's preparation against influenza in World War II is drawn from Paul, *History of Poliomyelitis,* 413–17; Thomas Francis Jr., "Vaccination against Influenza," *Bulletin of the World Health Organization* 8 (1953): 725–41; and John M. Wood and Michael S. Williams, "History of Inactivated Influenza Vaccines," in *Textbook of Influenza,* ed. Karl G. Nicholson, Robert G. Webster, and Alan J. Hay (London: Blackwell Sciences, 1998), 317–23.

31. Francis headed influenza research for the board throughout the war years and maintained his position into the postwar period, helping to form the Armed Forces Epidemiological Board (AFEB). The AFEB is a powerful entity that funds research and surveillance on infections that conceivably could threaten the United States and its military and makes recommendations of which vaccines to administer to the services.

32. S. R. Mostow et al., "Studies with Inactivated Influenza Vaccines Purified by Zonal Centrifugation," *Bulletin of the World Health Organization* 41 (1969): 525–30.

33. Unless otherwise noted, the following account of 1947 is drawn from Francis, "Vaccination against Influenza"; Wood and Wilson, "History of Inactivated Influenza Vaccines"; and A. M.-M. Payne, "The Influenza Programme of WHO," *Bulletin of the World Health Organization* 8 (1953): 755–74.

34. Edwin Kilbourne, interview by author, 20 January 2004.

35. Payne, "Influenza Programme of WHO," 756.

36. It was subsequently termed a "major intrasubtypic antigenic change" because the change from the earlier form was much more dramatic change than genetic drift, but the new strain did not incorporate novel hemagglutinin or neuraminidase antigens, as a viral shift would cause. See Edwin D. Kilbourne et al., "The Total Influenza Vaccine Failure of 1947 Revisited: Major Intrasubtypic Antigenic Change Can Explain Failure of Vaccine in a Post-World War II Epidemic," *Proceedings of the National Academy of Sciences* 99, no. 16 (6 Aug. 2002): 10748–52.

37. For the NIH, see Harden, *Inventing the NIH,* 179–91; for the NSF, see J. Merton England, *A Patron for Pure Science: The National Science Foundation's Formative Years, 1945–57* (Washington, D.C.: National Science Foundation, 1982); and for "grand expectations," see James T. Patterson, *Grand Expectations: The United States, 1945–1974* (New York: Oxford University Press, 1996).

38. Andrewes's idea of global surveillance began to form with the global spread of influenza B in 1945–46. Unless otherwise noted, information on the creation of the World Influenza Surveillance System is drawn from Payne, "Influenza Programme of WHO"; C. H. Andrewes, "Epidemiology of Influenza," *Bulletin of the World History Organization* 8 (1953): 595–612; John M. Watson, "Surveillance of Influenza," in *Textbook of Influenza,* ed. Karl G. Nicholson, Robert G. Webster, and Alan J. Hay (London: Blackwell Sciences, 1998), 207–16; and Alan W. Hampson and Nancy J. Cox, "Global Surveillance for Pandemic Influenza: Are We Prepared?" in *Options for the Control of Influenza III: Proceedings of the Third International Conference on Options for the Control of Influenza, Cairns, Australia, 4–9 May, 1996,* ed. Lorena E. Brown, Alan W. Hampson, and Robert G. Webster (Amsterdam: Elsevier, 1996), 50–59.

39. Payne appears to have found merit in the U.S. complaints that Andrewes ignored American contributions; in a letter from 7 April 1952 marked "Private and Confidential," he stated: "You will have guessed from previous communication that I too

felt that he [Andrewes] had not sufficiently referred to the American work. With regard to his criticism of your Weekly Communicable Disease Summaries, I personally find them of the greatest value and I do not regard his criticisms as being fully justifiable." Payne identified the origin of the bad blood as stemming from the original 1947 virologist meeting in Copenhagen, when the group detailing duties in the new World Influenza Centre "neglected to take into account the laboratory set up and the United States Influenza Commission" (A. M.-M. Payne to Dr. Dorland Davis, National Microbiology Institute, National Institutes of Health, letter dated 7 April 1952, WHO Archives, WHO 2 DC Infl. 6 R. I. C., microfiche, located at the World Health Organization Archives, Geneva, Switzerland [hereafter cited as WHO Archives, Geneva]).

40. "Proposal for the Setting Up of a Committee on Influenza," 3 April 1947, *United Nations World Health Organization Interim Commission,* WHO 1 481–1-1, microfiche, WHO Archives, Geneva.

41. "Informal Meeting on Influenza, 21–22 April 1954," 2 D. C. Infl. 6, W.I.C., microfiche, WHO Archives, Geneva.

42. The topic of functionalism has long generated debate in the field of international relations. For a sample of this voluminous literature, see Ernst B. Haas, Mary Pat Williams, and Don Babai, *Scientists and World Order: The Uses of Technical Knowledge in International Organizations* (Berkeley: University of California Press, 1977); Ernst B. Haas, *When Knowledge Is Power: Three Models of Change in International Organizations* (Berkeley: University of California Press, 1990); Robert W. Cox and Harold K. Jacobson, *The Anatomy of Influence: Decision Making in International Organizations* (New Haven, Conn.: Yale University Press, 1973); Akira Iriye, *Global Community: The Role of International Organizations in the Making of the Contemporary World* (Berkeley: University of California Press, 2002); Robert W. Cox with Timothy J. Sinclair, *Approaches to World Order* (Cambridge: Cambridge University Press, 1996); James E. Dougherty and Robert L. Pfaltzgraff Jr., *Contending Theories of International Relations: A Comprehensive Survey,* 4th ed. (New York: Longman, 1997); and A. J. R. Groom and Paul Taylor, eds., *Frameworks for International Co-operation* (New York: St. Martin's, 1990).

43. To be fair to Andrewes, however, the system of surveillance he devised was technically sophisticated, and only a relative handful of laboratories possessed the skills and material to operate within it—an imbalance still not completely solved in the present day.

44. See Jessica Wang, *American Science in an Age of Anxiety: Scientists, Anticommunism, and the Cold War* (Chapel Hill: University of North Carolina Press, 1999).

Chapter 4. Setbacks

1. Events surrounding the 1957 "Asian" flu pandemic provide many elements similar to later responses to influenza pandemics and the scientific study of the underlying virus, making a close study of those events particularly relevant to pandemic preparation both in 1976 and in the present day. Unless otherwise noted, the following information about the discovery of Asian flu is drawn from Maurice Hilleman, "Six Decades of Vaccine Development—A Personal History," *Nature Medicine Vaccine Supplement* 4, no. 5 (May 1998): 507–14; Elizabeth W. Etheridge, *Sentinel for Health: A History of the Centers for Disease Control* (Berkeley: University of California Press, 1992), 80–81; and Paul

A. Offit, *Vaccinated: One Man's Quest to Defeat the World's Deadliest Diseases* (New York: Smithsonian Books, 2007), 1–19.

2. Hilleman qtd. in Offit, *Vaccinated,* 13.

3. Hale to Payne, telegram dated 5 May 1957, I2/418/12, 1, microfiche, WHO Archives, Geneva.

4. Andrewes to A. M.-M. Payne, telegram dated 6 May 1957, I2/418/12, 1, microfiche, WHO Archives, Geneva.

5. Dr. C. Mani, regional director, SEARO, to Dr. W. Timmerman, ADG-CTS WHO, letter dated 21 May 1957, I2/418/12, 2, microfiche, WHO Archives, Geneva.

6. The following discussion of Hilleman's identification of the 1957 virus comes from Offit, *Vaccinated,* 13–16, unless otherwise noted.

7. Copy of a statement from the U.S. surgeon general to the *Journal of the American Medical Association,* received 17 June 1957, I2/418/12, 4, microfiche, WHO Archives, Geneva.

8. The following timeline of information is drawn from a document entitled "1957 Influenza Immunization Sequence of Events," box 10, file labeled "Background and History 5. 1957 Epidemic," RG 442, NARA SE Region.

9. The 1955 budget for the office within the HEW department charged with licensing vaccines (the Laboratory of Biologics Control) was $327,000; this supported a staff of forty-five, of whom only ten were physicians or scientists. Shaken by the mismanaged Cutter incident, when live polio virus was inadvertently injected into children receiving Jonas Salk's killed polio vaccine, the laboratory was renamed the Division of Biologic Standards, and the workforce swelled to 150 physicians and scientists working on vaccines. See Paul Offit, *The Cutter Incident: How America's First Polio Vaccine Led to the Growing Vaccine Crisis* (New Haven, Conn.: Yale University Press, 2005), generally and, for budget and staffing figures, 59, 178. The federal government's polio program, in which the government encouraged manufacturers to produce and voluntarily distribute the vaccine through private physicians, set the model for the 1957 flu vaccine program. For discussions of the polio campaigns, see David M. Oshinsky, *Polio: An American Story* (Oxford: Oxford University Press, 2005); Richard Carter, *Breakthrough: The Saga of Jonas Salk* (New York: Trident, 1965); and Aaron E. Klein, *Trial by Fury: The Polio Vaccine Controversy* (New York: Scribner's, 1972).

10. The following discussion of the USPHS decision-making process is drawn from a report titled "Influenza 1957" and prepared by Hod Ogden, who was the information officer for the U.S. Public Health Service in 1957. Hod Ogden appears to have written "Influenza 1957" in late 1958. The report, which details the public health response in 1957, caught the eye of Donald Berreth, who was the director of the Office of Information at the CDC in 1976. Berreth circulated the report in May 1976. See director, Office of Information, to influenza committee, memorandum dated 18 May 1976, subject "Influenza 1957," box 10, file labeled "Background and History 5. 1957 Flu Epidemic," RG 442, NARA SE Region.

11. W. Palmer Dearing, qtd. in Ogden, "Influenza 1957," 45–46, RG 442, NARA SE Region.

12. Ogden, "Influenza 1957."

13. See Daniel Carpenter, *Reputation and Power: Organizational Image and Pharmaceuti-*

cal Regulation at the FDA (Princeton, N.J.: Princeton University Press, 2010), 73–117; for Cutter, see Offit, *Cutter Incident*.

14. "Addendum to Memorandum to All Influenza Centres of 22 May 1957," unsigned memorandum dated 24 May 1957, I2/418/12, 1, microfiche, WHO Archives, Geneva.

15. Maurice Hilleman and Harry M. Meyer, "Far East Influenza Viruses," dated 27 May 1957 and attached to Maurice Hilleman to Dr. A. M.-M. Payne, letter dated 28 May 1957, I2/418/12, 2, microfiche, WHO Archives, Geneva.

16. I have been unable to locate reports associated with this test beyond references to it in the Hod Ogden report. The summary of this "dry run" is thus drawn from Ogden, "Influenza 1957," 41–42.

17. It is unclear, but these were probably the same six U.S. manufacturers that produced vaccine for the 1957 Asian flu pandemic.

18. Kelley Lee, *Historical Dictionary of the World Health Organization* (Lanham, Md.: Scarecrow, 1998), chronology, xxiii–xliii.

19. In an attempt to trace the 1957 pandemic for future lessons, the WHO solicited a report from its member states on how each nation responded to Asian flu. Dozens of nations responded with summaries, including schedules of vaccination production. These have been collected in the WHO Archives. Sometimes the planned responses of nation-states came as a surprise to the WHO. When India reported it was beginning vaccine preparation on 21 May 1957, an unnamed reader marked the lines with an exclamation point. See C. Mani to Dr. Timmerman (ADG-CTS WHO), letter dated 21 May 1957, I2/418/12, 2, microfiche, WHO Archives, Geneva.

20. Claude Hannoun, who later came to be the director of the WHO's collaborating center for respiratory viruses in France, remembers making just such vaccines at the Pasteur Institute in Paris in 1957. Hannoun recalls that events of that year convinced the Pasteur Institute to get back into the business of producing vaccines and also spurred the development of the vaccine manufacturer Merieux, which through a combination of growth and merger is now the world's largest manufacturer of vaccines, operating under the name Sanofi Pasteur (Claude Hannoun, interview by author, 23 Aug. 2007).

21. "Minutes of an Informal Meeting on Influenza" (Geneva), 11 July 1957, 4, I2/418/12, 7, microfiche, WHO Archives, Geneva.

22. Professor Zhdanov, deputy minister of health, to Dr. Payne, chief of the section of epidemic and endemic disease, WHO, letter dated 11 March 1958, I2/418/12, 25, microfiche, WHO Archives, Geneva. My thanks to Helen Hundley for translating this document.

23. See the special supplement on Alexander Langmuir, *American Journal of Epidemiology* 144, no. 8, suppl., especially William H. Foege, "Alexander D. Langmuir: His Impact on Public Health," S11–S15; William Schaffner and F. Marc LaForce, "Training Field Epidemiologists: Alexander D. Langmuir and the Epidemic Intelligence Service," S16–S22; and Stanley O. Foster and Eugene Gangarosa, "Passing the Epidemiological Torch from Farr to the World: The Legacy of Alexander Langmuir," S65–S73.

24. For discussions of the CDC and the role the EIS played in tracking the acciden-

tal, artificially produced polio outbreak, see Etheridge, *Sentinel for Health*; Offit, *Cutter Incident*; and Oshinsky, *Polio*.

25. Henderson, who went on to have an extraordinarily prominent career in public health, was one of those two-year draftees of the CDC. In the summer of 1957 he was nearing the end of his service and preparing for his residency training in upstate New York. As Henderson describes it, Langmuir called him and said, "'Look, I haven't had a vacation since I came here, and you're going off, so I'm going to take a holiday this summer, and nothing's going to interrupt that." According to Henderson, when he protested that he did not know what to do about a possible flu pandemic, Langmuir assured him that he (Henderson) could figure something out. When he departed for vacation, Langmuir tossed off a common injunction to Henderson: "You call me, and you owe me a bottle of whiskey, and if you don't, I'll owe you one." Left to his own devices, Henderson crafted a surveillance system for flu that served as a model for future disease surveillance efforts at the CDC. As he remembered the events, when Langmuir returned from vacation, he followed through on his promised bottle of whiskey (D. A. Henderson, interview by author, 26 July 2007).

26. Unless otherwise noted, the following discussion of Asian flu in the summer of 1957 is drawn from CDC reports that have been collected and bound at the National Library of Medicine (Bethesda, Md.); Ogden, "Influenza 1957"; and the Henderson interview, 26 July 2007.

27. Although it is tempting to look for connections to other localized outbreaks—in this case, two scouts from Tangipahoa Parish were hospitalized on their return from Valley Forge—it is unnecessary. Nearby New Orleans is a bustling port, and several summer camps in that area reported outbreaks, too.

28. The summary of Surgeon General Burney's introduction comes from U.S. Public Health Service, *Proceedings, Special Conference of Influenza, Surgeon General Public Health Service with State and Territorial Health Officials, August 27–28, 1957* (Washington, D.C.: U.S. Department of Health, Education, and Welfare, n.d.), 1–5.

29. The document says "60 million cc," but that is most certainly an error.

30. Ogden, "Influenza 1957," 81–82.

31. CDC Influenza Report, no. 10 (8 Aug. 1957), National Library of Medicine, Bethesda, Md.

32. "1957 Influenza Immunization Sequence of Events," box 10, file labeled "Background and History 5. 1957 Epidemic," RG 442, NARA SE Region.

33. Etheridge, *Sentinel for Health*, 84.

34. Ibid.

35. Wire service account of the 28 September 1957 medical panel in San Francisco collected from "Panel Hits Mass Need of Flu Shots," *Los Angeles Times*, 29 September 1957, 5; "Mass Flu Immunization Seen Needless by Experts," *Hartford Courant*, 29 September 1957, 22, col. 1; "Mass Vaccine Not Needed Panel Says," *Washington Post and Times Herald*, 29 September 1957, B1; "Cast a Dubious Eye at Vaccine for Asia Flu," *Chicago Daily Tribune*, 29 September 1957, 6–7.

36. Michael Hattwick to J. Donald Millar, memorandum dated 7 March 1977, subject "Influenza Vaccine Distribution and Usage 1957–1975," box 3, binder titled "In-

fluenza Immunization Pre Swine Flu," tab "Distribution, Administration of Vaccine 1957–1975 (Hattwick)," RG 442, NARA SE Region.

37. The discussion of the discovery of Hong Kong flu comes from W. Charles Cockburn, P. J. Delon, and W. Ferreira, "Origins and Progress of the 1968–69 Hong Kong Influenza Epidemic," *Bulletin of the World Health Organization* 41 (1969): 345. I have been unable to find the *Times* of London story in either microfilm collections or the virtual archive maintained by the newspaper itself. For the exchange of telegrams between Cockburn and Chang, see folio labeled "Information on Influenza Incidences (1 July 1968–30 June 1969)," I2/442/2 (1968–69), jacket no. 1, WHO Archives, Geneva.

38. See Walter R. Dowdle, Marion T. Coleman, Elmer C. Hall, and Violeta Knez, "Properties of the Hong Kong Virus: 2. Antigenic Relationship of the Hong Kong Virus Hemagglutinin to That of Other Human Influenza A Viruses," *Bulletin of the World Health Organization* 41 (1969): 419–24; and J. L. Schulman and E. D. Kilbourne, "Independent Variation in Nature of the Hemagglutinin and Neuraminidase Antigens of Influenza Virus: Distinctiveness of the Hemagglutinin Antigen of Hong Kong/68 Virus," *Proceedings of the National Academy of Science* 63 (1969): 326–33.

39. Production figures adapted from a chart in Roderick Murray, "Production and Testing in the USA of Influenza Virus Vaccine Made from the Hong Kong Variant in 1968–69," *Bulletin of the World Health Organization* 41 (1969): 496.

40. V. M Zdhanov and I. V. Antonova, "The Hong Kong Influenza Virus Epidemic in the USSR," *Bulletin of the World Health Organization* 41 (1969): 386.

Chapter 5. The Forecast Calls for Pandemics

1. See K. David Patterson, *Pandemic Influenza 1700–1900: A Study in Historical Epidemiology* (Totowa, N.J.: Rowman and Littlefield, 1986); Gerald F. Pyle, *Applied Medical Geography* (Washington, D.C.: V. H. Winston, 1979); and Gerald F. Pyle, *The Diffusion of Influenza: Patterns and Paradigms* (Totowa, N.J.: Rowman and Littlefield, 1986).

2. The official role of expert committees is not always well defined even to the experts involved, as Dr. F. Assaad (director, Division of Communicable Diseases, WHO) made clear to Dr. George Galasso (National Institutes of Health) in a discussion related to influenza in 1983. Assaad emphasized, "The official positions of WHO are only those laid down by the decisions of our governing bodies—i.e. the Executive Board of WHO and the World Health Assembly. When the Organization publishes the report of a technical meeting . . . it is always made plain that the views expressed are those of the experts concerned and do not necessarily represent the decisions or the stated policy of the Organization. Technical meetings advise and guide the Director-General and the Secretariat but their reports are not official statements by WHO. Their advice, of course, helps the WHO Secretariat to give guidance when this is requested by countries" (Assaad to Galasso, letter dated 15 December 1983, file labeled "WHO Informal Consultation on the Clinical Use of Amantadine/Rimantadine in Influenza, Vienna, Austria, 26–28/8/1983," I2/181/3, WHO Archives, Geneva). The general information about the WHO and expert committees is drawn from Fraser Brockington, *World Health,* 2d ed. (Boston: Little, Brown, 1968); Francis W. Hoole, *Politics and Budgeting in the World Health Organization* (Bloomington: Indiana University Press, 1976); and Amos

Yoder, *The Evolution of the United Nations System,* 3d ed. (Washington, D.C.: Taylor and Francis, 1997).

3. Description of experts meetings is drawn from Walter Dowdle, former director of the CDC's virology division, e-mail to author, 25 March 2007; and David Tyrrell and Michael Fielder, *Cold Wars: The Fight against the Common Cold* (New York: Oxford University Press, 2002), 170–76.

4. "Minutes of an Informal Meeting on Influenza, Geneva, 11 July 1957," I2/418/12-7, microfiche, 7, WHO Archives, Geneva. Kaplan, of course, was not the first to pursue the link between animal and human influenza. As was discussed, Shope believed he had uncovered the Spanish flu strain from the swine population of the U.S. Midwest. In addition, it appears that the United States Public Health Service was involved in researching swine influenza viruses for possible use in human influenza vaccine prior to December 1949. For reference to this research, see W. I. B. Beveridge to Dr. C. H. Andrewes, quoting James H. Steele, chief of the USPHS's veterinary division, letter dated 14 December 1949, WHO 2., DC Infl. 6, W.I.C. 1, microfiche, WHO Archives, Geneva.

5. The merits of the recycling theory are a matter of some dispute among influenza experts. The noted influenza virologist Edwin Kilbourne says, "I think the evidence is pretty good it has happened. It's serologic evidence but it's good. If you think of it, the recycling theory, that is based on a human life span—what used to be human lifetime, that's about it" (Edwin Kilbourne, interview by author, 20 Jan. 2004). But Walter Dowdle, another prominent influenza expert, has challenged the evidence that was used to construct the recycling theory; see W. R. Dowdle, "Influenza A Virus Recycling Revisited," *Bulletin of the World Health Organization* 77, no. 10 (Oct. 1999): 820–28. Dowdle argues that the evidence does not substantiate the predictive pattern of influenza recycling.

6. J. Mulder, "Asiatic Influenza in the Netherlands," *Lancet* 270, no. 6990 (17 Aug. 1957): 334; and J. Mulder, N. Masurel, E. M. Deggars, and P. J. Webbers, "Pre-Epidemic Antibody against 1957 Strain of Asiatic Influenza: In Serum of Older People Living in the Netherlands," *Lancet* 271, no. 7025 (19 Apr. 1958): 810–14.

7. A. M.-M. Payne to "All Influenza Centres and Observers," memorandum dated 21 June 1957, subject "Supplement to My Memorandum of 19 June 1957," I2/418/12-4, microfiche, WHO Archives, Geneva.

8. F. M. Davenport et al., "Further Observations on the Relevance of Serologic Recapitulations of Human Infection with Influenza Viruses," *Journal of Experimental Medicine* 120 (1964): 1087–97.

9. Thomas Francis Jr., "On the Doctrine of Original Antigenic Sin," *Proceedings of the American Philosophical Society* 104, no. 6 (15 Dec. 1960): 572–78.

10. See, for example, F. M. Davenport, E. Minuse, A. V. Hennessy, and T. Francis Jr., "Interpretations of Influenza Antibody Patterns of Man," *Bulletin of the World Health Organization* 41 (1969): 453–60; N. Masurel, "Serological Characteristics of a 'New' Serotype of Influenza A Virus: The Hong Kong Strain," ibid., 461–68; Hideo Fukumi, "Interpretation and Significance of Hong Kong Antibody in Old People Prior to the Hong Kong Influenza Epidemic," ibid., 469–73.

11. For a full discussion of the reasons behind the new naming system, see Walter R. Dowdle, Marion T. Coleman, Elmer C. Hall, and Violeta Knez, "Properties of the Hong Kong Influenza Virus: 2. Antigenic Relationship of the Hong Kong Virus Hemagglutinin to that of Other Human Influenza A Viruses," *Bulletin of the World Health Organization* 41 (1969): 419–24.

12. The following discussion of the recycling theory and the way it was understood following the 1968 Hong Kong flu is drawn from Fred M. Davenport, "Prospects for the Control of Influenza," *American Journal of Nursing* 69, no. 9 (Sept. 1969): 1908–11; and Davenport, Minuse, Hennessy, and Francis, "Interpretations of Influenza," 453–60.

13. The following discussion of the eleven-year-cycle theory is drawn from Edwin Kilbourne, "Epidemiology of Influenza," in *Influenza Viruses and Influenza,* ed. Kilbourne (New York: Academic, 1975), 483–538; and "Specific Immunity in Influenza— Summary of Influenza Workshop III," *Journal of Infectious Diseases* 127, no. 2 (Feb. 1973): 220–23 (see chart on 221 for a comprehensive description of this theory).

14. The eleven-year-cycle theory has not stood the test of time. Both 1946 and 1929 were subsequently determined not to be epidemic years, and thirty-two years passed before the novel H1N1 swine flu strain reset that clock from the 1977 Russian flu. No discernible pattern in influenza pandemics has been determined.

15. An embryonic form of the eleven-year-cycle explanation can be found in an article by Francis where he wrote, "It appears then that about ten years were required for virus of a family to circulate in the population so extensively as to build up immunity to the point that virus of that group did not find ready susceptibles in which to propagate" (Francis, "On the Doctrine," 547).

16. For the announcement of the process, see Edwin Kilbourne, "Future Influenza Vaccines and the Use of Genetic Recombinants," *Bulletin of the World Health Organization* 41 (1969): 643–45; for a step-by-step account of the process in action, see Harold M. Schmeck Jr., "Race for the Swine Flu Vaccine Began in a Manhattan Lab," *New York Times,* 21 May 1976, B1, 3.

17. Researchers and manufacturers wanted to avoid the possibility that a mammal virus might accidentally be injected into the population. In 1960 Maurice Hilleman had discovered a new virus (which he dubbed Simian Virus 40, or S.V. 40) in monkey kidney cells used to produce polio vaccine. Hilleman found viable S.V. 40 virus in both killed (Salk) and live (Sabin) polio vaccine. More worrying was the fact that S.V. 40 was found to cause cancer when injected into baby hamsters. Fortunately, long-term studies of the millions of people who received the two types of vaccines did not, and do not, reveal elevated cancer rates, and subsequent processes removed S.V. 40 from vaccines after 1963. The whole experience has served as a strong caution against using mammalian-line cells for vaccine production. See B. H. Sweet and M. R. Hilleman, "The Vacuolating Virus, S. V. 40," *Proceedings of the Society for Experimental Biology and Medicine* 105 (1960): 420–27; Paul Offit, *Vaccinated: One Man's Quest to Defeat the World's Deadliest Diseases* (New York: Smithsonian Books, 2007), 95–97; and David M. Oshinsky, *Polio: An American Story* (Oxford: Oxford University Press, 2005), 279–82.

18. For the "wars" on poverty and cancer, see James T. Patterson, *Grand Expectations: The United States, 1945–1974* (New York: Oxford University Press, 1996). For the CDC, see Elizabeth W. Etheridge, *Sentinel for Health: A History of the Centers for Dis-*

ease Control (Berkeley: University of California Press, 1992). Background material here comes from David Sencer, interview by author, 9 May 2007; J. Donald Millar, interview by author, 22 May 2007.

19. According to Alex Langmuir, then director of the CDC, the intense promotion of influenza vaccine use by the CDC in the early 1960s achieved a "rather large volume of use." Unfortunately, in the eyes of Langmuir, this increased usage occurred mostly among employees in the industrial sector rather than individuals in the high-risk population. Langmuir had strong doubts about the usefulness of this vaccine push in benefiting the public and about the effectiveness of influenza vaccines in general. See Alex Langmuir qtd. in "Sessions I-VIII: Open Discussion," in *Proceedings of the International Conference on the Application of Vaccines against Viral, Rickettsial, and Bacterial Disease of Man, 14–18 December 1970* (Washington, D.C.: Pan American Health Organization, 1971), 614.

20. D. A. Henderson, interview by author, 26 July 2007.

21. See Francis A. Ennis, "Production and Distribution of Vaccine Following Emergence of a New Viral Strain," in *Influenza: Virus, Vaccines and Strategy: Proceedings of a Working Group on Pandemic Influenza, Rougemount, January 1976,* ed. Philip Selby (London: Academic, 1976), 245–52.

22. This and the following discussion of French vaccine production come from an interview I conducted on 23 August 2007 with Claude Hannoun, who headed a French laboratory designated as a WHO reference collaborating center for respiratory viruses 1970 to 1995.

23. Unless otherwise noted, information about manufacturing in the United Kingdom is from an interview I conducted on 30 October 2007 with Ian Furminger, former head of research and development and production at Evans Medical, the Glaxo subsidiary that produced virtually all influenza vaccine for the U.K. market in the 1970s.

24. Joseph W. G. Smith, "Vaccination Strategy," from *Influenza: Virus, Vaccines, Strategy: Proceedings of a Working Group on Pandemic Influenza, Rougemount, January 1976,* ed. Philip Selby (London: Academic, 1976), 271–94.

25. J. Donald Millar, interview by author, 22 May 2007.

26. Figures and information about Japanese policy are drawn from a letter and a report from Hideo Fukumi, at Japan's National Institute of Health, to W. Charles Cockburn, Chief Medical Officer, virus diseases, World Health Organization, received 27 July 1973, file folder labeled "Information on Influenza Incidence 1/7/1972–30/6/1973 (72–73)," jacket no. 2, I2/442/2, WHO Archives, Geneva.

27. "Influenza Virus Polypeptides and Antigens—Summary of Influenza Workshop I," *Journal of Infectious Diseases* 125, no. 4 (Apr. 1972): 447–56; "Immunologic Methodology in Influenza Diagnosis and Research—Summary of Influenza Workshop II," *Journal of Infectious Diseases* 126, no. 2 (Aug. 1972): 219–30; "Specific Immunity in Influenza—Summary of Influenza Workshop III," *Journal of Infectious Diseases* 127, no. 2 (Feb. 1973): 220–36; "Epidemiology of Influenza—Summary of Influenza Workshop IV," *Journal of Infectious Diseases* 128, no. 3 (Sept. 1973): 361–86; "Influenza Vaccines—Summary of Influenza Workshop V," *Journal of Infectious Diseases* 129, no. 6 (June 1974): 750–71; "Animal Influenza: Its Significance in Human Infection—Summary of Influenza Workshop VI," *Journal of Infectious Diseases* 131, no. 5 (May 1975): 602–12; "Ge-

netics, Replication, and Inhibition of Replication of Influenza Viruses—Summary of Influenza Workshop VII," *Journal of Infectious Diseases* 132, no. 6 (Dec. 1975): 713–23; "Antiviral Agents in Influenza—Summary of Influenza Workshop VIII," *Journal of Infectious Diseases* 134, no. 5 (Nov. 1976): 516–27.

28. Walter Dowdle, interview by author, 26 May 2005.

29. The January 1976 Rougemount conference is of particular interest because, unbeknownst to the conference delegates, they would be able to directly assess pandemic preparedness in the ensuing weeks. The workshop was being held at the same time that the novel swine influenza strain was circulating at Fort Dix, New Jersey.

30. Discussion of surveillance capabilities comes from the summary discussion including Chairman W. R. Dowdle as recorded by *rapporteur* J. W. G. Smith, "Surveillance and Early Warning," in *Influenza: Virus, Vaccine, and Strategy: Proceedings of a Working Group on Pandemic Influenza, Rougemount, January 1976,* ed. Philip Selby (London: Academic, 1976), 89–92. The general discussion followed the first session and presumably included all twenty-eight participants.

31. Unless otherwise noted, the following discussion of vaccination strategies is drawn from Smith, "Vaccination Strategy," 271–94.

32. For example, some research programs had to be discontinued due to government cutbacks. Geoffrey Schild, of the Medical Research Council, told Charles Cockburn, director of the WHO's division of communicable diseases, that the MRC could not continue to fund studies of seabird colonies in northern Norway (as part of the influenza ecology series) because of "the considerable restrictions of [its] current budget"; see Schild to Cockburn, letter dated 14 December 1973, file labeled "CTS Agreement with the Medical Research Council, London, In Respect of a Field Study on the Ecology of Avian Influenza Viruses," I2/181/2 (1), WHO Archives, Geneva. Walter Dowdle would later express the hope that the "energy shortage in Britain [had] not affected [Schild's] laboratories as much as the press might" have reported (Walter Dowdle, WHO International Influenza Center for the Americas, to Geoffrey Schild, World Influenza Centre, National Institute for Medical Research, letter dated 7 January 1974, file labeled "Information on Influenza Incidence 1/7/73–30/6/74," jacket 1, I2/442/2 [73–74], WHO Archives, Geneva).

33. For example, Walter Dowdle and Marion Coleman reported that because antigenic drift was occurring at a more rapid pace, it might signal an imminent pandemic shift in the virus, since a similar pattern had been observed in 1957 and 1968. See WHO International Influenza Center for the Americas to "All Laboratories Collaborating with the World Health Organization International Influenza Center for the Americas," memorandum dated July 1974, file labeled "Information on Influenza Incidence-1/7/73–30/6/74," jacket no. 2, I2/442/2 (73–74), WHO Archives, Geneva. A similar point about a possible imminent pandemic shift was made by Charles Cockburn. While lobbying to keep Geoffrey Schild as the head of the World Influenza Centre in London, despite Schild's taking new duties in another government laboratory, Cockburn wrote that he was "very reluctant to lose [Schild's] services . . . at a time when the influenza virus [was] showing signs of very considerable antigenic instability which may be an indication of the appearance of a new sub-type in the not too distant future"

(Charles Cockburn to Sir John Gray, secretary of the Medical Research Council, letter dated 6 June 1975, file labeled "Designation and Activities of the WHO Collaborating Centre for Reference and Research on Influenza Virus-Virus Reference Laboratory, Central Public Health Laboratory London and Division of Virology, National Institute for Medical Research, London U.K.," jacket no. 2, I2/286/2, WHO Archives, Geneva).

34. From a report summarizing NIAID research on acute respiratory disease, prepared January 1976, box 5, book 32, "1976 Correspondence from National Institute of Allergy and Infectious Diseases," received in response to Freedom of Information request 28820, in possession of the author.

35. Maurice Hilleman, director, virus and cell biology research, Merck Institute for Therapeutic Research, to John Seal, acting deputy director, National Institute of Allergy and Infectious Diseases, letter dated 14 January 1976, box 6, book 42, "Workshops/Meetings and Fact Sheets," received in response to Freedom of Information request 28820, in possession of author. Emphasis Hilleman's. Hilleman had been predicting a late 1970s influenza pandemic since 1970 at least. See Hilleman qtd. in "Sessions I-VIII: Open Discussion," in *Proceedings of the International Conference on the Application of Vaccines against Viral, Rickettsial, and Bacterial Disease of Man, 14–18 December 1970* (Washington, D.C.: Pan American Health Organization, 1971), 614.

36. Although the remark is frequently attributed to Surgeon General Stewart, there is some question whether he actually said such a thing. The official historian of the USPHS, John Parascandola, can find no citation for the quotation, and Dr. Stewart did not recall uttering such a statement. But Dr. Stewart does not refute the possibility that he stated his views on infectious diseases in this or a similar manner. The fact that Dr. Stewart acknowledges he might have said such a thing illustrates the early 1970s public health community's wide acceptance of the notion that infectious diseases would continue to be a declining threat to human health. See FAQs at http://lhncbc.nlm.nih.gov/adb/phsHistory/faqs.html (accessed 29 Oct. 2008); B. Milstein, "Hygeia's Constellation: Navigating Health Futures in a Dynamic and Democratic World," in Syndemics Prevention Network, Centers for Disease Control, http://www.index/mongraph/syndemics/gov.cdc.htm (accessed 29 Oct. 2008); and Christopher M. Sassetti and Eric Rubin, "The Open Book on Infectious Diseases," *Nature Medicine* 13, no. 3 (Mar. 2007): 279–80.

37. See James Colgrove, *State of Immunity: The Politics of Vaccination in Twentieth-Century America* (Berkeley: University of California Press, 2006), especially chapters 3 and 4, 113–85, for a discussion of the power and limits of vaccination in the 1950s through the 1970s; see Arthur Allen, *Vaccine: The Controversial Story of Medicine's Greatest Lifesaver* (New York: Norton, 2007), 160–250, for polio and measles vaccination programs during the same time period. As Stern and Markel point out, many of these criticisms echo vaccine difficulties that go all the way back to the era of Jenner and the first vaccine. See Alexandra Minna Stern and Howard Markel, "The History of Vaccines and Immunization: Familiar Patterns, New Challenges," *Health Affairs* 24, no. 3 (May–June 2005): 611–21.

38. Michael A. W. Hattwick, chief of the respiratory and special pathogens branch,

of the CDC's Bureau of Epidemiology, to Pascal J. Imperator, first deputy commissioner of the City of New York's department of health, letter dated 19 February 1976, box 34, file labeled "Reading File, 1976," RG 442, NARA SE Region.

39. For the growth of the CDC, see Elizabeth Etheridge, *Sentinel for Health: A History of the Centers for Disease Control* (Berkeley: University of California Press, 1992).

40. Sencer interview, 9 May 2007.

41. For budget figures, see Victoria A. Harden, *Inventing the NIH: Federal Biomedical Research Policy, 1887–1937* (Baltimore, Md.: Johns Hopkins University Press, 1986), 183; for Congress, see Stephen P. Strickland, *Politics, Science, and Dread Disease: A Short History of United States Medical Research Policy* (Cambridge, Mass.: Harvard University Press, 1972), 109–33.

42. David Sencer defined control simply as "prevent death" (Sencer interview, 9 May 2007).

43. Etheridge, *Sentinel for Health*, 248.

Chapter 6. "Chance Favors the Prepared Mind"

1. International researchers were meeting in Switzerland on 26–28 January 1976; see Philip Selby, ed., *Influenza: Virus, Vaccines, and Strategy, Proceedings of a Working Group on Pandemic Influenza, Rougemount, January 1976* (London: Academic, 1976). National Institute of Allergy and Infectious Diseases (NIAID) officials were openly speculating whether they should accelerate research on live-virus vaccines to prepare for the "anticipated pandemic due to a new variant of influenza quite possibly occurring within the next five years" (acting deputy director, NIAID [John Seal], memorandum "for the record" dated 20 January 1976, subject "Discussion of Potential for Live Attenuated Influenza A Vaccine for General Use in the United States," obtained via Freedom of Information request, case no. 28820, to National Institute of Allergy and Infectious Diseases, in possession of author). Goldfield had jokingly prophesized that the unidentified strains were swine when he sent them on to Atlanta; see Lawrence Wright, "Sweating out the Swine Flu Scare," *New Times,* 11 June 1976, 30.

2. Unless otherwise noted, the following discussion of the collection of influenza samples from Fort Dix and their delivery to the CDC in Atlanta is drawn from Martin Goldfield et al., "Influenza in New Jersey in 1976: Isolation of Influenza A/New Jersey/76 Virus at Fort Dix," *Journal of Infectious Disease* 136, suppl. (Dec. 1977): S347–55; Wright, "Sweating," 29–36; and Walter Dowdle and (probably) Gary Noble, loose laboratory notes stored with Walter Dowdle's laboratory notebook, box 32, unlabeled folder, T-1 (1), RG 442, NARA SE Region.

3. Sencer recalled it as a Tuesday evening when interviewed, but it must have been Thursday, the day the virus was typed (David Sencer, interview by author, 9 May 2007).

4. Unless otherwise noted, the following discussion of the 14 February 1976 meeting is drawn from Sencer interview, 9 May 2007; Walter Dowdle, interview by author, 26 May 2005; Richard E. Neudstadt and Harvey V. Fineberg, *The Swine Flu Affair: Decision-Making on a Slippery Disease* (Washington, D.C.: U.S. Department of Health, Education, and Welfare, 1978), 5–9; Arthur Silverstein, *Pure Politics and Impure Science* (Baltimore, Md.: Johns Hopkins University Press, 1981), 24–27; Wright, "Sweating,"

29–36; and acting deputy director, NIAID (John Seal), memorandum "for the record" dated 17 February 1976, subject "Influenza Meeting at CDC, Saturday, February 14, 1976," box 32 unlabeled folder T-1 (1), RG 442, NARA SE Region.

5. Originally formed as part of the 1902 Biologics Control Act, the Hygienic Laboratory of the Public Health and Marine Hospital Service was charged with licensing manufacturers for the production of serums, antitoxins, and vaccines. In 1930 the Hygienic Laboratory was renamed the National Institute of Health (changed to the National Institutes of Health in 1948), and the unit was titled the Division of Biologics Standardization. Following a Senate investigation prompted by supporters of Ralph Nader, the division was taken from the NIH and moved to the Food and Drug Administration, where it was reorganized and christened the Bureau of Biologics in 1972. It eventually morphed into its current responsibilities and roles under the heading of the Center for Biologics Evaluation and Research. The organization's mandate remains the regulation and licensing of manufacturers and ensuring the safety and quality of biological products used by the public. For an overview of the unit's history, see http://www.fda.gov/AboutFDA/WhatWeDo/History/FOrgsHistory/CBER/ucm135758.htm (accessed 12 Oct. 2011).

6. Gary Noble qtd. in Wright, "Sweating," 33.

7. Anonymous participant qtd. in ibid., 33

8. Walter Dowdle, laboratory notes dated 13–17 February, "Discussion [with] Dr. Russell," box 32, unlabeled folder T-1 (1), RG 442, NARA SE Region.

9. *Morbidity and Mortality Weekly Report* 25, no. 6, box 31, folder titled "Swine Flu HEW/CDC Memos [Dowdle 4]," RG 442, NARA SE Region.

10. Quotations from Seal, memo "for the record," subject "Influenza Meeting, February 14, 1976," 3–4.

11. Dr. Eleanor Shore, notes, "ACIP meeting February 5–6, 1976," box 35, file labeled "Advisory Committee on Immunization Practices Meeting February 5–6, 1976," RG 442, NARA SE Region.

12. Quotation from Seal, memo "for the record," subject "Influenza Meeting, February 14, 1976," 10.

13. "Quickly" is a relative term. According to David Sencer, the "sero-survey" of the personnel at Fort Dix took an inordinately long time because of bureaucratic changes in the military: "In the old days . . . they could have just gone in and done it, [but] in 1976 they needed to get command, line command decisions, not just medical decisions. They had to go to the Pentagon and go back down to the commanding officer at Fort Dix. . . . It took quite a while. Normally, three years before that, they would have had the sero-survey done in a couple of days, but this took almost six weeks" (Sencer interview, 9 May 2007).

14. "Developing a National Plan for Influenza Program, 3–19–76," item 3-d, box 31, folder labeled "Swine Flu Bob 3/25/76, Swine Flu Events 3/1–30/76 [Dowdle 2]," RG 442, NARA SE Region.

15. David J. Sencer to "State Health Officials," Intrafax telegram dated 18 February 1976, box 44, binder labeled "Flu-1," tab "Feb. 18 Advisory to States," RG 442, NARA SE Region.

16. Unless otherwise noted, the following quotations come from H. Bruce Dull,

"Statement on Influenza—Thursday, February 19, 1976," box 27, file labeled "Influenza-A/Swine Background Material," RG 442, NARA SE Region.

17. Harold M. Schmeck Jr., "U.S. Calls Flu Alert on Possible Return of Epidemic's Virus," *New York Times,* 20 February 1976, p. 1, col. 3.

18. Assorted press clippings from box 44, binder labeled "Flu-1," tab "Press Coverage," RG 442, NARA SE Region.

19. T.K. (?) to H.F. (Harvey Fineberg) and R.E.N. (Richard E. Neustadt), memorandum dated 28 July 1977, subject "Evening News Coverage of Swine Flu, as abstracted in *Vanderbilt Television News Archives Index and Abstracts,*" box 44, file labeled "Press Briefing 10/12/76–1977," 1, RG 442, NARA SE Region.

20. David M. Rubin, "Remember Swine Flu?" *Columbia Journalism Review* 16, no. 2 (July–Aug. 1977), 43. See also David M. Rubin and Val Hendry, "Swine Influenza and the News Media," *Annals of Internal Medicine* 87 (Dec. 1977): 769–74.

21. Charles S. Taylor, UPI bulletin dated 7 May 1976, box 35, folder labeled "Advisory Committee on Immunization Practices Meeting of May 6–7, 1976," RG 442, NARA SE Region.

22. Unless otherwise noted, the following discussion of the 20 February 1976 meeting is drawn from "Centers for Disease Control, Bureau of Biologics, National Institute of Allergy and Infectious Diseases, Influenza Workshop, February 20, 1976," transcript, obtained from the U.S. Department of Health and Human Services via Freedom of Information request F02–17965 and in possession of author.

23. I have been unable to find a list of the meeting attendees, but thirty-three different people are recorded as speaking on the transcript.

24. Arthur Silverstein stated that in this meeting "a perceptible escalation had taken place in the fears and concerns of the scientists and public health officials in attendance. For reasons not entirely clear, the mood seemed to have changed from 'What if . . ?' to 'Well, here it is!'" (Silverstein, *Pure Politics,* 27). I agree there was an escalation in "fears and concerns" of the scientists and public health officials, but I see more "Well, here it is!" in the 14 February meeting than Silverstein acknowledges.

25. Harry Meyer, 20 February 1976 Influenza Workshop transcript, 9.

26. Walter Dowdle, 20 February 1976 Influenza Workshop transcript, 47–48.

27. Edwin Kilbourne, 20 February 1976 Influenza Workshop transcript, 79.

28. The problems of live-virus vaccines will be discussed in chapter 9.

29. Maurice Hilleman, 20 February 1976 Influenza Workshop transcript, 97–104.

30. Harry Meyer, 20 February 1976 Influenza Workshop transcript, 116.

31. Shope had collected the material from a sick pig and then passed it through a succession of chicken eggs and pigs before finally storing it as a reference sample. The strain's last passage had been through a host labeled "1976." The vaccine manufacturing firm Parke, Davis inadvertently began production using this strain instead of the A/New Jersey/76 strain. Parke, Davis produced forty-three lots before this error was detected. The Bureau of Biologics rejected these lots, and Parke, Davis was forced to stop production and restart with the proper seed stock, creating a significant delay. The federal government denied reimbursement to Parke, Davis for this error, ruling the mistake was the firm's, not the CDC's. See letter dated 24 August 1977, "Decision Disallowing Request of Parke, Davis and Company for Reimbursement of Costs In-

curred in the Production of A/Swine/1976/31 (Shope-like) Vaccine Under Letter Contract CDC 200–76–0426," box 2, binder labeled "Swine Flu Vaccine Contract (And Related Issues) Volume III," tab "Parke Davis Shope Vaccine Issue," RG 442, NARA SE Region.

32. Dowdle noted, "Possible use of [?] 1976/31 strain as vaccine, at least to start. Fred [Davenport] to describe at meeting on Friday" (Walter Dowdle, handwritten notes, notebook titled "Ft. Dix Log Book Feb. '76," box 32, unlabeled folder T-1 [1], RG 442, NARA SE Region).

33. Ibid.

34. See influenza program officer, IDB, NIAID (Franklin J. Tyeryer), memorandum "for the record" dated 1 March 1976, subject "Meeting on Influenza at BoB/FDA on February 27, 1976," box 32, unlabeled folder T-1 (1), RG 442, NARA SE Region.

35. Remarkably, however, it was not the strain that was used in producing the 40 million doses that were injected into the American public. Even though contemporary and retrospective critics attacked the program and the vaccine, and numerous lawsuits were subsequently filed asserting the vaccine had damaged their clients, no one noticed that the vaccine strain was different from the widely tested X-53 except for a passing reference in a CBS *Sixty Minutes* report. The vaccine was developed by Edwin Kilbourne, who dubbed it X-53a. The X-53a strain was a "second-generation, better-yielding swine vaccine that had never been field-tested. It was a different recombinant than the one used in the preliminary field trials [i.e., X-53]." As Kilbourne described it, "I don't want to emphasize how different they are, because antigenically they are almost identical, but in terms of growth capacity, one grew eight- to thirty-two-fold better in production" (Kilbourne, interview by author, 20 Jan. 2004). Manufacturers would certainly have recognized that the strain X-53a would have a higher yield, but it went unremarked that the strain had not been field-tested for possible reactions. George J. Galasso, chief of the NIAID's infectious disease branch, told the director of the NIAID (coincidentally, on the same day that the NIAID hosted a meeting reporting on the results of field tests using X-53) of reports that "X-53A high yield recombinant was found to be acceptable for vaccine production seed (A/NJ/76) based on studies at BoB and CDC and distributed to manufacturers." He asserted, "It is anticipated that this will increase the vaccine yield twofold." See Galsasso to director, NIAID, memorandum dated 21 June 1976, subject "The NIAID Weekly Progress Report on the National Influenza Immunization Program-Report no. 8," box 20, binder labeled "Swine Flu Reports, Misc. Early Reports to HEW, White House Biweekly Reports to Asst. Secretary, Secretary," tab "7/1/76," RG 442, NARA SE Region.

36. E. D. Kilbourne et al., "Correlated Studies of a Recombinant Influenza-Virus Vaccine. I. Derivation and Characterization of Virus and Vaccine," *Journal of Infectious Diseases* 124 (1971): 449–62.

37. Edwin Kilbourne, "Centers for Disease Control, Bureau of Biologics, National Institute for Allergy and Infectious Diseases Influenza Workshop March 25, 1976," transcript, 40–41, box 32, unlabeled folder T-1 (2), RG 442, NARA SE Region.

38. Edwin Kilbourne to Dr. John Seal, letter dated 24 February 1976, box 31, file labeled "Swine Flu HEW/CDC Memos (Dowdle 4 [in pencil])," RG 442, NARA SE Region.

39. Dr. Jordan and Walter Dowdle, "Centers for Disease Control, Bureau of Biologics, National Institute for Allergy and Infectious Diseases Influenza Workshop March 25, 1976," transcript, 47, box 32, unlabeled folder T-1 (2), RG 442, NARA SE Region.

40. Walter Dowdle's laboratory notebook reveals six small epidemics or clusters of unidentified influenza-like illnesses between 19 February and 16 March 1976. Any one of these could have been the emerging swine flu pandemic the public health experts feared. For example, on 19 February a large outbreak of influenza-like disease occurred in Mexico City, and forty specimens were sent for typing. On Monday, 23 February, two unidentified specimens from the Mayo Clinic were sent. On Tuesday, 24 February, the U.S. Air Force collected specimens from an outbreak at Brooks Air Force Base. On Thursday, 26 February, Fred Davenport relayed information that the WHO had reported at least one death of a child in the USSR and possible cases in Puerto Rico. On Monday, 1 March, Idaho reported a high death rate in an old-age home from an epidemic that had begun February 5 and said that it would send samples. On Tuesday, 16 March, Trinidad reported an influenza epidemic. See Walter Dowdle, notes, "Ft. Dix Log Book Feb. '76," box 32, unlabeled folder T-1 (1), RG 442, NARA SE Region.

41. Walter Dowdle, handwritten notes on Charles Hoke Jr. et al., "Influenza Surveillance Summary, Prepared for Advisory Committee on Immunization Practices, March 10, 1976," chart labeled "Pneumonia-Influenza Deaths in 121 United States Cities," box 32, unlabeled folder T-1 (3), RG 442, NARA SE Region.

42. The discussion of surveillance in New Jersey in February and March 1976 is drawn from Goldfield et al., "Influenza in New Jersey," S347–55, especially tables 3 and 4, unless otherwise noted.

43. Unless otherwise noted, the following discussion of seroarchaeology and the epidemiological investigation of the camp is from Colonel Top's discussion, "Center for Disease Control, Bureau of Biologics, National Institute of Allergy and Infectious Diseases Influenza Workshop March 25, 1976," transcript, 13–20, box 32, unlabeled folder T-1 (2), RG 442, NARA SE Region.

44. See chart, "Influenza—A/Swine Serologic Survey—Fort Dix, 17–27 Feb. 76," box 21, folder labeled "Swine Flu—Ft. Dix, etc.," RG 442, NARA SE Region. The CDC would screen some number of blood samples submitted for marriage licenses for antibodies to the new flu strain.

45. Dowdle, Notebook titled "Ft. Dix Log Book Feb. '76," box 32, unlabeled folder T-1 (1), RG 442, NARA SE Region.

46. Unless otherwise noted, the following discussion of the CDC's investigation is drawn from "Center for Disease Control, Bureau of Biologics, National Institute of Allergy and Infectious Diseases Influenza Workshop March 25, 1976," transcript, 20–25, box 32, unlabeled folder T-1 (2), RG 442, NARA SE Region.

47. I have been unable to find Fayettesville on any map of Pennsylvania or through Internet searches using Google, Yahoo, and Mapquest (searches conducted 8 July 2003). There is, however, a Fayetteville listed in rural central Pennsylvania near the Maryland border. This seems the likely location. It is possible that the letter s has been dropped from the town name since 1976, but I suspect that the name was initially misspelled and the error subsequently repeated throughout the documents.

48. See period articles, including E. D. Kilbourne, "Recombination of Influenza A Viruses of Human and Animal Origin," *Science* 160 (1968): 74–76; R. G. Webster and W. G. Laver, "Studies on the Origin of Pandemic Influenza I," *Virology* 48 (1972): 433–44; W. G. Laver and R. G. Webster, "Studies on the Origin of Pandemic Influenza II," *Virology* 48 (1972): 445–55; and W. G. Laver and R. G. Webster, "Studies on the Origins of Pandemic Influenza III," *Virology* 51 (1973): 383–91. The term "mixing vessel" is drawn from a later article: C. Scholtissek, H. Burger, O. Kistner, and K. F. Shortridge, "The Nucleoprotein as a Possible Factor in Determining Host Specificity of Influenza H3N2 Viruses," *Virology* 147 (1985): 287–94.

49. The study involved using the "Delphi technique," in which a small number of experts were quizzed to estimate the probability of a fall pandemic. The experts were then shown the anonymous responses of their colleagues and asked whether they would like to revise their estimate. See Stephen C. Schoenbaum, Barbara J. McNeil, and Joel Kavet, "The Swine-Influenza Decision," *New England Journal of Medicine* 295, no. 14 (Sept. 1976): 759–65. Unfortunately, in 1976 experts on influenza lacked the proper tools to assess the likelihood of a virus spreading. David Sencer later recalled that when he met with the secretary and staff of the Department of Health, Education, and Welfare, they insistently asked him, "What are the probabilities?" and the best he could answer was, "We do not know" (Sencer interview, 9 May 2007). Even today public health experts refuse to estimate the probability that a given flu strain will cause a pandemic because of the unpredictability resulting from recombination, where two viruses swapping genetic attributes can create a highly transmissible novel strain.

Chapter 7. An Act of Will

1. Richard E. Neudstadt and Harvey V. Fineberg, *The Swine Flu Affair: Decision-Making on a Slippery Disease* (Washington, D.C.: U.S. Department of Health, Education, and Welfare, 1978), 10. In a book generally critical of Sencer and the decision-making process of the "Swine Flu Affair," Neustadt and Fineberg also temper this compliment by stating Sencer was an "able and wily autocrat" (ibid.). Silverstein's description can be found in Arthur Silverstein, *Pure Politics and Impure Science* (Baltimore, Md.: Johns Hopkins University Press, 1981), 34.

2. Kilbourne was dismayed to see his op-ed piece, a sober suggestion that the nation prepare for the national disaster of an influenza pandemic, bear a hyperbolic headline; see Edwin D. Kilbourne, "Flu to Starboard! Man the Harpoons! Fill 'em with Vaccine! Alert the Captain! Hurry!" *New York Times*, 13 February 1976, p. 33, col. 1.

3. The following discussion of the ACIP is drawn from David Sencer, interview with author, 9 May 2007, unless otherwise noted.

4. The following discussion of and quotations from the 27 February 1976 staff meeting at the CDC come from Walter Dowdle's handwritten notes, marked "Friday staff meeting," in notebook labeled "Ft. Dix Log Book, Feb. '76," Box 32, unlabeled folder T-1 (1), RG 442, NARA SE Region.

5. The Board for the Investigation and Control of Influenza and Other Epidemic Diseases in the Army was renamed the Army Epidemiological Board in 1946. It was later retitled the Armed Forces Epidemiological Board in 1949, and oversight of it

was moved to the Department of Defense in 1953. The board's research function was stripped in a widespread committee reorganization program undertaken in 1972, and the reorganized AFEB retained the role of providing expert recommendations to assistant secretary of defense for health affairs and the surgeon generals of the military services on matters of health. See http://www.health.mil/dhb/AFEB-History.cfm (accessed 12 Oct. 2011).

6. David Sencer, assistant surgeon general, to Mr. Gar Kaganowich, undated letter, box 31, file labeled "Swine Flu BoB 3/25/76 Swine Flu Events 3/1–30/76 (Dowdle 2 [in pencil])," RG 442, NARA SE Region.

7. Unless otherwise noted, the following discussion of the 9 March 1976 meeting at the CDC and the 10 March 1976 ACIP meeting is drawn from Neustadt and Fineberg, *Swine Flu Affair,* 10–11; Silverstein, *Pure Politics,* 28–30; Lawrence Wright, "Sweating Out the Swine Flu Scare," *New Times,* 11 June 1976, 34–35; and Philip M. Boffey, "Anatomy of a Decision: How the Nation Declared War on Swine Flu," *Science* 192 (14 May 1976): 639–40.

8. The ACIP committee comprised Dr. E. Russell Alexander, a professor in and the chair of the Department of Epidemiology and International Health at the University of Washington; Dr. William Elsea, commissioner of health for the Fulton County Health Department; Dr. E. Charlton Prather, staff director for the Health Program Office in the Florida Department of Health and Rehabilitative Services; Dr. Eleanor Shore, assistant to the president of Harvard Medical School; and Dr. Reuel Stallones, dean of the School of Public Health at the University of Texas. (Two members were absent: Dr. Elizabeth Barrett-Connor, an assistant professor of epidemiology and medicine in the Department of Community Medicine at the University of California–San Diego, and Dr. Lonnie Burnett, a professor in the Department of Gynecology and Obstetrics and the director of the Fertility Control Center at Johns Hopkins Hospital.) See "Advisory Committee on Immunization Practices Meeting of March 10, 1976, Expected Attendees," box 35, folder labeled "Advisory Committee on Immunization Practices Meeting of March 10, 1976," RG 442, NARA SE Region. Although the meeting was open to all members of the media, apparently only Harold Schmeck from the *New York Times* attended (Sencer interview, 9 May 2007).

9. Sencer interview, 9 May 2007.

10. In addition to relying on published accounts of the meeting, the following discussion of the debates at the 10 March 1976 ACIP meeting are drawn from two sets of extensive and largely parallel handwritten notes from this meeting: J. Lyle Conrad, director, Field Services Division, CDC, handwritten notes, "ACIP Flu—3/10/76," box 37, file labeled "ACIP Flu Meeting—March 1976," RG 442, NARA SE Region; and Donald Berreth, CDC public information officer, notes attached to minutes for 3/10/76 ACIP meeting, box 45, G-1, "Box 5 Swine Flu Action," RG 442, NARA SE Region. Although Berreth is not listed among the attendees, the location of these notes in his files and references to gearing up for public information strongly suggest his attendance.

11. Edwin Kilbourne, the source of the "peanuts" comment, was apparently drawing on the data of Joel Kavet, who estimated that for the United States, the combined

direct and indirect costs of the 1968 pandemic were $3.8 billion; see "Survey of Economic Data 1968 Influenza—Joel Kavet," box 5, notebook labeled "Chronology of Decision Making," tab "Economic Costs," RG 442, NARA SE Region.

12. Reuel Stallones qtd. in Conrad's notes. Stallones summed up his thoughts for Neustadt and Fineberg in a subsequent interview, stating, "This was an opportunity to pay something back to society for the good life I've had as a public health doctor. Society has done a lot for me—this is sheer do-goodism" (qtd. in Neustadt and Fineberg, *Swine Flu Affair*, 12).

13. Although a certain amount of caution is suggested in reviewing minutes drawn up three weeks after such an important meeting—especially in the light of the decisions made during the intervening period—the summary of the meeting penned by Sencer follows closely the notes taken by some of the other participants. See "Department of Health, Education, and Welfare, Center for Disease Control, Summary Minutes of Meeting March 10, 1976," over the signature of David Sencer, box 42, folder labeled "Summary Minutes ACIP Meeting 3/10/76," RG 442, NARA SE Region; Donald Berreth, notes attached to minutes for 3/10/76 ACIP meeting, box 45, G-1, "Box 5 Swine Flu Action," RG 442, NARA SE Region; and Walter Dowdle's handwritten notations of "agreement" on "Influenza Surveillance Summary, Prepared for Advisory Committee on Immunization Practices, March 10, 1976," box 32, unlabeled folder T-1 (3), RG 442, NARA SE Region.

14. Some attendees of the meeting recalled that a trivalent vaccine was also discussed (to protect against A/Victoria, A/New Jersey, and B/Hong Kong), a fact borne out by Conrad's notes and a report by the WHO observers but not contained in the minutes. See "Report of the Meeting of the Advisory Committee on Immunization Practices, Center for Disease Control, Atlanta, Georgia, U.S. A., 10 March 1976, Prepared by Dr. P. Bres, Chief Medical Officer, Virus Diseases, WHO, Geneva, and Dr. G. Schild, N. I. B. S. C., London," box 32, unlabeled folder T-1 (3), RG 442, NARA SE Region.

15. Walter Dowdle, handwritten notes, "Influenza Surveillance Summary, Prepared for Advisory Committee on Immunization Practices, March 10, 1976," box 32, unlabeled Folder T-1 (3), RG 442, NARA SE Region. The interpretation of Walter Dowdle's views here, drawn from his notes and records, differs from the standard version proposed by Neustadt and Fineberg. They characterize Dowdle as "cool to claims that a swine virus . . . would shortly arise and sweep around the world" and suggest that he reluctantly went along with the decisions of the CDC hierarchy (Neustadt and Fineberg, *Swine Flu Affair*, 10). Dowdle himself characterized his role as a "good civil servant," saying that his job was "to give the data" and present "the facts at the meetings" (Dowdle, interview by author, 26 May 2005). I agree that Dowdle was not one of the scientists who touted the connection to 1918, saw the program as a chance to "give back," or promoted some of the myriad other reasons to justify the program. However, I differ on Dowdle's support for the program. The crucial fact for Dowdle was that the disease spread from person to person. Once that fact was determined, as it had been by 24 February, the decision was clear. Swine flu represented a potential pandemic, and the only current preventative strategy was immunization. Dowdle expressed his irrita-

tion with delay here and in other places. As I will show, Dowdle unsuccessfully sought to have this important factor of human transmission incorporated in the "WHO Consultation on Influenza (7–8 April 1976)," which he coauthored. The logic of immunization was incontrovertible.

16. Donald Berreth, handwritten notes, "March 10, 1976 Advisory Committee Meeting," box 45, "G-1 Box 5 Swine Flu Action," attached to minutes from 10 March 1976 ACIP meeting, RG 442, NARA SE Region.

17. Sencer interview, 9 May 2007.

18. The following quotations come from this document. See "FY 1977 Influenza Immunization Initiative," dated 11 March 1976, box 20, file labeled "Meetings 20. National Immunization Conference NIH—November 12–14, 1976," RG 442, NARA SE Region. The two-page document was discovered in an archive box I assigned to David Sencer. Sencer does not recall drafting the document (or "option paper," as he referred to it), but he joked, "That's a good piece of paper. I'd sign off on it again" (Sencer interview, 9 May 2007). Sencer was able to confirm that the handwritten notations on the paper were not his, and he could not identify the author of the handwritten additions.

19. The discussion of the 12 March 1976 AFEB meeting is drawn from Walter Dowdle's handwritten notes. See "Mar. 12, 1976 Meeting of Armed Forces Epidemiological Bd.," box 32, unlabeled folder T-1 (3), RG 442, NARA SE Region.

20. The "action memo," as it came to be called, can be found in the appendix of Neustadt and Fineberg's *Swine Flu Affair.* My discussion largely parallels their interpretation. The following quotations are from this document.

21. First emphasis added; second in the original.

22. Neustadt and Fineberg, *Swine Flu Affair,* 14.

23. David Sencer, transcript of testimony at the National Commission for the Protection of Human Subjects of Biomedical and Behavioral Research, 17 August 1976, 10, box 15, binder labeled "Swine Flu Informed Consent Guidelines and Forms September 1976," blank tab, RG 442, NARA SE Region.

24. See, for example, "Sequence of Events, Dowdle/Berreth 5/14/76," box 31, file labeled "Swine Flu Editorials/WHO Events/PERT [Dowdle 5 (in pencil)]," and box 10, unlabeled folder; "Sequence of events National Influenza Immunization Program February 1976–1977," box 28, unlabeled folder H-5 (8); "Chronology of Major Activities on Swine Influenza—1976," box 27, folder labeled "Swine Flu," all items in RG 442, NARA SE Region. For Sencer's date, see "Calendar of Events—Given by Dr. Sencer," attachment to "Final Report to Congress," box 19, binder labeled "Swine Flu Reports, Final Reports to Congress," tab "Final Report to Congress"; and J. Lyle Conrad, notes from the meeting quoting "DJS," box 37, file labeled "Programs and Projects FY 1977 National Influenza Immunization Program (NIIP)," both items in RG 442, NARA SE Region.

25. Neustadt and Fineberg, *Swine Flu Affair,* 30. However, this unverified information was recalled a significant amount of time after the phone calls and after the perceived "failure" of the program.

26. The confusion about whether all members were contacted by phone stems from a comment by Etheridge, who stated, "Sencer called the ACIP members and reached most of them, but not Alexander," citing a 1987 interview with Walter Dowdle as her

source. This must be read with caution, however, as no other source (including Alexander) asserts this, and the interview was conducted more than a decade after the events. See Elizabeth W. Etheridge, *Sentinel for Health: A History of the Centers for Disease Control* (Berkeley: University of California Press, 1992), 251. Sencer quotations are from his 9 May 2007 interview with the author.

27. This escalation did not pass unnoticed by those in the scientific community. Walter Dowdle circled and put a question mark next to "strong" in the first document he saw ratcheting up the pandemic potential of the new strain. See Dowdle's notation on his copy of "Preliminary Draft-March 23, 1976, Recommendation of the Public Health Service Advisory Committee on Immunization Practices," box 32, unlabeled folder T-1 (2), RG 442, NARA SE Region.

28. Sencer interview, 9 May 2007.

29. The following discussion and quotations are drawn from Neustadt and Fineberg, *Swine Flu Affair,* 17–23, unless otherwise noted.

30. See Alfred W. Crosby Jr., *Epidemic and Peace, 1918* (Westport, Conn.: Greenwood, 1976), especially chapter 15, "An Inquiry into the Peculiarities of Human Memory," 311–25. In another remarkable coincidence, Crosby's newly published book came to the attention of Secretary Mathews, who distributed it to HEW staff and personally gave a copy to President Ford. Crosby's book was later circulated throughout the organization of the National Influenza Immunization Program. See Neustadt and Fineberg, *Swine Flu Affair,* 19, for delivery to Ford. For distribution through the NIIP, see "DJS [Sencer] Briefing on Flu 4/27," in Dennis Tolsma, handwritten notes, box 38, file labeled "Influenza Staff Meeting Notes—Dtolsma," RG 442, NARA SE Region; and J. Donald Millar's 9 June 1976 letter to "Immunization Project Directors Regional Offices," in which he stated, "Enclosed is a copy of 'Epidemic and Peace, 1918,' by Alfred Crosby, Jr. This is a very good documentation of the 1918–19 influenza pandemic and should make interesting reading as you prepare for the forthcoming immunization campaign" (box 1, binder labeled "NIIP Reading File," RG 442, NARA SE Region).

31. The following quotations are drawn from this memorandum, which is published in an appendix to Neutstadt and Fineberg's *Swine Flu Affair,* 156. David Sencer recalls that there was another document drafted by James Cavanaugh, deputy chief of staff in the Ford administration, but I have been unable to locate such a document (Sencer interview, 9 May 2007).

32. Randall L. Woods to Margarita White, memorandum dated 22 March 1976, subject *"Swine Virus Expectations,"* White House Central Files, subject HE Health 1/1/76 (General) to HE 1 Disease 7/22/76 (executive), box 2, folder HE1 4/1/75–3/31/76, Gerald Ford Library, Ann Arbor Michigan (hereafter cited as Ford Library).

33. Jack Marsh to Bill Baroody, memorandum dated 23 March 1976, box labeled "Counselors to the President, John Marsh files, 1974–77," general subject file "Strip Mining-Public Opinion Mail," box 32, folder "Swine Flu 3/76–11/76," Ford Library.

34. Mrs. Harry W. Lewis to President Ford, letter dated 19 April 1976, in folder labeled "James M. Cannon, executive director and assistant to the president for domestic affairs, Sunshine Bill to taxes," October 7–December 31, 1975, box no. 34, file labeled "Swine Flu April 13–May 31, 1976," Ford Library.

35. This charge has had resiliency: two of the scientists from outside the United

States expressed to me in interviews that they thought "politics" played a role in the U.S. decision (Claude Hannoun, interview by author, 23 August 2007; Ian Furminger, interview by author, 30 October 2007).

36. Concerning this point, I am in substantial agreement with Neustadt and Fineberg, *Swine Flu Affair,* and Arthur Silverstein, *Pure Politics.* The following account of President Ford's staff meetings on swine flu is drawn from Silverstein, *Pure Politics,* 44–47.

37. Etheridge, *Sentinel for Health,* 252.

38. Accounts of the meeting are widely available including, Silverstein, *Pure Politics,* 48–49; and Wright, "Sweating," 35. The most detailed, however, remains Neustadt and Fineberg, *Swine Flu Affair,* 26–29.

39. Wright, "Sweating," 35.

40. President Ford, "The President's Remarks Announcing Actions to Combat the Influenza," *Weekly Compilation of Presidential Documents* 12, no. 13 (24 Mar. 1976): 483–84.

41. For the White House fact sheet, see "The White House Fact Sheet Swine Influenza Immunization Program," 24 March 1976, box 46, file labeled "Press Briefing Statement by Theodore Cooper M.D."; and box 44, binder labeled "Flu-1," tab "March 14–20," both in RG 442, NARA SE Region.

42. See "Centers for Disease Control, Bureau of Biologics, National Institute for Allergy and Infectious Diseases Influenza Workshop March 25, 1976 (transcript)," box 32, unlabeled folder T-1 (2), RG 442, NARA SE Region.

43. See Dr. Jordan's comments (87) and Dr. Meyer's comments (123) in ibid.

44. For the memorandum, see box 45, file labeled "Freedom of Information Act Related to the Guillain-Barre Syndrome"; box 32, unlabeled folder, "T-1 (2)"; and box 44, binder labeled "Flu-1," tab "March 14–20," all items in RG 442, NARA SE Region.

45. See Jane Gregory and Steve Miller, *Science in Public: Communication, Culture, and Credibility* (New York: Plenum, 1998).

Chapter 8. A Different Interpretation Emerges

1. "Constitution of the World Health Organization," available at http://apps.who.int/gb/bd/PDF/bd47/EN/constitution-en.pdf (accessed 21 Sept. 2011).

2. United Nations, *Yearbook of the United Nations,* vol. 30 (New York: Office of Public Information, United Nations, 1979), 975. For smallpox eradication, see F. Fenner et al., *Smallpox and Its Eradication* (Geneva: World Health Organization, 1988). The director of the program, D. A. Henderson, and many of the fieldworkers were United States Public Health Service employees who were "loaned" to the WHO.

3. Dr. F. Assaad, WHO virus medical officer, qtd. by Walter Dowdle, handwritten notes for the 7–8 April 1976 WHO Consultation on Influenza meeting held in Geneva, box 32, unlabeled folder, T-1 (3), RG 442, NARA SE Region.

4. Walter Dowdle, handwritten notes, loose pages dated 13–17 February 1976; ibid., loose pages dated 17 February 1976, both items in box 32, unlabeled folder T-1 (1), RG 442, NARA SE Region. Dowdle transposed the numbers in his notes, calling the strain A/NJ/8/67.

5. Sir John Skehel, interview by author, 6 September 2007. The relationship between the laboratories of Mill Hill and Atlanta was such that the members would stay

at each other's houses while attending meetings or conferences on one side of the Atlantic or the other.

6. Paul Bres's statement is recorded in J. Lyle Conrad's handwritten notes from 10 March 1976 ACIP meeting, box 37, file labeled "ACIP Flu Meeting-March 1976," RG 442, NARA SE Region.

7. The following quotations are drawn from "Report of the Meeting of the Advisory Committee on Immunization Practices, Center for Disease Control, Atlanta, Georgia, U.S.A., 10 March 1976, Prepared by Dr. P. Bres, Chief Medical Officer, Virus Diseases, WHO, Geneva, and Dr. G. Schild, N.I.B.S.C., London," box 32, unlabeled folder T-1 (3), RG 442, NARA SE Region. Curiously, no mention of the report was found in the WHO archives.

8. The following summary of U.K. research studies is from "G. C. Schild, Vaccine Studies in the UK" (underlined in original), box 32, unlabeled folder, loose papers, RG 442, NARA SE Region.

9. In his logbook, right after the entry noting the "Planning Meeting" on 19 March 1976, Dowdle wrote, "Called Cockburn" (Walter Dowdle, handwritten notes, box 32, "Ft. Dix Log Book Feb. '76," RG 442, NARA SE Region).

10. Claude Hannoun also said that although his laboratory was on the mailing list for the WHO's *Weekly Epidemiological Record* and the CDC's *Morbidity and Mortality Weekly Report,* both were "chronically two . . . or three weeks behind the situation" (Hannoun, interview by author, 23 Aug. 2007). For von Magnus's query about the epidemiological information, see "Correspondence dated March 31, 1976, from Herdis von Magnus, Director, WHO Collaborating Centre for Virus Reference and Research, to Dr. John A. Bryan, Department of Health, Education, and Welfare, Centre for Disease Control," box 34, unlabeled file, RG 442, NARA SE Region. It is likely that national health organizations further removed from Geneva than France or Denmark were even more poorly informed.

11. For television coverage, see T.K. (?) to H.F. (Harvey Fineberg) and R.E.N. (Richard E. Neustadt), memorandum dated 28 July 1977, subject "Evening News Coverage of Swine Flu as Abstracted in *Vanderbilt Television News Archive Index and Abstracts,*" 25 March 1976, box 44, file labeled "Press Briefing 10/12/76–1977," RG 442, NARA SE Region; for print coverage, see Harold M. Schmeck Jr., "Test of Flu Vaccine Expected in April," *New York Times,* 26 March 1976, p. 14, col. 3. I have been unable to determine who spoke of being "surprised." For what it is worth, John Skehel speculated that either Fakhry Assaad or Paul Bres was the source; in any event, the staff at WHO headquarters was so small that there would have been only a handful of people competent in the area to field questions from the media.

12. "But after some careful diplomacy ('We had to beat the hell out of them,' explains an ACIP adviser), WHO recognized the wisdom of the decision" (Lawrence Wright, "Sweating Out the Swine Flu Scare," *New Times,* 11 June 1976, 38).

13. For media reports of the WHO endorsement, see T.K. (?) to H.F. (Harvey Fineberg) and R.E.N. (Richard E. Neustadt), undated memorandum, subject "Evening News Coverage of Swine Flu as Abstracted in *Vanderbilt Television News Archive Index and Abstracts,*" 27 March 1976 , box 44, file labeled "Press Briefing 10/12/76–1977," RG 442, NARA SE Region. When Assistant Secretary for Health Theodore Cooper was

testifying before a Senate appropriations committee on 6 April, he was asked, "What caused WHO's change from 'surprise' to support?" Dr. Cooper replied, "The first wire service story on WHO reaction to President Ford's announcement of the vaccine campaign was based on an interview with a WHO official who was unfamiliar with the investigation and meetings preceding that announcement. Thus he was caught by 'surprise.' The subsequent WHO affirmation of support for U.S. policy came from a WHO official who had attended the March 10 meeting in Atlanta of the Advisory Committee on Immunization Practices, and during the meeting voiced agreement with the recommendation of that Committee" (Theodore Cooper speaking before the Senate Subcommittee of the Committee on Appropriations, *Preventative Health Services and Employment Programs Emergency Supplemental Appropriations,* Hearing on H.J. Res. 890, 94th Cong., 2d sess., 6 April 1976, 30).

14. For example, NBC news reported on 24 February 1976 that the "WHO feels epidemic unlikely." See T.K. to H.F. (Harvey Fineberg) and R.E.N. (Richard E. Neustadt), undated memorandum, subject "Evening News Coverage of Swine Flu as Abstracted in *Vanderbilt Television News Archive Index and Abstracts,*" 24 February 1976, box 44, file labeled "Press Briefing 10/12/76–1977," RG 442, NARA SE Region. "Close Watch on New Flu Strain," WHO press release no. 16, dated 26 March 1976, can be found both at WHO Archives, Geneva, and at box 44, unlabeled binder, tab "March 28–April 1," RG 442, NARA SE Region. The following quotations are from this press release.

15. See, for example, J. Lyle Conrad's handwritten notes from a CDC influenza program meeting held on 26 May: "Is surveill[ance] any better now? *no.* Brush fires always occur. It's *possible* we've stumbled on the first—but not likely" (box 37, file labeled "ACIP Flu Meeting March 1976," RG 442, NARA SE Region).

16. Walter Dowdle, e-mail to author, 25 March 2007. For another description of the format of expert meetings at the WHO, see David Tyrrell and Michael Fielder, *Cold Wars: The Fight against the Common Cold* (New York: Oxford University Press, 2002), 170–76.

17. This and the following quotations are from David Perlman, "The Flu Shot Program Poses a Dilemma," *San Francisco Chronicle,* penciled notation "S. F. Chronicle, 4/5," box 44, unlabeled binder, blank tab, RG 442, NARA SE Region.

18. See "List of Participants," attached to "Draft Agenda," box 32, unlabeled folder T-1 (3), RG 442, NARA SE Region.

19. The following quotations from Dr. Bernard are drawn from a document labeled "Opening of the Consultation on Influenza, Geneva, 7–8 April 1976, By Dr. L. Bernard Assistant Director General," box 32, unlabeled folder T-1 (3), RG 442, NARA SE Region, unless otherwise noted.

20. The following discussion is drawn from Kelley Lee, *Historical Dictionary of the World Health Organization* (Lanham, Md.: Scarecrow, 1998), 12–25; Virginia Berridge, Kelly Loughlin, and Rachel Herring, "Historical Dimensions of Global Health Governance," in *Making Sense of Global Health Governance: A Policy Perspective,* ed. Kent Buse, Wolfgang Hein, and Nick Drager (Basingstoke, U.K.: Palgrave Macmillan, 2009), 28–46; Fiona Godlee, "WHO in Retreat: Is It Losing Its Influence?" *British Medical Journal*

39, no. 6967 (3 Dec. 1994): 1491–95; Socrates Litsios, "The Christian Medical Commission and the Development of the World Health Organization's Primary Health Care Approach," *American Journal of Public Health* 94, no. 11 (Nov. 2004): 1884–93; and Italian Global Health Watch, "From Alma Ata to the Global Fund: The History of International Health Policy," *Social Medicine* 3, no. 1 (Jan. 2008): 36–48.

21. Lee, *Historical Dictionary,* 16.

22. Ibid., 13.

23. Walter Dowdle, e-mail to author, 25 March 2007. Unless otherwise noted, the following discussion of the 7–8 April 1976 meeting is drawn from Walter Dowdle's handwritten notes of the meeting, "World Health Organization Consultation on Influenza Geneva, 7 and 8 April 1976, Report to the Director-General (Vir/76.4)," box 32, unlabeled folder, T-1 (3), RG 442, NARA SE Region.

24. The following discussion of Millar's background and biography is drawn from J. Donald Millar, interview by author, 22 May 2007.

25. The following discussion of Claude Hannoun's recollection of the 7–8 April 1976 meeting in Geneva is from Claude Hannoun, interview by author, 23 August 2007.

26. Hannoun recollected that the person who spoke at the WHO 7–8 April 1976 meeting was a military man in uniform and recalled the name Franklin Top. Only Dowdle and Millar are recorded as experts from the United States, however, and no other meeting attendees interviewed remember military personnel attending. Hannoun came to the United States to work in Robert Channock's infectious diseases laboratory at the NIH shortly after the WHO meeting. He worked on live-virus vaccines with Brian Murphy and attended several meetings about the Swine Flu Program. It is likely that he conflated the WHO meeting with one of these meetings where Colonel Top would have presented the epidemiological evidence from Fort Dix. While working in the United States, Hannoun continued a long-running tradition among research scientists. He was a "volunteer" for swine flu vaccination studies conducted in May 1976 and was pleased to recall that he developed high titers of A/New Jersey antibodies, meaning he would likely have been protected against a swine flu pandemic. Hannoun correctly recalled a phrase frequently cited by U.S. health officials to justify the swine flu decision: they had decided to "gamble with money rather than with human life." For examples of U.S. officials using that phrase, see J. Donald Millar's statements recorded in "Comments to the Assembled Delegates at the 34th Annual Meeting of the US-Mexican Border Public Health Association in Hermosillo, Sonora Mexico, on Wednesday, March 31, 1976 on Swine Influenza," box 32, unlabeled Folder T-1 (3), RG 442, NARA SE Region. Indeed, some U.S. health officials feared that the frequent use of a phrase with the negative connotation of gambling might offend members of fundamentalist communities. One of them, Dennis Tolsma, the program analysis officer at the Office of Program Planning and Evaluation, suggested the phrase "risking money" instead; see Dennis Tolsma to Don Berreth, memorandum, subject "core speech," box 38, FY 1976–77, file labeled "Programs and Projects NIIP-Publicity," RG 442, NARA SE Region.

Chapter 9. WHO Decides

1. Unless otherwise noted, the following discussion of the afternoon session is drawn from Walter Dowdle, handwritten notes, box 32, unlabeled folder, T-1 (3), RG 442, NARA SE Region.

2. Schild's description of the resulting infections differed slightly from that in the published conclusions. In the latter, the clinical reactions were noted as "1 case was nil, 1 case very mild, 3 cases as mild and 1 case as moderate." See A. S. Beare and J. W. Craig, "Virulence for Man of a Human Influenza-A Virus Antigenically Similar to 'Classical' Swine Viruses," *Lancet* 308, no. 7975 (3 July 1976): 4–5.

3. Sir John Skehel, interview by author, 6 October 2007.

4. Walter Dowdle, interview by author, 26 May 2005. This point was made by the eminent influenza expert Edwin Kilbourne, too, who noted that emphasizing the lack of severity of infection among the six volunteers was "nonsense, nonsense. . . . It's not the same as sitting next to a cot with somebody sneezing in your face" (Kilbourne, interview by author, 20 Jan. 2004).

5. Kilbourne interview, 20 January 2004.

6. Dowdle interview, 26 May 2005.

7. Emphasis in the original. Unless otherwise noted, the following quotations and summary of discussion are drawn from Walter Dowdle's notes, box 32, unlabeled folder, T-1 (3), RG 442, NARA SE Region.

8. Dowdle ascribed these quotes to a "Dr. Cho." He most likely meant Dr. Chang Yi-hao, from the vaccine department of the Peking Institute of Biological Products. But it also could be Dr. Kuo Yuan-chi, from the Institute of Epidemiology at the Chinese Academy of Medical Sciences, Peking.

9. Acting deputy director, NIAID (John Seal), memorandum "for the record" dated 20 January 1976, subject "Discussion of Potential for Live Attenuated Influenza A Vaccines for General Use in the United States"; Maurice Hilleman to John Seal, letter dated 14 January 1976; Maurice Hilleman to John Seal, letter dated 4 February 1976. All items obtained from the National Institute of Allergy and Infectious Diseases via Freedom of Information Act request, FOI Case No. 28820, in possession of author.

10. The quotation is from an 11 March 1958 report, "Scientific Plan to Study Flu in 1957–58," that the Soviet influenza expert Zhdanov sent to Dr. Payne. See Professor Zhdanov, deputy minister of health [USSR], to Dr. Payne, chief, section of e[ndemic] and e[pidemic] diseases, World Health Organization, memorandum dated 11 March 1958, I2/418/12, 25 (microfiche), WHO Archives, Geneva. Another communication mentions the Soviets' use of live-virus vaccines: "During this epidemic of influenza we have carried out [a] rather large program of immunization with live attenuated influenza virus vaccine, [and] more than 10 millions of population are already immunized" (V. Zhdanov, director, USSR influenza center, to Dr. A. M. M. Payne, chief, section of e[ndemic] and e[pidemic] diseases, World Health Organization, letter dated November 1957 [received 12 Dec. 1957], I2/418/12, 23 [microfiche], WHO Archives, Geneva). I thank Helen Hundley for translating both documents from Russian to English.

11. In 1972, D. A. J. Tyrrell, at the Clinical Research Centre in the United Kingdom, headed a collaborative WHO study on the effectiveness and safety of various

live-virus vaccines. Although indicating that they would do so, the Soviets never sent a sample of their inactivated live-virus vaccine, eventually requesting a "modern killed Western vaccine produced in the USA or England" to perform their own field studies. Although the study coordinators thanked the Soviets for the data they provided in a 1976 letter, the WHO was not able to independently test the vaccine for safety and efficacy. See I2/445/6, file labeled "Collaborative Study on Live Influenza Vaccine Strains," unnumbered jacket, box A.526, WHO Archives, Geneva. Quotation is from A. A. Smorodintsev, State Research Institute of Influenza, Leningrad, to W. Chas. Cockburn, chief medical officer of the WHO's virus division, letter dated 25 January 1974, at ibid.

12. Dr. A. S. Beare, "Visit to the Department of Epidemiology, School of Public Health, University of Michigan under the auspices of the World Health Organization," report attached to A. S. Beare, Medical Research Council and Department of Health and Social Security, MRC Common Cold Unit, to Dr. W. C. Cockburn, Virus Diseases Unit, letter dated 5 July 1972, I2/445/6, folder labeled "Collaborative Study on Live Influenza Vaccine Strains," box A.526, WHO Archives, Geneva.

13. "Report to the Director-General on an Informal Consultation on International Collaboration in Research on Live Influenza Virus Vaccines, Geneva, 4 and 5 October 1971," I2/445/6, folder labeled "Collaborative Study on Live Influenza Vaccine Strains," box A.526, WHO Archives, Geneva. There is no way to tell from this source, what, if any, importance was attached to this observation at this time.

14. G. C. Schild to Walter Dowdle, letter dated 19 July 1974; G. C. Schild to W. C. Cockburn, letter dated 19 July 1974. Both in I2/442/2 (73–74), file labeled "Information on Influenza Incidence 1/7/73–30/6/74," jacket no. 2, box A.0525, WHO Archives, Geneva.

15. For Dowdle's exclamation points, see handwritten notes, box 32, unlabeled folder, T-1 (3), RG 442, NARA SE Region; for justification for "extreme caution," see Walter R. Dowdle, "Influenza Pandemic Periodicity, Virus Recycling, and the Art of Risk Assessment," *Emerging Infectious Diseases* 12, no. 1 (Jan. 2006): 38. See also Walter Dowdle, "The 1976 Experience," *Journal of Infectious Diseases* 176, suppl. 1 (Aug. 1997): S69–72.

16. W. G. Laver, "Report on Visit to China, September 9–October 4, 1972," I2/181/15, microfiche, WHO Archives, Geneva.

17. "Global Distribution of Influenza Vaccines, 2000–2003," *Weekly Epidemiological Record* 40 (1 Oct. 2004): 366–67. David Fedson estimates that the 2000 production rate was more than twice that of 1990, and there is no evidence to suggest that there has been a significant change in the nations producing vaccine (Fedson, unpublished observation). See David S. Fedson, "Preparing for Pandemic Vaccination: An International Policy Agenda for Vaccine Development," *Journal of Public Health Policy* 26, no. 1 (2005): 8.

18. World Health Organization, *International List of Availability of Vaccines,* tab "Influenza," BLG/76.1, located at the World Health Organization Library and Information Networks for Knowledge (hereafter WHO Library), Geneva.

19. Dowdle interview, 26 May 2005; Hideo Fukumi to Dr. W. Chas. Cockburn, chief medical officer, virus diseases, World Health Organization, letter dated 20 July 1973, enclosing a report titled "Recent Influenza Epidemic of the New Type B in

Japan," I2/442/2 (72–73), file labeled "Information on Influenza Incidence 1/7/1972–30/6/1973," jacket 2, box A.0525, WHO Archives, Geneva; Claude Hannoun, interview by author, 23 August 2007; J. Lyle Conrad to "Director, Immunization Division Bureau of State Services," letter dated 23 April 1976, box 37, file labeled "Swine Influenza National Influenza Immunization Program (NIIP) 1976—Correspondence," RG 442, NARA SE Region. For what it is worth, Hannoun thinks that the estimate of SCALVO's production is "probably" a high figure but "not impossible."

20. David Sencer, interview by author, 9 May 2007.

21. Ian Furminger, interview by author, 30 October 2007.

22. D. A. Henderson, interview by author, 26 July 2007.

23. Unless otherwise noted, the following quotations and summary are from "Consultation on Influenza, Report—First Draft, Recommendations," with Dowdle's penciled notes, box 32, unlabeled folder T-1 (3), RG 442, NARA SE Region.

24. M. F. Warburton to Dr. W. Chas. Cockburn, letter dated 9 July 1965; Cockburn to Dr. M. F. Warburton, Commonwealth Serum Laboratories, letter dated 15 July 1965, both items at I2/286/4 (64–65), 1, microfiche, WHO Archives, Geneva.

25. Unfortunately, the first draft of the consultation report included only the "Conclusions and Recommendations" section. Presumably the additional information existed at one time, for the "Conclusion and Recommendations" section was paginated 11 and 12. Therefore, I cannot compare what changes may have been made in the characterization of the information. Unless otherwise noted, the following quotations are taken from this later draft, "Consultation on Influenza Geneva 7 and 8 April 1976, Draft Final Report," box 32, unlabeled folder T-1 (3), RG 442, NARA SE Region.

26. The original sentence read (with the excised words in bold) "The appearance of a new strain of influenza A at Fort Dix, New Jersey, in the USA in February this year caused **some** concern **about its spread from man-to-man because of its antigenic relationship to the swine influenza–like virus which caused the 1918 pandemic**" ("Opening of the Consultation on Influenza, Geneva, 7–8 April 1976, by Dr. L. Bernard, Assistant Director General," box 32, unlabeled folder T-1 (3), RG 442, NARA SE Region).

27. Unless otherwise noted, the following quotations and summary are drawn from World Health Organization, "Consultation on Influenza, Geneva, 7 and 8 April 1976," Report to the Director-General, Vir/76.4, the WHO Library, Geneva.

28. The first draft of the press release was attached to the draft final report in Walter Dowdle's files. The following quotations and summary are from the draft of the press release attached to "Consultation on Influenza Geneva 7 and 8 April 1976, Draft Final Report," box 32, unlabeled folder T-1 (3), RG 442, NARA SE Region.

29. "Experts' Recommendations on New Flu Strain," WHO press release 21, 8 April 1976, WHO Library, Geneva.

30. Dowdle interview, 26 May 2005.

31. J. Donald Millar, interview by author, 22 May 2007; J. Donald Millar, notes faxed to author, 24 May 2007.

32. D. A. Henderson to Professor Richard E. Neustadt, letter dated 12 March 1979. Copy sent via e-mail from David Sencer, 9 May 2007.

Chapter 10. A Program Begins and Ends and an Epidemic Appears

1. J. Donald Millar qtd. in "Swine Flu Highly Infectious in Test," *Dallas Times Herald,* 25 April 1976, A-41, box 46, scrapbook, RG 442, NARA SE Region; Michael Hattwick qtd. in Donald Berreth, CDC public information officer, "Notes from Flu Meeting-Thursday-April 22, 1976," typescript, box 44, unlabeled binder, blank tab, RG 442, NARA SE Region; Dennis Tolsma, handwritten notes labeled "Flu Mtg., 4/22," box 38, file labeled "Influenza Staff Meeting Notes-DTolsma," RG 442, NARA SE Region; Walter Dowdle qtd. in Berreth, "Notes from Flu Meeting-Thursday-April 22, 1976."

2. Director, virology division (Dowdle), to assistant director for program (H. Bruce Dull), memorandum dated 2 July 1976, subject "Draft of a Working Proposal," box 36, unlabeled folder J-1 (6), RG 442, NARA SE Region; "Items Ignored by the GAO Investigation," signed by J. Donald Millar, box 21, unlabeled folder, RG 442, NARA SE Region. Some critics had charged that the vaccine was insufficiently tested, but that was incorrect (although technically true, since the more productive X-53a strain was injected, not the extensively tested X-53 strain). Walter Dowdle points out that reactogenicity tests for influenza vaccines are rarely run on humans. Instead, rabbits are used for the test, which determine whether the antigens, or outer coat of the vaccine, are a close match with the prevailing strain. With the Swine Flu Program, there was a chance for field trials, but, Walter Dowdle said, "that was not the usual thing, very unusual" (Dowdle, interview by author, 26 May 2005). As late as 2001, the vaccine trials undertaken in 1976 qualified as the "largest, most intensive series of influenza vaccine trials ever conducted"; see John M. Wood, "Developing Vaccines against Pandemic Influenza," *Philosophical Transactions of the Royal Society of London,* ser. B, 356 (2001): 1953–60.

3. The Advisory Committee on Immunization Practices is also known as IPAC. See "Summary Minutes of Meeting, June 22, 1976," box 36, unlabeled file, J-1 (6), RG, NARA SE Region; and director, virology division (Dowdle), to assistant director of program (Dull), memo, "Draft of a Working Proposal."

4. Later clinical trials determined that a two-dose schedule using split virus vaccines (in which the viral shell is partially disrupted by chemical action) was necessary to provide adequate protection. The resulting delay in studying the problems of dose schedule and reaction rates meant that the recommendation for children between the ages of three and seventeen was not made until 15 November 1976. In addition, because of problems at the manufacturer making monovalent split-virus vaccine (Parke, Davis), only enough vaccine for four million children was available by December—and only a small percentage of children in this age group ever received the vaccine. See Assistant Secretary for Health (Theodore Cooper) to the Honorable Spencer Johnson, undated memorandum, subject "Biweekly Status Report on the National Influenza Immunization Program (NIIP), for the Period Ending November 15, 1976," box 20, binder labeled "Swine Flu Reports, Early Reports to HEW White House, Biweekly Reports to Asst. Secretary, Secretary," tab "11/14/76," RG 442, NARA SE Region.

5. Senator Kennedy was persuaded to abandon combining swine flu vaccine with other childhood immunizations such as measles or mumps because there was no data

on possible reactogenic complications to multiple vaccinations in children. For the hearings, see U.S. Congress, House Committee on Interstate and Foreign Commerce, Subcommittee on Health and the Environment, *Hearings on Proposed National Swine Flu Vaccination Program,* 94th Cong., 2d sess., 31 March 1976; and U.S. Congress, Senate Committee on Labor and Public Welfare, Subcommittee on Health, *Hearings on Swine Flu Immunization Program, 1976,* 94th Cong., 2d sess., 1 April and 5 August 1976. For an insightful account of the political maneuvering in ratifying and authorizing the program, see Arthur J. Viseltear, "A Short Political History of the 1976 Swine Influenza Legislation," in *History, Science, and Politics: Influenza in America, 1918–1976,* ed. June E. Osborn (New York: Prodist, 1977), 29–58.

6. Assistant secretary for health (Theodore Cooper) to the Honorable Spencer Johnson, undated memorandum, subject "Biweekly Status Report on the National Influenza Immunization Program (NIIP), for the Period Ending June 15, 1976," box 20, binder labeled "Swine Flu Reports, Early Reports to HEW White House, Biweekly Reports to Asst. Secretary, Secretary," tab "6/15/76," RG 442, NARA SE Region.

7. The following discussion of the Cutter incident and its legal impact is drawn from Paul A. Offit, *The Cutter Incident: How America's First Polio Vaccine Led to the Growing Vaccine Crisis* (New Haven, Conn.: Yale University Press, 2005), 88 and passim.

8. Unless otherwise noted, the following discussion of court cases on vaccination programs is drawn from "Liability Lawsuits," box 7, binder labeled "March 1977 Influenza Policy and Program Development," tab "Lawsuits," RG 442, NARA SE Region; assistant director for program, CDC (H. Bruce Dull), to Charles M. Gozonsky, memorandum dated 11 November 1974, subject "Reyes v. Wyeth," loose papers in boxes containing material on the Swine Flu Program, internally labeled "1–6," box 4, Centers for Disease Control, Atlanta, Georgia.

9. At the trial, experts testified that the chance of acquiring polio in that area if not vaccinated was 1 in 3,000 and the chance of acquiring vaccine-induced polio was 1 in 5.88 million. They could not determine how the child was infected, however. See director, Division of Health Protection, OPDP, to director, OPDP, memorandum dated 22 January 1976, subject "CDC Proposal to Relieve Vaccine Manufacturers of Financial Liability for Vaccine-Associated Disability," 2, box 8, folder labeled "CDC Liability Proposal," RG 442, NARA SE Region.

10. Harry Meyer, director of the FDA's Bureau of Biologics, told Bruce Dull that 95 percent of vaccines used in the United States during 1960 were produced by eleven firms. Since that time, he said, "five of these companies have either dropped out of biologics production or have made management decisions to close out" (Meyer to Dull, letter dated 1 December 1975, box 8, folder labeled "CDC Liability Proposal," RG 442, NARA SE Region).

11. Assistant director for program (Dull) to Gozonsky, memo, "Reyes v. Wyeth."

12. The following discussion of the liability issue is drawn from Viseltear, "Short Political History," 42–51; Richard Neustadt and Harvey Fineberg, *The Swine Flu Affair: Decision-Making on a Slippery Disease* (Washington, D.C.: U.S. Department of Health, Education, and Welfare, 1978), 48–56; and Arthur M. Silverstein, *Pure Politics and Impure Science: The Swine Flu Affair* (Baltimore, Md.: Johns Hopkins University Press, 1981), 88–97.

13. Canadian production estimates from Harry M. Meyer, director, Bureau of Biologics, Food and Drug Administration, to deputy assistant secretary for health, memorandum dated 9 April 1976, subject "Production Estimates of A/Swine-Like Influenza Virus Vaccines," box 44, unlabeled binder, tab "March 28–April 3," RG 442, NARA SE Region.

14. Dr. John Abbott, LCDC Health Protection Branch, Health and Welfare Canada, to Dr. David J. Sencer, telegram dated 31 March 1976, box 27, file labeled "A/Swine-WHO and Foreign Statements," RG 442, NARA SE Region; Walter Dowdle, notes, "Center for Disease Control, Bureau of Biologics, National Institute of Allergy and Infectious Diseases Influenza Workshop, 25 March 1976," box 32, unlabeled folder T-1 (2), RG 442, NARA SE Region.

15. John J. Witte, memorandum "for the record" dated 25 May 1976, box 5, unlabeled binder, tab "Cooperation State Dept.-International," subtab "Canada Flu," RG 442, NARA SE Region; Ian Furminger, interview by author, 30 October 2007. Furminger remembers the Canadian vaccine purchase well, for he was called into court to testify about the vaccine. Evans had sold it in bulk to the Canadian firm Connaught Laboratories. Connaught proceeded to bottle the vaccine for individual doses. The process of bottling the material denatured the proteins, causing some precipitation in the bottom of the containers. When the material was delivered to Canadian health officials, they refused the shipment. As Furminger recalls, the refusal of the shipment occurred right after the United States had halted its program because of a possible causal connection between swine flu vaccine and Guillain-Barré syndrome. He suspects that Canadian officials were looking for any excuse to halt the program. Furminger was called to testify that Evans Medical had delivered the vaccine in good shape to Connaught Laboratories.

16. The following discussion of Legionnaires' disease is from Allen B. Weisse, *Medical Odysseys: The Different and Sometimes Unexpected Pathways to Twentieth Century Medical Discoveries* (New Brunswick, N.J.: Rutgers University Press, 1991); Gordon Thomas and Max Morgan Witts, *Anatomy of an Epidemic* (Garden City, N.Y.: Doubleday, 1982); David W. Fraser et al., "Legionnaires' Disease: Description of an Epidemic of Pneumonia," *New England Journal of Medicine* 297, no. 22 (1 Dec. 1977): 1189–97; and Joseph E. McDade et al., "Legionnaires' Disease: Isolation of a Bacterium and Demonstration of Its Role in Other Respiratory Diseases," *New England Journal of Medicine* 297, no. 22 (1 Dec. 1977): 1197–1203.

17. Remarkably, in late August the CDC would also be involved in another unusual infectious outbreak. The CDC was invited to Zaire to help seek the cause of a mysterious hemorrhagic fever outbreak. It eventually discovered the virus, which the investigators named "Ebola," after a local river. For the CDC, 1976 embodied the Chinese blessing/curse: may you live in interesting times.

18. The following account of the passing of liability legislation is drawn from Viseltear, "Short Political History," 42–51; Neustadt and Fineberg, *Swine Flu Affair,* 48–56; and Silverstein, *Pure Politics,* 88–97.

19. See U.S. Department of Health, Education, and Welfare, press release dated 2 June 1976, box 32, unlabeled folder T-1 (4), RG 442, NARA SE Region. The department refused to pay for the mistaken production and denied Parke, Davis's claims that

the CDC was at fault for providing the firm with contaminated seed stock. See John L. Williams, contracting officer, contracts and purchases branch, HEW procurement and grants office, to Dr. Robert Adams, Parke, Davis, letter dated 24 August 1977, box 2, binder labeled "Swine Flu Vaccine Contract (and Related Issues), Volume III," tab "Parke, Davis Shope Vaccine Issue," RG 442, NARA SE Region.

20. Figures from *Morbidity and Mortality Weekly Report* 25, no. 41 (22 Oct. 1976): 331; see also Silverstein, *Pure Politics,* 110–12; Neustadt and Fineberg, *Swine Flu Affair,* 65–69; and T.K. (?) to H.F. (Harvey Fineberg) and R.E.N. (Richard Neustadt), memorandum dated 28 July, subject "Evening News Coverage of Swine Flu as abstracted in *Vanderbilt Television News Archive Index and Abstracts,"* box 44, file labeled "Press Briefing 10/12/76–1977," RG 442, NARA SE Region.

21. Death rate figures from *Morbidity and Mortality Weekly Report* 25, no. 41 (22 Oct. 1976): 331; public attitude numbers from U.S. Comptroller General, *The Swine Flu Program: An Unprecedented Venture in Preventive Medicine,* report to Congress (Washington, D.C.: Department of Health, Education, and Welfare, 1977), 56 (fig. 1).

22. Figures from assistant secretary for health (Theodore Cooper) to the Honorable Spencer Johnson, undated memorandum, subject "Biweekly Status Report on the National Influenza Immunization Program (NIIP), for the Period Ending December 1, 1976," box 20, binder labeled "Swine Flu Reports, Early Reports to HEW White House, Biweekly Reports to Asst. Secretary, Secretary," tab "12/1/76," RG 442, NARA SE Region.

23. Discussion of the condition contemporary to 1976 in "Statement on Guillain-Barre, 12/14/76," box 15, binder labeled "Swine Flu GBS and Vaccination Moratorium Misc. Documents-Chronological December 14 1976 January 30, 1977," tab "Draft Press Statement CDC-December 14 1976," RG 442, NARA SE Region; National Institute of Neurological Disorders and Stroke, National Institutes of Health, "Guillain-Barré Syndrome Fact Sheet," http://www.ninds.nih.gov/disorders/gbs/detail_gbs. htm (accessed 22 Sept. 2011); for the association with lightning, see June E. Osborn, "Epilogue—The Costs and Benefits of the National Immunization Program of 1976," in *History, Science, and Politics: Influenza in America 1918–1976,* ed. Osborn (New York: Prodist), 64.

24. For the chronology of GBS events, see director, Surveillance and Assessment Center National, Influenza Immunization Program (Michael Hattwick), to J. Donald Millar, memorandum dated 23 December 1976, subject "Chronology of Investigation of Guillain-Barre Syndrome," box 15, binder labeled "Swine Flu GBS and Vaccination Moratorium Misc. Documents-Chronological December 14 1976 January 30, 1977," tab "Summary of Investigation Update International Dec. 23, 1976," RG 442, NARA SE Region.

25. Figures drawn from director, Centers for Disease Control, to special assistant to the assistant secretary of health, telegram, subject "Biweekly Status Reports on the National Influenza Immunization Program (NIIP), for the Period Ending December 15, 1976," box 20, binder labeled "Swine Flu Reports Early Reports to HEW White House Biweekly Reports Ast. Secretary, Secretary," tab "12/15/76," RG 442, NARA SE Region; graph from "Summary Report on Influenza Virus Vaccine Use, February 7, 1977," fig. 1, box 21, "Misc. Folder," RG 442 NARA SE Region.

NOTES TO PAGES 186–189

26. "Statement by Theodore Cooper, Assistant Secretary for Health, Press Briefing 12/16/76," box 15, binder labeled "Swine Flu GBS and Vaccination Moratorium Misc. Documents-Chronological December 14 1976 January 30, 1977," tab "Cooper Press Release December 16, 1976," RG 442, NARA SE Region.

27. For the Institute of Medicine investigation, see Kathleen Stratton, Donna A. Alamario, Theresa Wizemann, and Marie C. McCormick, eds., *Immunization Safety Review: Influenza Vaccines and Neurological Complications* (Washington, D.C.: National Academies, 2004). For epidemiological debate over the relationship between swine flu vaccines and GBS, see contrasting articles and letters in the *Archives of Neurology* 42 (Nov. 1985), especially Leonard T. Kurland et al., "Swine Influenza Vaccine and Guillain-Barré Syndrome: Epidemic or Artifact?" 1089–90; Charles M. Poser, "Swine Influenza Vaccination: Truth and Consequences," 1090–92; and Vladimir Hachinski, "The Swine Influenza Vaccination Controversy," 1092. See also letters to the editor in response and replies, *Archives of Neurology* 43 (Oct. 1986): 979–82. Also see A. D. Langmuir et al., "An Epidemiologic and Clinical Evaluation of Guillain-Barré Syndrome Reported in Association with the Administration of Swine Influenza Vaccines," *American Journal of Epidemiology* 119, no. 6 (June 1984): 841–79; a letter to the editor, with response from authors, in *American Journal of Epidemiology* 121, no. 4: 620–23; and Peter James Dyck to Michael Gregg, letter dated 28 December 1976, box 15, binder labeled "Swine Flu and GBS Moratorium Chronological Misc. Document-December 14, 1976 January 30, 1977," tab "Letter from Dyke [sic]-Review of Cases Investigation Forum, Dec. 28, 1976," RG 442, NARA SE Region.

28. Richard E. Neustadt and Harvey Fineberg, *The Epidemic That Never Was: Policy-Making and the Swine Flu Scare* (New York: Vintage, 1982), xxiv–xxv. The book is a reprint of *The Swine Flu Affair* with a new introduction. Another possible interpretation is that the mistakenly identified association, and the subsequent request that others look for the same association, made it more likely that physicians would attribute such symptoms to GBS if the patient had been vaccinated. The result would be an inflated total of GBS cases associated with influenza vaccine, especially in a difficult-to-identify condition such GBS, for which there was no accepted diagnostic standard.

29. The account of Cooper's resignation and Sencer's firing comes from Silverstein, *Pure Politics,* 130; that of Sencer's tenure at the CDC comes from David Sencer, interview by author, 9 May 2007; Califano remark is from "Press Conference HEW Secretary, Joseph A. Califano, Jr., February 8, 1977," box 9, folder labeled "Meeting Concerning Influenza Virus Vaccine Use, Washington, D.C., Feb. 8, 1977," RG 442, NARA SE Region. Interestingly, the announcement of Sencer's resignation is not recounted in Califano's book; see Joseph A. Califano Jr., *Governing America: An Insider's Report from the White House and the Cabinet* (New York: Simon and Schuster, 1981).

30. "Summary Report on Influenza Virus Vaccine Use, February 7, 1977, Addendum," box 21, "Misc. Folder," RG 442, NARA SE Region.

31. "Chronology of Decisionmaking and Related Events, 1978–1979 Influenza Policy," box 5, notebook labeled "Chronology of Decision Making-Congressional Tab," RG 442, NARA SE Region.

32. M. S. Pereira and J. J. Skehel, "Report of the World Influenza Centre for the Period April 1977 to May 1978 Inclusive," I2/181/3, folder labeled "CTS Agreement

within the Public Health Laboratory Service Board, London UK, in Respect of Identifying of Influenza Strains Research on Influenza Virus, Supply of Strains to National Influenza Centres," box A.2139, WHO Archives, Geneva.

33. Alan P. Kendal, Gary R. Noble, John J. Skehel, and Walter R. Dowdle, "Antigenic Similarity of Influenza A (H1N1) Viruses from Epidemics in 1977–1978 to 'Scandinavian' Strains Isolated in Epidemics of 1950–1951," *Virology* 89 (1978): 632–36; Pereira and Skehel, "Report of the World Influenza Centre, April 1977 to May 1978."

34. Public Health Service, Department of Health, Education, and Welfare, "Summary Report on Influenza Virus Vaccine Use, February 7, 1977," 2, box 21 "Misc. Folder," RG 442, NARA SE Region; Comptroller General, *Swine Flu Program,* 48. Several of those involved in the program claimed that they would still make the same decision in similar circumstances when interviewed two years after the fact. David Sencer said, "Placed in a similar position again I would certainly have made the same recommendations as I did then," and June Osborn, an adviser from the University of Wisconsin, said, "I have never been able to come up with a better rationale." When asked whether he would have made the same decision, Edward Kilbourne replied, "Absolutely, unequivocally." See Nicholas Wade, "1976 Swine Flu Campaign Faulted yet Principals Would Do It Again," *Science* 202, no. 4320 (24 Nov. 1978): 849–52. Edwin Kilbourne's belief in the correctness of the decision remains unchanged: "I've said before and I've been quoted on this: I would do nothing different . . . given the facts . . . and *not* on the basis that this is 1918 all over again: the basis that this is a new antigenic strain coming into a largely nonimmune population, that we had to be ready. . . . I have no regrets" (Kilbourne, interview by author, 20 Jan. 2004).

35. The literature on this conflict in WHO goals and methods has become substantial. See, among other works, a series of articles from Fiona Godlee, an assistant editor at the *British Medical Journal,* including "WHO at the Crossroads: Will It Embrace the Necessary Reforms?" *British Medical Journal* 306, no. 6886 (1 May 1993): 1143–44; "WHO's Special Programmes: Undermining from Above," *British Medical Journal* 310, no. 6973 (21 Jan. 1995): 178–82; "WHO Reform and Global Health: Radical Restructuring Is the Only Way Ahead," *British Medical Journal* 314, no. 7091 (10 May 1997): 1359–60; and a response to Goodlee's series from Ilona Kickbusch, "World Health Organisation: Change and Progress," *British Medical Journal* 310, no. 6993 (10 June 1995): 1518–20. See also Kelley Lee, *Historical Dictionary of the World Health Organization* (Lanham, Md.: Scarecrow, 1998), 16–36; Derek Yach and Douglas Bettcher, "The Globalization of Public Health, I: Threats and Opportunities," *American Journal of Public Health* 88, no. 5 (May 1998): 735–38; Derek Yach and Douglas Bettcher, "The Globalization of Public Health, II: The Convergence of Self-Interest and Altruism," *American Journal of Public Health* 88, no. 5 (May 1998): 738–41; Theodore M. Brown, Marcos Cueto, and Elizabeth Fee, "The World Health Organization and the Transition from International to Global Public Health," *American Journal of Public Health* 96, no. 1 (Jan. 2006): 62–72; Gill Walt and Kent Buse, "Global Cooperation in International Public Health," in *International Public Health: Diseases, Program, System, and Policies,* 2d ed., ed. Michael H. Merson, Robert E. Black, and Anne J. Mills (Sudbury, Mass.: Jones and Bartlett, 2006), 649–80; Laurie Garrett, "The Challenge of Global Health," *Foreign Affairs* 86, no. 1 (Jan.–Feb. 2007): 14–38; Ruth Bonita, Alec Irwin, and Robert Beagle-

hole, "Promoting Public Health in the Twenty-First Century: The Role of the World Health Organization," in *Globalization and Health,* ed. Ichiro Kawachi and Sara Wamala (Oxford: Oxford University Press, 2007), 268–83; and Kent Buse, Wolfgang Hein, and Nick Drager, eds., *Making Sense of Global Health Governance: A Policy Perspective* (Basingstoke, U.K.: Palgrave Macmillan, 2009).

Chapter 11. The Continuing Lessons of Influenza's History

1. See Dorothy Bonn, "Isolation of New Flu-Virus Strain May Presage Pandemic," *Lancet* 350, 9079 (6 Sept. 1997): 717; Kennedy F. Shortridge, "Poultry and the Influenza H5N1 Outbreak in Hong Kong, 1997: Abridged Chronology and Virus Isolation," *Vaccine* 17 (1999): S26–29; and Rene Snacken, Alan P. Kendal, Lars R. Haaheim, and John M. Woods, "The Next Influenza Pandemic: Lessons from Hong Kong 1997" *Emerging Infectious Diseases* 5, no. 2 (Mar.–Apr. 1999): 195–203.

2. China first reported an outbreak of "atypical pneumonia" to the WHO on 11 February 2003, though the SARS infection actually broke out in late November 2002, the delay perhaps due to politics: "In China, in contrast with many other settings globally, scientific inquiry and dissemination of results to the international community are subject to institutional interference. The SARS pandemic has shown that virulent pathogens are beholden to no political philosophy or edict" (Robert F. Breiman et al., "Role of China in the Quest to Define and Control Severe Acute Respiratory Syndrome," *Emerging Infectious Diseases* 9, no. 9 [Sept. 2003], available at http://www.cdc.gov/ncidod/EID/vol9no9/03–0390.htm [accessed 31 Oct. 2004]). As David Heymann, the WHO's executive director, communicable diseases, stated, "The SARS experience . . . made one lesson clear early in its course: inadequate surveillance and response capacity in a single country can endanger national populations and the public health security of the entire world. As long as national capacities are weak, international mechanisms for outbreak alert and response will be needed as a global safety net that protects other countries when one nation's surveillance and response systems fail" (David L. Heymann and Guenael Rodier, "Global Surveillance, National Surveillance, and SARS," *Emerging Infectious Diseases* 10, no. 2 [Feb. 2004], available at http://www.cdc.gov/ncidod/EID/vol10no2/013–1038.htm [accessed 31 Oct. 2004]).

3. Quotation from Marc Santora, "Private Doctors in Frantic Quest for Flu Vaccine," *New York Times,* 21 October 2004, p. 2, col. 1. See also Denise Grady, "Before Shortage of Flu Vaccine, Many Warnings," *New York Times,* 17 Oct. 2004, p. 1, col. 1; and Scott P. Layne, "Human Influenza Surveillance: The Demand to Expand," *Emerging Infectious Diseases* 12, no. 4 (April 2006): 562–68.

4. See WHO, Department of Communicable Disease Surveillance and Response, "WHO Consultation on Priority Public Health Interventions before and during an Influenza Pandemic," *Weekly Epidemiological Record* 79, no. 11 (12 Mar. 2004): 107–8; Michael G. Baker and David P. Fidler, "Global Public Health Surveillance under New International Health Regulations," *Emerging Infectious Diseases* 12, no. 7 (July 2006): 1058–65; Rebecca Katz, "Use of Revised International Health Regulations during Influenza A (H1N1) Epidemic, 2009," *Emerging Infectious Diseases* 15, no. 8 (Aug. 2009): 1165–70; and World Health Organization, "WHO Pandemic Influenza Draft Protocol for Rapid Response and Containment" (updated draft 30 May 2006), available at

http://www.who.int/csr/disease/avian_influenza/guidelines/protocolfinal30_05_06a.
pdf (accessed 22 Sept. 2011).

5. For information on the WHO phases and alert levels for pandemic influenza,
see http://www.who.int/csr/disease/avian_influenza/phase/en/index.html (accessed 22
Sept. 2011).

6. For example, compare the "Cover Your Cough" placards distributed by the
USPHS with similar public health exhortations to protect against the Spanish flu by
not spitting. For printable "cover your cough" posters, see http://www.cdc.gov/flu/
protect/covercough.htm (accessed 11 Sept. 2009).

7. For unused vaccine, see Mike Stobbe, "Millions of Vaccine Doses to Be Burned,"
wire service (AP) article, 1 July 2010. For conspiracy, see Mark Honigsbaum, "Was
Swine Flu Ever a Real Threat?" (2 Feb. 2010); Imogen Foulkes, "WHO Faces Questions over Swine Flu Policy," 20 May 2010, BBC News Europe, http://www.bbc.
co.uk/news/10128604.

8. David W. Barry, Ronald E. Mayner, Jules M. Meisler, and Edward B. Seligmann
Jr., "Evaluation and Control of Vaccines for the National Influenza Immunization Pro-
gram," *Journal of Infectious Diseases* 136, suppl., *Clinical Studies of Influenza Vaccines: 1976*
(December 1977): S407–14.

9. In a letter to David Sencer, E. Russell Alexander suggested that Sencer consider
stockpiling the vaccine and awaiting more evidence of the pandemic before beginning
administration of the shots. This became known as the "half a hog" letter from Alexander's closing: "with personal regards from your 'half-a-hog' colleague." The comment was in response to Sencer's artless announcement that he was ready to go "whole
hog" on the vaccination program at the 10 March 1976 ACIP meeting. See Alexander
to Sencer, letter dated 7 April 1976, box 35, folder labeled "Advisory Committee on
Immunization Practices Meeting on May 6–7 (1976)," RG 442, NARA SE Region. For
the report rejecting the stockpiling option, see Walter R. Dowdle, Philip S. Brachman,
Harold M. Mauldin, and Dennis D. Tolsma to director, Bureau of State Services (Millar), memorandum dated 7 June 1976, subject "Stockpiling of Monovalent Influenza A/
New Jersey/76 Influenza Vaccine,," box 44, file labeled "National Swine Flu Immunization Program of 1976 (PL-94.380) #2," RG 442, NARA SE Region.

10. Dennis Tolsma, handwritten notes from 3/24, box 38, file labeled "Influenza
Staff Meeting Notes, DTolsma," RG 442, NARA SE Region.

11. Statement from Dr. Margaret Chan, director general of the World Health
Organization, "World Now at the Start of 2009 Influenza Pandemic," dated 11 June
2009, available at http://who.int/mediacentre/news/statements/2009/h1n1_pandemic_
phase6_20090611/en/index.html (accessed 22 June 2009); Donald G. McNeil, "Virus's
Tangled Genes Straddle Continents, Raising a Mystery about Its Origins," *New York
Times,* 30 April 2009, A12; F. Dawood et al., "Emergence of a Novel Swine-Origin
Influenza A (H1N1) Virus in Humans," *New England Journal of Medicine* 360, no. 25 (18
June 2009): 2605–15; and Shinde et al., "Triple-Reassortant Swine Influenza A (H1) in
Humans in the United States, 2005–2009," *New England Journal of Medicine* 360, no. 25
(18 June 2009): 2616–25.

12. See Edwin Kilbourne, "Influenza Pandemics: Can We Prepare for the Unpredictable?" *Viral Immunology* 17, no. 3 (2004): 350–57.

13. See Alfred Crosby, *Epidemic and Peace, 1918* (Westport, Conn.: Greenwood, 1976); and Carol R. Byerly, *Fever of War: The Influenza Epidemic in the U.S. Army during World War I* (New York: New York University Press, 2005).

14. This, of course, was not a new observation. René and Jean Dubos were making the seed and soil argument in the 1950s in regard to tuberculosis; see René and Jean Dubos, *The White Plague: Tuberculosis, Man and Society* (Boston: Little, Brown, 1952).

BIBLIOGRAPHY

Archival Sources

Centers for Disease Control, Atlanta, Georgia

Centers for Disease Control, files on the Swine Flu Program, accession number 442-00-0058, boxes internally labeled 1–6.

National Archive and Records Administration, Southeast Region, East Point, Georgia

Centers for Disease Control, Swine Flu Immunization Program Files. FRC accession number 442-91-0075, RG 442.

World Health Organization, Geneva, Switzerland

Influenza. First-, second-, and third-generation files.

Correspondence and Memorandums

Bureau of Biologics (BoB), U.S. Food and Drug Administration. 1976. "Records Related to the Swine Flu Program." "Feb. 20, 1976 Meeting BoB at Bethesda with Army, CDC, NIAID, and Press"; "March 25, 1976 a.m. Meeting at BoB." Received via Freedom of Information Act request, F02-17965.

Centers for Disease Control. 1976. "Swine Flu Program of 1976." Assorted memorandums and correspondence. Received via Freedom of Information Act Request, no. 06-0781.

National Institutes of Health, National Institute of Allergy and Infectious Diseases (NIAID). 1976. "Swine Flu Program of 1976." Assorted memorandums and correspondence. Received via Freedom of Information Act Request, no. 28820.

World Health Organization, "Consultation on Influenza, Geneva, 7 and 8 April 1976, Report to the Director-General," Vir/76.4. Received via e-mail from the World Health Organization.

Interviews

Walter Dowdle, 26 May 2005.
Ian Furminger, 30 October 2007.
Claude Hannoun, 23 August 2007.
D. A. Henderson, 26 July 2007.
Edwin Kilbourne, 20 January 2004.
J. Donald Millar, 22 May 2007.
David Sencer, 9 May 2007.
Kennedy Shortridge, 17 and 19 June 2011.
Sir John Skehel, 6 June 2007.

Published Sources

Allen, Arthur. *Vaccine: The Controversial Story of Medicine's Greatest Lifesaver.* New York: Norton, 2007.

Andrewes, C. H. "Epidemiology of Influenza." *Bulletin of the World Health Organization* 8 (1953): 595–612.

"Animal Influenza: Its Significance in Human Infection—Summary of Influenza Workshop VI." *Journal of Infectious Diseases* 131, no. 5 (May 1975): 602–12.

"Antiviral Agents in Influenza—Summary of Influenza Workshop VIII." *Journal of Infectious Diseases* 134, no. 6 (Nov. 1976): 516–27.

Arnold, David. "Introduction." In *Imperial Medicine and Indigenous Societies,* edited by David Arnold, 1–26. Manchester, U.K.: Manchester University Press, 1988.

———. *Warm Climates and Western Medicine: The Emergence of Tropical Medicine, 1500–1900.* Amsterdam: Rodopi, 1996.

Baker, Michael G., and David P. Fidler. "Global Public Health Surveillance under New International Health Regulations." *Emerging Infectious Diseases* 12, no. 7 (July 2006): 1058–65.

Balinska, Marta Aleksandra. "Assistance and Not Mere Relief: The Epidemic Commission of the League of Nations, 1920–1923." In *International Health Organizations and Movements, 1918–1939,* edited by Paul Weindling, 81–108. Cambridge: Cambridge University Press, 1995.

Barry, David W., Ronald E. Mayner, Jules M. Meisler, and Edward B. Seligmann Jr. "Evaluation and Control of Vaccines for the National Influenza Immunization Program." *Journal of Infectious Diseases* 136, suppl., *Clinical Studies of Influenza Vaccines: 1976* (Dec. 1977): S407–14.

Barry, John M. *The Great Influenza: The Epic Story of the Deadliest Plague in History.* New York: Viking, 2004.

Beare, A. S., and J. W. Craig. "Virulence for Man of a Human Influenza-A Virus Antigenically Similar to 'Classical' Swine Viruses." *Lancet* 308, no. 7975 (3 July 1976): 4–5.

Begley, Sharon L. "Failure of the 1976 Swine Flu Drive." *Yale Journal of Biology and Medicine* 50 (1977): 645–57.

Berridge, Virginia, Kelly Loughlin, and Rachel Herring. "Historical Dimensions of Global Health Governance." In *Making Sense of Global Health Governance: A*

Policy Perspective, edited by Kent Buse, Wolfgang Hein, and Nick Drager, 30–34. Basingstoke, U.K.: Palgrave Macmillan, 2009.

Beveridge, W. I. B. *Influenza: The Last Great Plague, an Unfinished Story of Discovery.* New York: Prodist, 1977.

Birn, Anne-Emanuelle, Yogan Illay, and Timothy H. Holtz. *Textbook of International Health: Global Health in a Dynamic World.* 3d ed. New York: Oxford University Press, 2009.

Boffey, Phillip. "Anatomy of a Decision: How the Nation Declared War on Swine Flu." *Science* 192 (14 May 1976): 636–41.

Bonita, Ruth, Alec Irwin, and Robert Beaglehole. "Promoting Public Health in the Twenty-First Century: The Role of the World Health Organization." In *Globalization and Health,* edited by Ichiro Kawachi and Sara Wamala, 268–83. Oxford: Oxford University Press, 2007.

Bonn, Dorothy. "Isolation of New Flu-Virus Strain May Presage Pandemic." *Lancet* 350, no. 9079 (6 Sept. 1997): 717.

Brandt, Allan M. *No Magic Bullet: A Social History of Venereal Disease in the United States since 1880.* New York: Oxford University Press, 1987 [1985].

Bray, R. S. *Armies of Pestilence: The Impact of Disease on History.* New York: Barnes and Noble Books, 1996.

Breiman, Robert F., Meirion R. Evans, Wolfgang Preiser, James Maguire, Alan Schnur, Ailan Li, Henk Bekedam, and John S. MacKenzie. "Role of China in the Quest to Define and Control Severe Acute Respiratory Syndrome." *Emerging Infectious Diseases* 9, no. 9 (Sept. 2003): 1037–41.

Bresalier, Michael. "Neutralizing Flu: Immunological Devices and the Making of a Virus Disease." In *Crafting Immunity: Working Histories of Clinical Immunology,* edited by Keton Kroker, Pauline M. H. Mazumdar, and Jennifer Keelan, 107–44. Aldershot, U.K.: Ashgate, 2008

Brockington, Fraser. *World Health.* 2d ed. Boston: Little, Brown, 1968.

Brown, Theodore M., Marcos Cueto, and Elizabeth Fee. "The World Health Organization and the Transition from International to Global Public Health." *American Journal of Public Health* 96, no. 1 (Jan. 2006): 62–72.

Buse, Kent, Wolfgang Hein, and Nick Drager, eds. *Making Sense of Global Health Governance: A Policy Perspective.* Basingstoke, U.K.: Palgrave Macmillan, 2009.

Byerly, Carol R. *Fever of War: The Influenza Epidemic in the U.S. Army during World War I.* New York: New York University Press, 2005.

Califano, Joseph A., Jr. *Governing America: An Insider's Report from the White House and the Cabinet.* New York: Simon and Schuster, 1981.

Carpenter, Daniel. *Reputation and Power: Organizational Image and Pharmaceutical Regulation at the FDA.* Princeton, N.J.: Princeton University Press, 2010.

Carter, Richard. *Breakthrough: The Saga of Jonas Salk.* New York: Trident, 1965.

"Cast a Dubious Eye at Vaccine for Asia Flu." *Chicago Daily Tribune,* 29 September 1957, 6–7.

Chadwick, Edwin. *Report on the Sanitary Condition of the Labouring Population of Gt. Britain.* Edited and with an introduction by Michael Flinn. Edinburgh: Edinburgh University Press, 1965 [1842].

Cockburn, W. Charles, P. J. Delon, and W. Ferreira. "Origins and Progress of the 1968–69 Hong Kong Influenza Epidemic." *Bulletin of the World Health Organization* 41 (1969): 345–48.

Coleman, William. *Death Is a Social Disease: Public Health and Political Economy in Early Industrial France.* Madison: University of Wisconsin Press, 1982.

Colgrove, James. *State of Immunity: The Politics of Vaccination in Twentieth-Century America.* Berkeley: University of California Press, 2006.

Cox, Robert W., and Harold K. Jacobson. *The Anatomy of Influence: Decision Making in International Organizations.* New Haven, Conn.: Yale University Press, 1973.

Cox, Robert W., with Timothy J. Sinclair. *Approaches to World Order.* Cambridge: Cambridge University Press, 1996.

Crawford, Dorothy. *The Invisible Enemy: A Natural History of Viruses.* Oxford: Oxford University Press, 2000.

Crosby, Alfred. *Epidemic and Peace, 1918.* Westport, Conn.: Greenwood. Subsequently reissued as *America's Forgotten Pandemic.* Cambridge: Cambridge University Press, 1989.

Curtin, Philip D. *Death by Migration: Europe's Encounter with the Tropical World in the Nineteenth Century.* Cambridge: Cambridge University Press, 1989.

———. *Disease and Empire: The Health of European Troops in the Conquest of Africa.* Cambridge: Cambridge University Press, 1998.

———. "The End of the 'White Man's Grave'? Nineteenth-Century Mortality in West Africa." *Journal of Interdisciplinary History* 21, no. 1 (Summer 1990): 63–88.

———. "Epidemiology and the Slave Trade." *Political Science Quarterly* 82 (2 June 1968): 191–216.

———. "'The White Man's Grave': Image and Reality, 1780–1850." *Journal of British Studies* 1, no. 1 (Nov. 1961): 94–110.

Davenport, Fred M. "Prospects for the Control of Influenza." *American Journal of Nursing* 69, no. 9 (Sept. 1969): 1908–11.

Davenport, F. M., A. V. Hennessy, J. Drescher, J. Mulder, and T. Francis Jr. "Further Observations on the Relevance of Serologic Recapitulations of Human Infection with Influenza Viruses." *Journal of Experimental Medicine* 120 (1964): 1087–97.

Davenport, F. M., E. Minuse, A. V. Hennessy, and T. Francis Jr. "Interpretations of Influenza Antibody Patterns of Man." *Bulletin of the World Health Organization* 41 (1969): 453–60.

Davies, Sara E. "Securitizing Infectious Disease." *International Affairs* 84, no. 2 (2008): 295–313.

Davis, Kingsley. *The Population of India and Pakistan.* Princeton, N.J.: Princeton University Press, 1951.

Dawood, Fatima S., Seema Jain, Lyn Finelli, Michael W. Shaw, Stephen Lindstrom, Rebecca J. Garten, Larisa V. Gubareva, Xiyan Xu, Carolyn B. Bridges, and Timothy M. Uyeki. "Emergence of a Novel Swine-Origin Influenza A (H1N1) Virus in Humans." *New England Journal of Medicine* 360, no. 25 (18 June 2009): 2605–15.

De la Rivière, René Dujarric. "La grippe, est-elle une maladie à virus filtrant?" [Is influenza a filtering virus disease?] *Comptes Rendus de L'Académie des Sciences* 167 (1918): 606–7.

Dougherty, James E., and Robert L. Pfaltzgraff. *Contending Theories of International Relations: A Comprehensive Survey.* 4th ed. New York: Longman, 1997.

Dowdle, W[alter]. R. "Influenza A Virus Recycling Revisited." *Bulletin of the World Health Organization* 77, no. 10 (Oct. 1999): 820–28.

———. "Influenza Pandemic Periodicity, Virus Recycling, and the Art of Risk Assessment." *Emerging Infectious Diseases* 12, no. 1 (Jan. 2006): 34–39.

———. "The 1976 Experience." *The Journal of Infectious Diseases* 176, suppl. 1 (Aug. 1997): S69–72.

Dowdle, Walter R., Marion T. Coleman, Elmer C. Hall, and Violeta Knez. "Properties of the Hong Kong Virus: 2. Antigenic Relationship of the Hong Kong Virus Hemagglutinin to That of Other Human Influenza A Viruses." *Bulletin of the World Health Organization* 41 (1969): 419–24.

Dubos, René, and Jean Dubos. *The White Plague: Tuberculosis, Man and Society.* Boston: Little, Brown, 1952.

Duffy, John. *The Sanitarians: A History of American Public Health.* Urbana: University of Illinois Press, 1990.

Duncan, Kirsty E. *Hunting the 1918 Flu: One Scientist's Search for a Killer Virus.* Toronto: University of Toronto Press, 2003.

Ellison, James G. "A Fierce Hunger: Tracing the Impacts of the 1918–19 Influenza in Southwest Tanzania." In *The Spanish Influenza Pandemic of 1918–19: New Perspectives,* edited by Howard Phillips and David Killingray, 221–29. London: Routledge, 2003.

England, J. Merton. *A Patron for Pure Science: The National Science Foundation's Formative Years, 1945–57.* Washington, D.C.: National Science Foundation, 1982.

Ennis, Francis A. "Production and Distribution of Vaccine Following Emergence of a New Viral Strain." In *Influenza: Virus, Vaccines, and Strategy; Proceedings of a Working Group on Pandemic Influenza, Rougemont, January 1976,* edited by Philip Selby, 245–52. London: Academic, 1976.

Enserink, Martin. "From Two Mutations, an Important Clue about the Spanish Flu." *Science* 315 (2 Feb. 2007): 582.

"Epidemiology of Influenza—Summary of Influenza Workshop IV." *Journal of Infectious Diseases* 128, no. 3 (Sept. 1973): 361–86.

Etheridge, Elizabeth W. *Sentinel for Health: A History of the Centers for Disease Control.* Berkeley: University of California Press, 1992.

Ewald, Paul. *Evolution of Infectious Disease.* New York: Oxford University Press, 1994.

Eyler, John M. *Victorian Social Medicine: The Ideas and Methods of William Farr.* Baltimore, Md.: Johns Hopkins University Press, 1979.

Fara, Patricia. *Newton: The Making of Genius.* New York: Columbia University Press, 2002.

Farley, John. *To Cast out Disease: A History of the International Health Division of the Rockefeller Foundation (1913–1951).* Oxford: Oxford University Press, 2004.

Fedson, David S. "Preparing for Pandemic Vaccination: An International Policy Agenda for Vaccine Development." *Journal of Public Health Policy* 26, no. 1 (2005): 4–29.

Fee, Elizabeth. *Disease and Discovery: A History of the Johns Hopkins School of Hygiene and Public Health, 1916–1939.* Baltimore, Md.: Johns Hopkins University Press, 1987.

Fenner, F., D. A. Henderson, I. Arita, Z. Jezek, and I. D. Ladnyi. *Smallpox and Its Eradication.* Geneva: World Health Organization, 1988.

Fernandez, Elizabeth. "The Virus Detective: Dr. John [*sic*] Hultin Has Found Evidence of the 1918 Flu Epidemic That Had Eluded Experts for Decades." *San Francisco Chronicle,* 17 February 2002, CM-8.

Fidler, David. *International Law and Infectious Diseases.* Oxford: Clarendon, 1999.

———. "Public Health and International Law: The Impact of Infectious Diseases on the Formation of International Legal Regimes, 1800–2000." In *Plagues and Politics: Infectious Disease and International Policy,* edited by Andrew T. Price-Smith, 262–84. Houndmills, U.K.: Palgrave, 2001.

Flexner, Abraham. *Medical Education in the United States and Canada: A Report to the Carnegie Foundation for the Advancement of Teaching.* New York, 1910.

Foege, William H. "Alexander Langmuir: His Impact on Public Health." *American Journal of Epidemiology* 144, no. 8, suppl. 8 (1996): S11–15.

Ford, Gerald. "The President's Remarks Announcing Action to Combat the Influenza." *Weekly Compilation of Presidential Documents* 12, no. 13 (24 Mar. 1976): 484–85.

Foster, Stanley O., and Eugene Gangarosa. "Passing the Epidemiological Torch from Farr to the World: The Legacy of Alexander Langmuir." *American Journal of Epidemiology* 144, no. 8, suppl. 8 (1996): S65–73.

Foulkes, Imogen. "WHO Faces Questions over Swine Flu Policy." *BBC News Europe,* 20 May 2010.

Francis, Thomas, Jr. "On the Doctrine of Original Antigenic Sin." *Proceedings of the American Philosophical Society* 104, no. 6 (15 Dec. 1960): 572–78.

———. "Vaccination against Influenza." *Bulletin of the World Health Organization* 8 (1953): 725–41.

Fraser, David W., Theodore R. Tsai, Walter Orenstein, William E. Parkin, H. James Beecham, Robert G. Sharrar, John Harris, et al. "Legionnaires' Disease: Description of an Epidemic of Pneumonia." *New England Journal of Medicine* 297, no. 22 (1 Dec. 1977): 1189–97.

Fukumi, Hideo. "Interpretation and Significance of Hong Kong Antibody in Old People Prior to the Hong Kong Influenza Epidemic." *Bulletin of the World Health Organization* 41 (1969): 469–73.

Gadsby, Patricia. "Fear of Flu: Pandemic Influenza Outbreaks." *Discover* 20, no. 1 (Jan. 1999): 82–89.

Garrett, Laurie. "The Challenge of Global Health." *Foreign Affairs* 86, no. 1 (Jan.–Feb. 2007): 14–38.

Garten, Rebecca J., C. Todd Davis, Colin A. Russell, Bo Shu, Stephen Lindstrom, Amanda Balish, Wendy M. Sessions, et al. "Antigenic and Genetic Characteristics of Swine-Origin 2009 A (H1N1) Influenza Viruses Circulating in Humans." *Science* 325 (10 July 2009): 197–201.

"Genetics, Replication, and Inhibition of Replication of Influenza Viruses—Summary of Influenza Workshop VII." *Journal of Infectious Diseases* 132, no. 6 (Dec. 1975): 713–23.

Gernhart, Gary. "A Forgotten Enemy: PHS's Fight against the 1918 Influenza Pandemic." *Public Health Reports* 114, no. 6 (Dec. 1999): 559–61.

"Global Distribution of Influenza Vaccines, 2000–2003." *Weekly Epidemiological Record,* no. 40 (1 Oct. 2004): 366–67.

Godlee, Fiona. "WHO at the Crossroads: Will It Embrace the Necessary Reforms?" *British Medical Journal* 306, no. 6886 (1 May 1993): 1143–44.

———. "WHO in Retreat: Is It Losing Its Influence?" *British Medical Journal* 309, no. 6967 (3 Dec. 1994): 1491–95.

———. "WHO Reform and Global Health: Radical Restructuring Is the Only Way Ahead." *British Medical Journal* 314, no. 7091 (10 May 1997): 1359–60.

———. "WHO's Special Programmes: Undermining from Above." *British Medical Journal* 310, no. 6973 (21 Jan. 1995): 178–82.

Goldfield, Martin, Joseph D. Bartley, W. Pizzuti, H. C. Black, R. Alton, and W. E. Halperin. "Influenza in 1976: Isolations of Influenza A/New Jersey/76 Virus at Fort Dix." *Journal of Infectious Disease* 136, suppl. (Dec. 1977): S347–55.

Grady, Denise. "Before Shortage of Flu Vaccine, Many Warnings." *New York Times,* 17 October 2004, p. 1, col. 1.

Gregory, Jane, and Steve Miller. *Science in Public: Communication, Culture, and Credibility.* New York: Plenum, 1998.

Groom, A. J. R., and Paul Taylor, eds. *Frameworks for International Co-operation.* New York: St. Martin's, 1990.

Haas, Ernst B. *When Knowledge Is Power: Three Models of Change in International Organizations.* Berkeley: University of California Press, 1990.

Haas, Ernst B., Mary Pat Williams, and Don Babai. *Scientists and World Order: The Uses of Technical Knowledge in International Organizations.* Berkeley: University of California Press, 1977.

Hachinski, Vladimir. "The Swine Influenza Vaccination Controversy." *Archives of Neurology* 42 (Nov. 1985): 1092.

Hamlin, Christopher. "State Medicine in Great Britain." In *The History of Public Health and the Modern State,* edited by Dorothy Porter, 132–64. Amsterdam: Rodopi, 1994.

Hampson, Alan W., and Nancy J. Cox. "Global Surveillance for Pandemic Influenza: Are We Prepared?" In *Options of the Control of Influenza III: Proceedings of the Third International Conference on Options of the Control of Influenza, Cairns, Australia, 4–9 May 1996,* edited by Lorena E. Brown, Alan W. Hampson, and Robert G. Webster, 50–59. Amsterdam: Elsevier, 1996.

Harden, Victoria. *Inventing the NIH: Federal Biomedical Research Policy, 1887–1937.* Baltimore, Md.: Johns Hopkins University Press, 1986.

Hatchett, Richard J., Carter E. Mecher, and Marc Lipsitch. "Public Health Interventions and Epidemic Intensity during the 1918 Influenza Pandemic." *Proceedings of the National Academy of Sciences* 104, no. 18 (1 May 2007): 7582–87.

Haynes, Douglas M. *Imperial Medicine: Patrick Manson and the Conquest of Tropical Disease.* Philadelphia: University of Pennsylvania Press, 2001.

Hays, J. N. *The Burdens of Disease: Epidemics and Human Response in Western History.* New Brunswick, N.J.: Rutgers University Press, 2000.

Headrick, Daniel. *The Tools of Empire: Technology and European Imperialism in the Nineteenth Century.* New York: Oxford University Press, 1981.

Heymann, David L., and Guenael Rodier. "Global Surveillance, National Surveillance, and SARS." *Emerging Infectious Diseases* 10, no. 2 (Feb. 2004): 173–75.

Hilleman, Maurice. "Six Decades of Vaccine Development—a Personal History." *Nature Medicine Vaccine Supplement* 4, no. 5 (May 1998): 507–14.

Hilts, Philip J. *Protecting America's Health: The FDA, Business, and One Hundred Years of Regulation.* New York: Knopf, 2003.

"Hong Kong Battling Influenza Epidemic." *New York Times,* 17 April 1957, 3.

Honigsbaum, Mark. "Was Swine Flu Ever a Real Threat?" *Daily Telegraph,* 2 Feb. 2010.

Hoole, Francis W. *Politics and Budgeting in the World Health Organization.* Bloomington: Indiana University Press, 1976.

Humphreys, Margaret. *Yellow Fever and the South.* Baltimore, Md.: Johns Hopkins University Press, 1992.

"Immunological Methodology in Influenza Diagnosis and Research—Summary of Influenza Workshop II." *Journal of Infectious Diseases* 126, no. 2 (Aug. 1972): 219–30.

"Influenza Vaccines—Summary of Influenza Workshop V." *Journal of Infectious Diseases* 129, no. 6 (June 1974): 750–71.

"Influenza Virus Polypeptides and Antigens—Summary of Influenza Workshop I." *Journal of Infectious Diseases* 125, no. 4 (Apr. 1972): 447–56.

Institute of Medicine. *Emerging Infections: Microbial Threats to Health in the United States.* Washington, D.C.: National Academies, 1992.

Iriye, Akira. *Cultural Internationalism and World Order.* Baltimore, Md.: Johns Hopkins University Press, 1997.

———. *Global Community: The Role of International Organizations in the Making of the Contemporary World.* Berkeley: University of California Press, 2002.

Italian Global Health Watch. "From Alma Ata to the Global Fund: The History of International Health Policy." *Social Medicine* 3, no. 1 (Jan. 2008): 36–48.

Jannetta, Ann. "Disease Dissemination in the Early Modern World: Connecting East and West." In *Higashi to Hishi No Iryo Bunka* [Medical culture east and west], edited by Yoshida Iadashis and Fukase Yasuaki, 390–410. Tokyo: Shibunkaku, 2001.

Johnson, Niall P. A. S., and Juergen Mueller. "Updating the Accounts: Global Mortality of the 1918–1920 'Spanish' Influenza Pandemic." *Bulletin of the History of Medicine* 76, no. 1 (2002): 105–15.

Johnson, Steven. *The Ghost Map: The Story of London's Most Terrifying Epidemic and How It Changed Science, Cities, and the Modern World.* New York: Riverhead, 2006.

Jones, Norman Howard. "The Organizational Problems between the Two World Wars." Pt. 1, *WHO Chronicle* 31 (1977): 391–403; pt. 2, 31 (1977): 449–60; pt. 3, 32 (1978): 26–38; pt. 4, 32 (1978): 63–75; pt. 5, 32 (1978): 114–25; "Epilogue," 32 (1978): 156–66.

———. "The World Health Organization in Historical Perspective." *Perspectives in Biology and Medicine* (Spring 1981): 467–82.

Jordan, Edwin O. *Epidemic Influenza: A Survey.* Chicago: American Medical Association, 1927.

Katz, Rebecca. "Use of Revised International Health Regulations during Influenza A (H1N1) Epidemic, 2009." *Emerging Infectious Diseases* 15, no. 8 (Aug. 2009): 1165–70.

Kelly, Eugene R. *The Commonwealth of Massachusetts, Annual Report of the Department of Public Health for the Year Ending November 30, 1920.* Boston: Wright and Patten, 1921.

Kendal, Alan P., Gary R. Noble, John J. Skehel, and Walter Dowdle. "Antigenic Similarity of Influenza A (H1N1) Viruses from Epidemics in 1977–1978 to 'Scandinavian' Strains Isolated in Epidemics of 1950–1951." *Virology* 89 (1978): 632–36.

Kickbusch, Ilona. "World Health Organisation: Change and Progress." *British Medical Journal* 310, no. 6993 (10 June 1995): 1518–20.

Kilbourne, Edwin. "Flu to the Starboard! Man the Harpoons! Fill 'em with Vaccine! Alert the Captain! Hurry!" *New York Times,* 13 February 1976, pp. 33, col. 1.

———. "Future Influenza Vaccines and the Use of Genetic Recombinants." *Bulletin of the World Health Organization* 41 (1969): 643–45.

———. *Influenza.* New York: Plenum Medical, 1987.

———. "Influenza Pandemics: Can We Prepare for the Unpredictable?" *Viral Immunology* 17, no. 3 (2004): 350–57.

———, ed. *Influenza Viruses and Influenza.* New York: Academic, 1975.

———. "Recombination of Influenza A Viruses of Human and Animal Origin." *Science* 160 (1968): 74–76.

Kilbourne, E[dwin] D., J. L. Schulman, G. C. Schild, G. Scholer, J. Swanson, and D. L. Bucher. "Correlated Studies of a Recombinant Influenza-Virus Vaccine. I. Derivation and Characterization of Virus and Vaccine." *Journal of Infectious Diseases* 124 (1971): 449–62.

Kilbourne, Edwin, Catherine Smith, Ian Brett, Barbara A. Pokorny, Bert Johansson, and Nancy Cox. "The Total Influenza Vaccine Failure of 1947 Revisited: Major Intrasubtypic Antigenic Change Can Explain Failure of Vaccine in a Post-World War II Epidemic." *Proceedings of the National Academy of Sciences* 99, no. 16 (6 Aug. 2002): 10748–52.

King, Nicholas B. "Security, Disease, Commerce: Ideologies of Postcolonial Global Health." *Social Studies of Science* 32, nos. 5–6 (Oct.–Dec. 2002): 763–89.

Klein, Aaron E. *Trial by Fury: The Polio Vaccine Controversy.* New York: Scribner's, 1972.

Kobasa, Darwyn, Steven M. Jones, Kyoko Shinay, John C. Kash, John Copps, Hideki Ebihara, Yasuko Hatta, et al. "Aberrant Innate Immune Response in Lethal Infection of Macaques with the 1918 Influenza Virus." *Nature* 445 (18 Jan. 2007): 319–23.

Kolata, Gina. *Flu: The Story of the Great Influenza Pandemic of 1918 and the Search for the Virus That Caused It.* New York: Farrar, Straus and Giroux, 1999.

———. "Study Shows Why the Flu Likes Winter." *New York Times,* 5 December 2007, p. 1, col. 1.

Kraut, Alan. *Silent Travelers: Germs, Genes, and the "Immigrant Menace."* New York: Basic Books, 1994.

Krieger, Nancy. "The Making of Public Health Data: Paradigms, Politics, and Policy." *Journal of Public Health Policy* 13, no. 4 (Winter 1992): 412–27.

Kuhn, Thomas. *The Structure of Scientific Revolutions.* 2d ed., enlarged. University of Chicago Press, 1970 [1962].

Kurland, Leonard T., Wigbert C. Wiederholt, James W. Kirkpatrick, Gilbert Potter, and Page Armstrong. "Swine Influenza Vaccine and Guillain-Barré Syndrome: Epidemic or Artifact?" *Archives of Neurology* 42 (Nov. 1985): 1089–90.

Langmuir, Alexander. "William Farr: Founder of Modern Concepts of Surveillance." *International Journal of Epidemiology* 5, no. 1 (1976): 13–18.

Langmuir, A[lexander] D., D. J. Bregman, L. T. Kurland, N. Nathanson, and M. Victor. "An Epidemiological and Clinical Evaluation of Guillain-Barré Syndrome Reported in Association with the Administration of Swine Influenza Vaccines." *American Journal of Epidemiology* 119, no. 6 (June 1984): 841–79.

Laver, W. G., and R. G. Webster. "Studies on the Origin of Pandemic Influenza II." *Virology* 48 (1972): 445–55.

———. "Studies on the Origin of Pandemic Influenza III." *Virology* 51 (1973): 383–91.

Layne, Scott P. "Human Influenza Surveillance: The Demand to Expand." *Emerging Infectious Diseases* 12, no. 4 (Apr. 2006): 562–68.

Lee, Kelley. *Historical Dictionary of the World Health Organization.* Lanham, Md.: Scarecrow, 1998.

Leffell, Mary S., Albert D. Donnenberg, and Noel R. Rose, eds. *Handbook of Human Immunology.* Boca Raton, Fla.: CRC, 1997.

Litsios, Socrates. "The Christian Medical Commission and the Development of the World Health Organization's Primary Health Care Approach." *American Journal of Public Health* 94, no. 11 (Nov. 2004): 1884–93.

Loo, Yueh-Ming, and Michael Gale Jr. "Fatal Immunity and the 1918 Virus." *Nature* 445 (18 Jan. 2007): 267–68.

Lowen, A. C., S. Mubareka, J. Steel, and P. Palese. "Influenza Virus Transmission Is Dependent on Relative Humidity and Temperature." *PLoS Pathology* 3 (10). Online journal. http://www.plospathogens.org/article/info:doi/10.1371/journal.ppat.0030151.

Macleod, Roy. "Introduction." In *Disease, Medicine, and Empire: Perspectives on Western Medicine and the Experience of European Expansion,* edited by Roy Macleod and Milton Lewis, 1–11. London: Routledge, 1988.

Markel, Howard. *Quarantine! East European Jewish Immigrants and the New York City Epidemics of 1892.* Baltimore, Md.: Johns Hopkins University Press, 1999.

———. *When Germs Travel: Six Major Epidemics That Have Invaded America since 1900 and the Fears They Have Unleashed.* New York: Pantheon, 2004.

Marsh, James A., and Marion D. Kendall, eds. *The Physiology of Immunity.* Boca Raton, Fla.: CRC, 1996.

Martindale, Diane. "No Mercy." *New Scientist* (14 Oct. 2000): 2929.

"Mass Flu Immunization Seen Needless by Experts." *Hartford Courant,* 29 September 1957, p. 22, col. 1.

"Mass Vaccine Not Needed Panel Says." *Washington Post and Times Herald,* 29 September 1957, B1.

Masurel, N. "Serological Characteristics of a 'New' Serotype of Influenza A Virus: The Hong Kong Strain." *Bulletin of the World Health Organization* 41 (1969): 461–68.

Matrosovich, Mikhail, Alexander Tuzikov, Nikolai Bovin, Alexandra Gambaryan, Alexander Klimov, Maria R. Castrucci, Isabella Donatelli, and Yoshihiro

Kawaoka. "Early Alteration of the Receptor-Binding Properties of H1, H2, and H3 Avian Influenza Virus Hemagglutinins after Their Introduction into Mammals." *Journal of Virology* 74, no. 18 (Sept. 2000): 8502–12.

McDade, Joseph E., Charles C. Shepard, David W. Fraser, Theodore R. Tsai, Martha A. Redus, Walter R. Dowdle, and the Laboratory Investigation Team. "'Legionnaires' Disease: Isolation of a Bacterium and Demonstration of Its Role in Other Respiratory Disease." *New England Journal of Medicine* 297, no. 22 (1 Dec. 1977): 1197–1203.

McNeil, Donald G. "Virus's Tangled Genes Straddle Continents, Raising a Mystery about Its Origins." *New York Times,* 30 April 2009.

McNeill, William H. *Plagues and Peoples.* New York: Anchor/Doubleday, 1976.

Merson, Michael H., Robert E. Black, and Anne J. Mills, eds. *International Public Health: Disease, Programs, Systems and Policies.* 2d ed. Sudbury, Mass.: Jones and Bartlett, 2006.

Milstein, B. "Hygeia's Constellation: Navigating Health Futures in a Dynamic and Democratic World." Syndemics Prevention Network, Centers for Disease Control. Internet file. http://www.index/monograph/syndemics/gov.cdc.htm.

Moran, Bruce T. *Distilling Knowledge: Alchemy, Chemistry and the Scientific Revolution.* Cambridge, Mass.: Harvard University Press, 2005.

Morse, Stephen S., ed. *Emerging Viruses.* New York: Oxford University Press, 1993.

———. *The Evolutionary Biology of Viruses.* New York: Raven, 1994.

———. "Pandemic Influenza: Studying the Lessons of History." *Proceedings of the National Academy of Sciences* 104, no. 18 (1 May 2007): 7313–14.

Mostow, S. R., S. C. Schoenbaum, W. R. Dowdle, M. T. Coleman, and H. S. Kaye. "Studies with Inactivated Influenza Vaccines Purified by Zonal Centrifugation." *Bulletin of the World Health Organization* 41 (1969): 525–30.

Mulder, J. "Asiatic Influenza in the Netherlands." *Lancet* 270, no. 6990 (17 Aug. 1957): 334.

Mulder, J., N. Masurel, E. M. Deggars, and P. J. Webbers. "Pre-Epidemic Antibody against 1957 Strain of Asiatic Influenza: In Serum of Older People Living in the Netherlands." *Lancet* 271, no. 7025 (19 Apr. 1958): 810–14.

Murray, Roderick. "Production and Testing in the USA of Influenza Virus Vaccine Made from the Hong Kong Variant in 1968–69." *Bulletin of the World Health Organization* 41 (1969): 495–96.

Neustadt, Richard E., and Harvey Fineberg. *The Epidemic That Never Was: Policy Making and the Swine Flu Scare.* New York: Vintage, 1982.

———. *The Swine Flu Affair: Decision-Making on a Slippery Disease.* Washington, D.C.: U.S. Department of Health, Education, and Welfare, 1978.

Nguyen-Van-Tam, Jonathan S. "Epidemiology of Influenza." In *Textbook of Influenza,* edited by Karl G. Nicholson, Robert G. Webster, and Alan J. Hay, 181–206. London: Blackwell Science, 1998.

Nicholson, Karl G., Robert G. Webster, and Alan J. Hay, eds. *Textbook of Influenza.* London: Blackwell Science, 1998.

Nicholson-Preuss, Mari Loreena. "Managing Morbidity and Mortality: Pandemic Influenza in France, 1889–90." Master's thesis, Texas Tech University, 2001.

Normile, Dennis. "Wild Birds Only Partly to Blame in Spreading H5N1." *Science* 312 (9 June 2006): 1451.

Offit, Paul. *The Cutter Incident: How America's First Polio Vaccine Led to the Growing Vaccine Crisis*. New Haven, Conn.: Yale University Press, 2005.

———. *Vaccinated: One Man's Quest to Defeat the World's Deadliest Diseases*. New York: Smithsonian Books, 2007.

Olsen, Bjorn, Vincent J. Munster, Anders Wallensten, Jonas Waldenstrom, Albert D. M. E. Osterhaus, and Ron A. M. Fouchier. "Global Patterns of Influenza A Virus in Wild Birds." *Science* 312 (21 Apr. 2006): 384–88.

Osborn, June E., ed. *History, Science, and Politics: Influenza in America 1918–1976*. New York: Prodist, 1977.

Oshinsky, David M. *Polio: An American Story*. Oxford: Oxford University Press, 2005.

Oxford, J. S. "The So-Called Great Spanish Influenza Pandemic of 1918 May Have Originated in France in 1916." *Philosophical Transactions of the Royal Society of London*, ser. B, Biological Sciences, no. 356 (2001): 1857–59.

Oxford, J. S., A. Sefton, R. Jackson, N. P. A. S. Johnson, and R. S. Daniels. "Who's That Lady?" *Nature Medicine* 5, no. 12 (Dec. 1999): 1351–52.

"Panel Hits Mass Need of Flu Shots." *Los Angeles Times,* 29 September 1957, 5.

Parsons, H. Franklin. *Further Report and Papers on Pandemic Influenza, 1889–92: Presented to Both Houses of Parliament by Command of Her Majesty*. London: Eyre and Spottiswoode, 1893.

———. *Report on the Influenza Epidemic of 1889–90: Presented to Both Houses of Parliament by Command of Her Majesty*. London: Eyre and Spottiswoode, 1891.

Patten, Christopher W. "Chronicle of Influenza Pandemics." In *Textbook of Influenza,* edited by Karl G. Nicholson, Robert G. Webster, and Alan J. Hay, 3–18. London: Blackwell Science, 1998.

Patterson, James T. *Grand Expectations: The United States, 1945–1974*. New York: Oxford University Press, 1996.

Patterson, K. David. *Pandemic Influenza 1700–1900: A Study in Historical Epidemiology*. Totowa, N.J.: Rowman and Littlefield, 1986.

Patterson, K. David, and Gerald F. Pyle. "The Geography and Mortality of the 1918 Influenza Pandemic." *Bulletin of the History of Medicine* 65 (1991): 4–21.

Paul, John R. *A History of Poliomyelitis*. New Haven, Conn.: Yale University Press, 1971.

Payne, A. M.-M. "The Influenza Programme of WHO." *Bulletin of the World Health Organization* 8 (1953): 755–74.

Pennisi, Elizabeth. "First Genes Isolated from the Deadly 1918 Flu Virus." *Science* 275 (21 Mar. 1997): 1739.

Phillips, Howard, and David Killingray, eds. *The Spanish Influenza Pandemic of 1918–19: New Perspectives*. London: Routledge, 2003.

Planck, Max. *The Philosophy of Physics*. New York: Norton, 1936.

Pollitzer, R. *Cholera*. Geneva: World Health Organization, 1959.

Poser, Charles M. "Swine Influenza Vaccination: Truth and Consequences." *Archives of Neurology* 42 (Nov. 1985): 1090–92.

Pyle, Gerald F. *Applied Medical Geography*. Washington, D.C.: V. H. Winston, 1979.

————. *The Diffusion of Influenza: Patterns and Paradigms.* Totowa, N.J.: Rowman and Littlefield, 1986.

Rosen, George. *A History of Public Health.* New York: MD Publications, 1958.

Rosenberg, Charles. *The Cholera Years: The United States in 1832, 1849, and 1866.* Chicago: University of Chicago Press, 1987 [1962].

Rosenkratz, Barbara Gutmann. *Public Health and the State: Changing Views in Massachusetts, 1842–1936.* Cambridge, Mass.: Harvard University Press, 1972.

Rozell, Ned. "Permafrost Preserves Clues to Deadly 1918 Flu." Article 1386, *Alaska Science Forum* (29 Apr. 1998). Internet file. http://www.gi.alaska.edu/Science Forum/ASF13/1386.html.

————. "Villager's Remains Lead to 1918 Flu Breakthrough." Article 1772, *Alaska Science Forum* (1999). Internet file. http://www.gi.alaska.edu/ScienceForum/ASF17/1772.html.

Rubin, David M. "Remember Swine Flu?" *Columbia Journalism Review* (July–Aug. 1977): 42–45.

Rubin, David M., and Val Hendry. "Swine Influenza and the News Media." *Annals of Internal Medicine* 87 (Dec. 1977): 769–74.

Santora, Marc. "Private Doctors in Frantic Quest for Flu Vaccine." *New York Times,* 21 October 2004, p. 2, col. 1.

Sassetti, Christopher, and Eric Rubin. "The Open Book on Infectious Diseases." *Nature Medicine* 13, no. 3 (Mar. 2007): 279–80.

Schaffner, William, and F. Marc LaForce. "Training Field Epidemiologists: Alexander D. Langmuir and the Epidemic Intelligence Service." *American Journal of Epidemiology* 144, no. 8, suppl. 8 (1996): S16–22.

Schmeck, Harold M., Jr. "Race for the Swine Flu Vaccine Began in a Manhattan Lab." *New York Times,* 21 May 1976, p. B1, col. 3.

————. "Test of Flu Vaccine Expected in April." *New York Times,* 26 March 1976, p. 14, col. 3.

————. "U.S. Calls Flu Alert on Possible Return of Epidemic's Virus." *New York Times,* 20 February 1976, p. 1, col. 3.

Schoenbaum, Stephen C., Barbara J. McNeil, and Joel Kavet. "The Swine-Influenza Decision." *New England Journal of Medicine* 295, no. 14 (Sept. 1976): 759–65.

Scholtissek, Christopher. "Genetic Reassortments of Human Influenza Viruses in Nature." In *Textbook of Influenza,* edited by Karl G. Nicholson, Robert G. Webster, Alan J. Hay, 120–25. London: Blackwell Science, 1998.

Scholtissek, C[hristopher], H. Burger, O. Kistner, and K. F. Shortridge. "The Nucleoprotein as a Possible Factor in Determining Host Specificity of Influenza H3N2 Viruses." *Virology* 147 (1985): 287–94.

Schulman, J. L., and Edwin Kilbourne. "Independent Variation in Nature of the Hemagglutinin and Neuraminidase Antigens of Influenza Virus: Distinctiveness of the Hemagglutinin Antigen of Hong Kong/68 Virus." *Proceedings of the National Academy of Science* 63 (1969): 326–33.

Schwartz, Harry. "Swine Flu Fiasco." *New York Times,* 21 December 1976, p. 33, col. 2.

Selby, Philip, ed. *Influenza: Virus, Vaccines, and Strategy; Proceedings of a Working Group on Pandemic Influenza, Rougemont, January 1976.* London: Academic, 1976,

"Sessions I-VIII: Open Discussion." In *Proceedings of the International Conference on the Application of Vaccines against Viral, Rickettsial, and Bacterial Disease of Man, 14–18 December 1970*, 611–18. Washington, D.C.: Pan American Health Organization, 1971.

Seytre, Bernard, and Mary Shaffer. *The Death of a Disease: A History of the Eradication of Poliomyelitis*. New Brunswick, N.J.: Rutgers University Press, 2005. Originally published as *Histoire de l'eradication de la poliomyélite*. Presses Universitaires de France, 2004.

Shanks, Niall, and Rebecca A. Pyles. "Evolution and Medicine: The Long Reach of 'Dr. Darwin.'" *Philosophy, Ethics, and Humanities in Medicine* 2, no. 4 (3 Apr. 2007): 4–18. Avaialable at http://www.ncbi.nlm.nih.gov/pmc/articles/PMC1852567/.

Shattuck, Lemuel, et al. *Report of the Sanitary Commission of Massachusetts*. Boston: Dutton and Wentworth, 1850.

Shinde, Vivek, Carolyn B. Fridges, Timothy M. Uyeki, Bo Shu, Amanda Balish, Xiyan Xu, Stephen Lindstrom, et al. "Triple-Reassortant Swine Influenza A (H1) in Humans in the United States, 2005–2009." *New England Journal of Medicine* 360, no. 25 (18 June 2009): 2616–25.

Shope, Richard. "Swine Influenza I: Experimental Transmission and Pathology." *Journal of Experimental Medicine* 54 (1931): 349–60.

———. "Swine Influenza II: A Hemophilic Bacillus from the Respiratory Tract of Infected Swine." *Journal of Experimental Medicine* 54 (1931): 361–72.

———. "Swine Influenza III: Filtration Experiments and Etiology." *Journal of Experimental Medicine* 54 (1931): 373–85.

Shortridge, Kennedy F. "Poultry and the Influenza H5N1 Outbreak in Hong Kong, 1997: Abridged Chronology and Virus Isolation." *Vaccine* 17 (1999): S26–29.

Silverstein, Arthur M. *Pure Politics and Impure Science: The Swine Flu Affair*. Baltimore, Md.: Johns Hopkins University Press, 1981.

Smith, Derek J. "Predictability and Preparedness in Influenza Control." *Science* 312 (21 Apr. 2006): 392–94.

Smith, Joseph W. G. "Vaccination Strategy." In *Influenza: Virus, Vaccines, and Strategy; Proceedings of a Working Group on Pandemic Influenza, Rougemont, January 1976*, edited by Philip Selby, 271–94. London: Academic, 1976.

Smith, Kerri. "Concern as Revived 1918 Flu Virus Kills Monkeys." *Nature* 445 (18 Jan. 2007): 237.

Snacken, Rene, Alan P. Kendal, Lars R. Haaheim, and John M. Wood. "The Next Influenza Pandemic: Lessons from Hong Kong, 1997." *Emerging Infectious Diseases* 5, no. 2 (Mar.–Apr. 1999): 195–203.

Soper, George A. "The Lessons of the Pandemic." *Science*, new ser., 49, no. 1274 (30 May 1919): 501–6.

"Specific Immunity in Influenza—Summary of Influenza Workshop III." *Journal of Infectious Diseases* 127, no. 2 (Feb. 1973): 220–23.

Starr, Paul. *The Social Transformation of American Medicine: The Rise of a Sovereign Profession and the Making of a Vast Industry*. New York: Basic Books, 1982.

Stern, Alexandra Minna, and Howard Markel. "The History of Vaccines and

Immunization: Familiar Patterns, New Challenges." *Health Affairs* 24, no. 3 (May June 2005): 611–21.

Stobbe, Mike. "Millions of Vaccine Doses to be Burned." Wire service (AP) story, 1 July 2010.

Stratton, Kathleen, Donna A. Alamario, Theresa Wizemann, and Marie C. McCormick, eds. *Immunization Safety Review: Influenza Vaccines and Neurological Complications.* Washington, D.C.: National Academies, 2004.

Strickland, Stephen P. *Politics, Science and Dread Disease: A Short History of United States Medical Research Policy.* Cambridge, Mass.: Harvard University Press, 1972.

"Surveillance and Early Warning, Discussion." In *Influenza: Virus, Vaccine, and Strategy; Proceedings of a Working Group on Pandemic Influenza, Rougemont, January 1976,* edited by Philip Selby, 89–92. London: Academic, 1976.

Sweet, B. H., and M. R. Hilleman. "The Vacuolating Virus, S.V. 40." *Proceedings of the Society for Experimental Biology and Medicine* 105 (1960): 420–27.

Taubenberger, Jeffrey K. "Genetic Characterisation of the 1918 'Spanish' Influenza Virus." In *The Spanish Influenza Pandemic of 1918–19: New Perspectives,* edited by Howard Phillips and David Killingray, 39–46. London: Routledge, 2003.

Taubenberger, Jeffrey K., and David M. Morens. "1918 Influenza: The Mother of All Pandemics." *Emerging Infectious Diseases* 12, no. 1 (Jan. 2006): 15–22.

Taubenberger, Jeffrey K., Ann H. Reid, Thomas A. Janczewski, and Thomas G. Fanning. "Integrating Historical, Clinical, and Molecular Genetic Data in Order to Explain the Origin and Virulence of the 1918 Spanish Influenza Virus." *Philosophical Transactions of the Royal Society of London,* ser. B, Biological Sciences, 356, no. 1416 (29 Dec. 2001): 1829–39.

Taubenberger, Jeffrey K., Ann H. Reid, Amy E. Krafft, Karen E. Bijwaard, and Thomas G. Fanning. "Initial Genetic Characterization of the 1918 'Spanish' Influenza Virus." *Science* 275 (21 Mar. 1997): 1793–96.

Thomas, Gordon, and Max Morgan Witts. *Anatomy of an Epidemic.* Garden City, N.Y.: Doubleday, 1982.

Thorne, R. Thorne. "Introduction by the Medical Office, to Local Government Board." In *Further Report and Papers on Pandemic Influenza, 1889–92: Presented to Both Houses of Parliament by Command of Her Majesty,* by H. Franklin Parsons, i–xi. London: Eyre and Spottiswoode, 1893.

Tumpey, Terrence M., Christopher F. Basler, Patricia V. Aguilar, Hui Zeng, Alicia Solorzano, David E. Swayne, Nancy J. Cox, Jacqueline M. Katz, Jeffrey K. Taubenberger, Peter Palese, and Adolfo Garcia-Sastre. "Characterization of the Reconstructed 1918 Spanish Influenza Pandemic Virus." *Science* 310 (7 Oct. 2005): 77–80.

Tumpey, Terence M., Taronna R. Maines, Neal Van Hoeven, Laurel Glaser, Alicia Solorzano, Claudia Pappas, Nancy J. Cox, David E. Swayne, Peter Palese, Jacqueline M. Katz, and Adolfo Garcia-Sastre. "A Two-Amino Acid Change in the Hemagglutinin of the 1918 Influenza Virus Abolishes Transmission." *Science* 315 (2 Feb. 2007): 655–59.

Tyrrell, David. "Discovery of Influenza Virus." In *Textbook of Influenza,* edited by

Karl G. Nicholson, Robert G. Webster, and Alan J. Hay, 19–26. London: Blackwell Sciences, 1998.

Tyrrell, David, and Michael Fielder. *Cold Wars: The Fight against the Common Cold.* New York: Oxford University Press, 2002.

United Nations. *Yearbook of the United Nations, 1976.* Volume 30. New York: Office of Public Information, United Nations, 1979.

U.S. Comptroller General. Report to the Congress. *The Swine Flu Program: An Unprecedented Venture in Preventive Medicine.* Washington, D.C.: Department of Health, Education, and Welfare, 1977.

U.S. Congress. House. Subcommittee of the Committee on Appropriations. *Departments of Labor and Health, Education, and Welfare Appropriations for 1977: Hearings before a Subcommittee of the Committee on Appropriations.* 94th Cong., 2d sess., n.d.

U.S. Congress. House. Subcommittee of the Committee on Appropriations. *Departments of Labor and Health, Education, and Welfare Appropriations for 1977: Testimony of Members of Congress and Other Interested Individuals and Organizations, Hearings before a Subcommittee of the Committee on Appropriations.* 94th Cong., 2d sess., n.d.

U.S. Congress. House. Subcommittee on Health and the Environment of the Committee on Interstate and Foreign Commerce. *Proposed National Swine Flu Vaccination Program.* 94th Cong., 2d sess., 31 March 1976.

U.S. Congress. House. Subcommittee on Health and the Environment of the Committee on Interstate and Foreign Commerce. *Swine Flu Immunization Program: Supplemental Hearings before the Subcommittee on Health and the Environment of the Committee on Interstate and Foreign Commerce.* 94th Cong., 2d sess., 28 June, 20, 23 July, and 13 September 1976.

U.S. Congress. Senate. Subcommittee of the Committee on Appropriations on H. J. Res. 890. *Preventive Health Services and Employment Programs Emergency Supplemental Appropriations: Hearing before a Subcommittee of the Committee on Appropriations on H. J. Res. 890.* 94th Cong., 2d sess., 6 April 1976.

U.S. Congress. Senate. Subcommittee of the Committee on Appropriations on H. R. 14232. *An Act Making Appropriations for the Departments of Labor and Health, Education, and Welfare and Related Agencies for the Fiscal Year Ending September 30, 1977, and for Other Purposes: Hearings before a Subcommittee of the Committee on Appropriations on H. R. 14232.* Part 8 (pages 5461–6721), "Department of Health, Education, and Welfare, Nondepartmental Witnesses, Department of Labor." 94th Cong., 2d sess., n.d.

U.S. Congress. Senate. Subcommittee on Appropriations. *Departments of Labor and Health Education, and Welfare and Related Agencies for Fiscal Year 1977: Hearings before a Subcommittee on Appropriations.* 94th Cong., 2d sess., 3 February 1976.

U.S. Congress. Senate. Subcommittee on Health of the Committee on Labor and Public Welfare. *Swine Flu Immunization Program, 1976.* 94th Cong., 2d sess., 1 April and 5 August 1976.

U.S. Public Health Service. *Proceedings, Special Conference of Influenza, Surgeon General Public Health Service with State and Territorial Health Officials, August 27–28, 1957.* Washington, D.C.: U.S. Department of Health, Education, and Welfare, n.d.

Viseltear, Arthur J. "A Short Political History of the 1976 Swine Influenza Legislation." In *History, Science, and Politics: Influenza in America, 1918–1976,* edited by June E. Osborn, 29–58. New York: Prodist, 1977.

Von Dietze, Erich. *Paradigms Explained: Rethinking Thomas Kuhn's Philosophy of Science.* Westport, Conn.: Praeger, 2001.

Wade, Nicholas. "1976 Swine Flu Campaign Faulted Yet Principals Would Do It Again." *Science* 202 (24 Nov. 1978): 849–52.

Walt, Gill, and Kent Buse. "Global Cooperation in International Public Health." In *International Public Health: Disease, Program, System, and Policies,* 2d ed., edited by Michael H. Merson, Robert E. Black, and Anne J. Mills, 649–80. Sudbury, Mass.: Jones and Bartlett, 2006.

Walters, F. P. *A History of the League of Nations.* London: Oxford University Press, 1952.

Wang, Jessica. *American Science in an Age of Anxiety: Scientists, Anticommunism, and the Cold War.* Chapel Hill: University of North Carolina Press, 1999.

Watson, Ian, producer. "The Next Pandemic." Transcript. Australian Broadcasting Corporation, 7 May 1998. Available at www.abc.net.au/quantrum/scripts98/9808/script.htm.

Watson, John. "Surveillance of Influenza." In *Textbook of Influenza,* edited by Karl G. Nicholson, Robert G. Webster and Alan J. Hay, 207–16. London: Blackwell Science, 1998.

Webster, Robert G., and William J. Bean Jr. "Evolution and Ecology of Influenza Viruses: Interspecies Transmission." In *Textbook of Influenza,* edited by Karl G. Nicholson, Robert G. Webster and Alan J. Hay, 109–19. London: Blackwell Science, 1998.

Webster, R[obert] G., and W. G. Laver. "Studies on the Origin of Pandemic Influenza I." *Virology* 48 (1972): 433–44.

Weindling, Paul, ed. *International Health Organizations and Movements, 1918–1939.* Cambridge: Cambridge University Press, 1995.

Weir, Lorna, and Eric Mykhalovskiy. *Global Public Health Vigilance: Creating a World on Alert.* New York: Routledge, 2010.

Weisse, Allen B. *Medical Odysseys: The Different and Sometimes Unexpected Pathways to Twentieth Century Medical Discoveries.* New Brunswick, N.J.: Rutgers University Press, 1991.

Winn, Washington C., Jr. "Influenza and Parainfluenza Viruses." In *Pathology of Infectious Diseases,* vol. 1, edited by Daniel H. Connor, 221–27. Stamford, Conn.: Appleton and Lange, 1997.

Wise, Darla J., and Gordon R. Carter. *Immunology: A Comprehensive Review.* Iowa City: Iowa State University Press, 2002.

Wood, John. "Developing Vaccines against Pandemic Influenza." *Philosophical Transactions of the Royal Society of London,* ser. B, 356 (2001): 1953–60.

Wood, John, and Michael S. Williams. "History of Inactivated Influenza Vaccines." In *Textbook of Influenza,* edited by Karl G. Nicholson, Robert G. Webster, and Alan J. Hay, 317–23. London: Blackwell Science, 1998.

World Health Organization. "WHO Pandemic Influenza Draft Protocol for Rapid Response and Containment." Updated draft 30 May 2006. Internet file. http://www.who.int/csr/disease/avian_influenza/guidelines/protocolfinal30_05_06a.pdf.

World Health Organization, Executive Board. "Influenza Pandemic Preparedness and Response: Report by the Secretariat." 115th Session, Agenda Item 4. 17, EB 115/44, 20 January 2005.

Wright, Donald R. *The World and a Very Small Place in Africa.* Armonk, N.Y.: M. E. Sharpe, 1997.

Wright, Lawrence. "Sweating Out the Swine Flu Scare." *New Times,* 11 June 1976, 28–38.

Yach, Derek, and Douglas Bettcher. "The Globalization of Public Health, I: Threats and Opportunities." *American Journal of Public Health* 88, no. 5 (May 1998): 735–38.

———. "The Globalization of Public Health, II: The Convergence of Self-Interest and Altruism." *American Journal of Public Health* 88, no. 5 (May 1998): 738–41.

Yoder, Amos. *The Evolution of the United Nations System.* 3d ed. Washington, D.C.: Taylor and Francis, 1997.

Zdhanov, V. M., and I. V. Antonova. "The Hong Kong Influenza Virus Epidemic in the USSR." *Bulletin of the World Health Organization* 41 (1969): 381–86.

Zinsser, Hans. *Rats, Lice and History.* Boston: Little, Brown, 1934.

INDEX